Stress, Personal Control and Health

This book results from the Concerted Action on Breakdown in Human Adaptation, part of the Medical and Health Research Programme of the Commission of the European Communities.

Stress, Personal Control and Health

Edited by

Andrew Steptoe
Department of Psychology,
St George's Hospital Medical School,
University of London, UK

and

Ad Appels
Department of Medical Psychology,
University of Limburg,
Maastricht,
The Netherlands

JOHN WILEY & SONS
Chichester • New York • Brisbane • Toronto • Singapore

in association with the Commission of the European Communities

Publication arrangements by
Commission of the European Communities,
Directorate-General Telecommunications, Information Industries and Innovation, Scientific and
Technical Communications Service, Luxembourg

Published by John Wiley & Sons Ltd.
Baffins Lane, Chichester, West Sussex PO19 1UD, UK

Library of Congress Cataloging-in-Publication Data

Stress, personal control, and health / edited by Andrew Steptoe and Ad
  Appels.
    p. cm.
  Includes bibliographies and index.
  ISBN 0 471 92388 5
  1. Medicine and psychology. 2. Stress (Psychology) 3. Control
  (Psychology) 4. Health. 5. Life Change Events. I. Steptoe,
  Andrew. II. Appels, A., 1938–   . III. Commission of the European
  Communities.
    [DNLM: 1. Health. 2. Internal–External Contro. 3. Stress,
  Psychological. WM 172 S91556]
  R726.5.S82 1989
  616'.0019—dc20
  DNLM/DLC
  for Library of Congress   89-14696
                            CIP

British Library Cataloguing in Publication Data

Stress, personal control and health.
  1. Man. Stress. Psychosocial aspects
  I. Steptoe, Andrew II. Appels, Ad
  155.9

  ISBN 0 471 92388 5

Typeset in Great Britain by Associated Publishing Services, Petersfield, Hampshire
Printed and bound in Great Britain by Biddles Ltd, Guildford and King's Lynn

Contents

List of contributors

AD APPELS, *Department of Medical Psychology, University of Limburg, Postbus 616, NL-6200 MD Maastricht, The Netherlands*

ARNOUD ARNTZ, *Department of Medical Psychology, University of Limburg, Postbus 616, NL-6200 MD Maastricht, The Netherlands*

GUNILLA BOHLIN, *Department of Clinical Psychology, University of Uppsala, PO Box 1225, S-752 41 Uppsala, Sweden*

BÉLA BOHUS, *Department of Animal Physiology, University of Groningen, Biologisch Centrum, Kerklaan 30, PO Box 14, 9750AA Haren, The Netherlands*

CHRISTOPHER COMBS, *Department of Psychology, Temple University, Weiss Hall, 13th Street & Cecil B. Moore Avenue, Philadelphia, Pennsylvania 19122 USA*

ROBERT DANTZER, *Psychobiologie des Comportements Adaptifs, INRA-INSERM 259, Domaine de Carreire, Rue Camille Saint-Saëns, F-33077 Bordeaux, France*

KELLY A. KELLY, *Department of Psychology, Northwestern University, 102 Swift Hall, Evanston, Illinois 60208, USA*

JAAP KOOLHAAS, *Department of Animal Physiology, University of Groningen, Biologisch Centrum, Kerklaan 30, PO Box 14, 9750AA Haren, The Netherlands*

HERBERT MATSCHINGER, *Central Institute for Mental Health, PO Box 122120, D6800, Mannheim, FRG*

SUZANNE M. MILLER, *Department of Psychology, Temple University, Weiss Hall, 13th Street & Cecil B. Moore Avenue, Philadelphia, Pennsylvania 19122 USA*

SUSAN MINEKA, *Department of Psychology, Northwestern University, 102 Swift Hall, Evanston, Illinois 60208, USA*

ARNE ÖHMAN, *Department of Clinical Psychology, University of Uppsala, PO Box 1225, S-752 41 Uppsala, Sweden*

JOHAN ORMEL, *Department of Psychiatry, University of Groningen, Academisch Ziekenhuis Groningen, Oostersingel 59, Postbus 30 001, 9700 RB Groningen, The Netherlands*

KATHARINE R. PARKES, *Department of Experimental Psychology, University of Oxford, South Parks Road, Oxford OX1 3UD, UK*

Keith Phillips, *Department of Psychology, Polytechnic of East London, The Green, Stratford, London E15 4LZ, UK*

Robbert Sanderman, *Department of Health Sciences, University of Groningen, Oostersingel 59, Postbus 30 001 9700 RB, Groningen, The Netherlands*

Anton J. M. Schmidt, *Department of Medical Psychology, University of Limburg, Postbus 616, NL-6200 MD, Maastricht, The Netherlands*

Johannes Siegrist, *Department of Medical Sociology, University of Marburg, Bunsenstrasse 2, D3550 Marburg, FRG*

Andrew Steptoe, *Department of Psychology, St George's Hospital Medical School, Cranmer Terrace, London SW17 0RE, UK*

Ellen Stoddard, *Department of Psychology, Temple University, Weiss Hall, 13th Street & Cecil B. Moore Avenue, Philadelphia, Pennsylvania 19122 USA*

S. Leonard Syme, *Department of Epidemiology, School of Public Health, University of California at Berkeley, 140 Warren Hall, Berkeley, California 94720, USA*

Töres Theorell, *National Institute for Psychosocial Factors and Health, Box 60210, S-104 01 Stockholm, Sweden*

Kenneth A. Wallston, *School of Nursing, Vanderbilt University, Nashville, Tennessee 37240, USA*

Preface

Personal control is being increasingly recognized as a central concept in the understanding of relationships between stressful experience, behaviour and health. Experimental investigations indicate that control over aversive stimulation has profound effects on automatic, endocrine and immunological responses, and may influence the pathological processes implicated in the development of cardiovascular disease, tumour rejection and proliferation, and the acquisition of gastrointestinal lesions. Clinically, control and lack of control have been identified as relevant to the experience of pain, anxiety and depression. In the field of psychosocial epidemiology, interesting observations are emerging that relate health to control over job parameters and other aspects of people's lives. The enhancement of personal control is also a common thread running through many intervention techniques, from behaviour therapy and preparation for stressful medical procedures to providing opportunities for self-determination among the institutionalized elderly, and increasing employee participation in decision making.

The aim of the present volume is to bring together contributors with diverse perspectives on stress, personal control and health. The disciplines represented include public health and epidemiology, medical sociology, social psychiatry, experimental and clinical psychology, nursing studies and animal physiology. This provides an opportunity for assessing the similarities and differences in the way in which control is invoked in a range of health-relevant issues. The current state of knowledge is summarized and opportunities for new integrative developments in research are highlighted.

The impetus for this book stemmed from the Concerted Action on the Quantification of Parameters for the Study of Breakdown in Human Adaptation. This initiative commenced in 1983 as part of the Medical and Health Research Programme of the Commission of the European Communities, and is concerned with research on breakdown in adaptation from a multidisciplinary perspective. Several of the contributors to this book are participants in the programme, and there have been wide-ranging discussions within the Concerted Action on the value of the concept of personal control. Research from six countries is represented in the volume, adding an international flavour to the multidisciplinary endeavour.

The book has been divided into three major sections, preceded by an introductory chapter and followed by a postscript. These sections reflect three broad areas in which research on control has been prominent. Section I is entitled 'Occupational aspects', and focuses on the role of control in job settings, and its influence on health. Section II, 'The clinical perspective', details the relationship of control with clinical problems such as pain, emotional disorders, heart disease and coping with stressful medical procedures. Finally, Section III, 'Mechanisms relating stress with control', describes the pathways through which control affects behaviour and psychobiological responses from an experimental perspective.

The editors wish to acknowledge the efforts of all the contributors to this volume, and hope that the compilation will be a valuable addition to the literature. Our thanks also go to Karyna Gilvarry and Margaret Reuben for their prompt and efficient clerical assistance.

ANDREW STEPTOE
AD APPELS

Introduction

CHAPTER 1

Control and health: a personal perspective

S. Leonard Syme
Department of Epidemiology, University of California at Berkeley, USA

The concept of control is of interest and importance to researchers in the health field for at least three reasons. First, it seems to provide a parsimonious integration that incorporates into one thought a variety of lesser and apparently unconnected ideas that up to now have been only of moderate interest. Second, the concept seems to have broad applicability: it has been invoked as an explanatory variable in experimental studies of both animals and humans, in clinical studies and in epidemiological research. As a result, this concept may be one of the few that transcends research boundaries and that may be useful in the development of interdisciplinary research. Third, the concept deals with behaviors that may be amenable to intervention: it involves behaviors which hopefully we can do something about. For at least these three reasons, the concept of control has in recent years increasingly been noted and mentioned in the literature in one form or another. In view of this growing interest, it now seems appropriate to examine the concept in more detail.

Four general issues are involved in such an examination. First, is there really anything to the idea? Is it worth further study? Second, if it is worthy of additional consideration, can we move closer toward a definition of what we mean by the term? At present, we use the term so vaguely that its usefulness is in question. Third, if we can define it, can we do so in a way that permits reliable and valid measurement? And fourth, if all of the foregoing is possible, what should the next steps be? Where do we go from here?

Stress, Personal Control and Health. Edited by A. Steptoe and A. Appels.
Published by John Wiley & Sons Ltd.
© ECSC–EEC–EAEC, Brussels–Luxembourg, 1989

CONTROL AS AN INTEGRATING CONCEPT

My introduction to the concept of control came about entirely by accident. I had for some years been interested in the fact that disease rates varied by socio-economic status: the lower the socio-economic status position, the higher the rate of virtually every disease and condition known to researchers (Antonovsky, 1967; Kitagawa and Hauser, 1973; Syme and Berkman, 1976). Most of the efforts to explain this well-known phenomenon had focused on such factors as inadequate medical care, unemployment, low income, racial factors, poor nutrition, poor housing and poor education. The difficulty with this approach was that these factors could not account for the existence of a *gradient* of disease rates by socio-economic status. It is not simply that people at the bottom of the socio-economic status hierarchy have higher rates of disease but that rates of disease increase *progressively* as one moves down from the top of the socio-economic status hierarchy to the bottom.

For example, in the work of Marmot and his colleagues (Marmot *et al.*, 1978), British civil servants in the highest social class grade (administrators) have the lowest rate of coronary heart disease, while those in the lowest grade have rates 4 times as high. Most interesting, however, is the fact that civil servants in the professional and executive grade and in the clerical grade have rates 2 times and 3.2 times as high as administrators, respectively. After account had been taken of such coronary heart disease risk factors as serum cholesterol, cigarette smoking, blood pressure, physical activity, obesity and glucose tolerance, this gradient of disease rates remained unchanged. While it might be possible to explain the high rates of coronary heart disease among less skilled manual workers in the British civil service in terms of such factors as income, education, housing and nutrition, these factors are unlikely to explain the difference in rates between administrators and professionals/executives, or clerical workers.

This gradient is not unique to British civil servants. It has been observed in a wide variety of populations in many different countries and it is not confined to a single disease entity or age group. This gradient has been observed for many body systems, including the digestive, genitourinary, respiratory, circulatory, nervous, infective and parasitic, blood and endocrine systems. It has been observed also for most malignancies, congenital anomalies, accidents, poisoning and violence, perinatal mortality, diabetes and musculoskeletal impairments (Susser *et al.*, 1985). It is very difficult to explain these gradients and, especially, to account for differences between those at the top of the hierarchy and those just one or two steps down from the top.

One hypothesis consistent with these data involves the concept of control. It could be postulated that the lower down one is in the socio-economic status hierarchy, the less control one has over the factors that affect life and living circumstances. Of course, this hypothesis is very general and it does not specify whether control involves money, power, information, prestige, experience or something else. While not precise, the hypothesis does at least direct attention to a general range of issues. In this sense, the concept of control can be seen as a 'sensitizing concept' that deserves further research and examination.

Whatever the merits of this hypothesis, it does fit the data regarding socio-economic status, whereas most other hypotheses do not and, furthermore, it is the only hypothesis I could develop to fit the facts. To me, the plausibility of the control hypothesis is strengthened by the fact that it is consistent also with many other research findings that have little or nothing specifically to do with socio-economic status.

It is important to recognize the dangers inherent in such a search of the literature to find support for a favored hypothesis. This activity is dangerous because it is virtually certain that such support will be found. Searches of this kind tend to give more weight to findings that are consistent with the hypothesis and less weight to those that are not. In spite of this, the existence of such supportive evidence does tend to increase the plausibility of the hypothesis and, as long as appropriate skepticism and caution is exercised, such searches can be worthwhile.

The first supportive evidence I came across involved the work on job stress that had been carried out by Karasek *et al.* (1981), Alfredsson *et al.* (1982) and Theorell *et al.* (1984) in Sweden and the United States. These investigators had shown that rates of coronary heart disease were higher among workers who experienced not only high job demand but low discretion and latitude for dealing with those demands. The work of these researchers is especially impressive because previous studies of job stress had for decades failed to establish a link between job pressures and health even though this issue had been examined intensively. When the concepts of control and discretion were included in the research, important findings at least emerged and in fact are now being replicated by others (House *et al.*, 1986; Haan and Aro, 1988). In our work on hypertension among San Francisco bus drivers, and in new studies of British civil servants, we also are now using this concept and it is proving to be a very useful tool.

As pleasing as it was to find support for the concept of control in the job stress literature, I was astonished to learn that it had already been studied very successfully for years by many psychologists and sociologists in the study of health and illness. My naivety on this is embarrassing: I had come across a great truth only to find that literally dozens of scholars had been working on this issue for many years. A partial listing of such usage will illustrate this point. Pearlin and his colleagues (1981) have studied the concept of 'mastery'; Bandura (1982) and O'Leary (1985), among others, have studied 'self-efficacy'; Rotter (1975) and Wallston and Wallston (1982) have studied 'locus of control'; Seligman (1975) 'learned helplessness'; Glass and Singer (1972) and Sherrod (1974) 'controll-ability'; Cohen (1980) 'predictability'; Burger (1985) 'desire for control'; Langer (1983), Rodin (1986) and Schulz (1976) 'sense of control'; Bauman and

Udry (1972) 'powerlessness'; Kobasa (1982) 'hardiness'; Libassi and Maluccio (1986) 'competence'; and so on. In addition, other scholars have used concepts that easily can be seen as related to the notion of control. For example, James *et al.* (1983) have suggested the importance of 'John Henryism' in accounting for the high rates of hypertension among poor blacks in the United States; by this term, James is referring to blacks who enthusiastically have accepted American middle-class goals relating to success and achievement but who by reason of poor education are not likely to reach these goals.

It is important not to over-interpret the fact that so many investigators have suggested the importance of control for health and well-being. In fact, few of these people are using the same term in exactly the same way; each use tends to have a special focus and each has been found of value in explaining different disease outcomes. For this reason, it is an exaggeration to claim that they are variations on one theme. On the other hand, it is intriguing that so many different scholars, from different backgrounds and with different research objectives, should come up with ideas that are so similar to one another.

There is more. The idea of control is not inconsistent with other major findings in social epidemiology. Everyone has a different list of 'major findings' but my listing includes mobility, social support, type A behavior, and stressful life events Syme (1986). The evidence on these factors suggests that each is associated with the higher incidence and prevalence of disease independently of other known risk factors. While these associations are fairly clear, the reasons for them are not. Each of these factors has been studied relatively independently of the others and, to my knowledge, no one has seriously attempted a search for commonalities. Seen from the perspective of control, however, it is possible to suggest that all of these factors are simply different facets or manifestations of control or of its absence.

With the caution appropriate for such ad hoc reasoning, we can suggest that social support is useful in helping to influence the events that affect our lives. This idea, of course, is an old one but its first and most elegant expression in modern writings comes from the work of John Cassel (1974). More recently, Pearlin *et al.* (1981) reported that people with confidants exhibited higher levels of self-esteem and personal control. Seeman and Syme (1987) have found also that people with high levels of social support are in a better position to control the events that impinge upon them. In this study of people undergoing coronary angiography, a comparison was made of the various components that are included in the concept of social support. Components studied were number of friends, number of close friends, frequency of seeing people, satisfaction with the quantity and quality of relationships, what one did for people, what people did for one, and so on. Comparing the predictive power of these various approaches, the most powerful one was the instrumental view of support. Compared to other definitions of social support, less coronary atherosclerosis was seen among people who could count on specific people to help them when they needed specific kinds of help (e.g., to borrow money, help with household repairs, advise with problems).

If social support is important as an aid in dealing with events that affect life, it is not difficult to see that mobility and stressful life events disturb control by interrupting social relationships. Mobility involving changes in jobs and places of residence inevitably affect social ties as do most of the important life events such as marriage, divorce or death of a loved one. However, if people can participate in some aspects of the disruption, the likelihood of disease consequences may be lessened. For example, when elderly persons are geographically relocated, the morbidity and mortality results usually seen are much less pronounced when they are given a choice about when and where to move or about various aspects of their new living arrangements (Krantz and Schulz, 1980). In the same spirit of ad hoc reasoning, it is possible to suggest that those exhibiting type A behavior have higher rates of coronary heart disease because of their continual but unsuccessful efforts to control events in their lives (Glass, 1977).

It is unnecessary to go on in this vein. Obviously, with some ingenuity and motivation, it is not difficult to weave a consistent story regarding control from almost any set of data. Enough perhaps has already been said to suggest that the concept does provide for the integration of a wide variety of apparently unconnected and independent observations. It is difficult to think of other concepts that do this as easily or simply. This is attractive because it is the aim of science to present facts in the simplest and most economical conceptual formulation.

CONTROL AS A TRANSCENDENT CONCEPT FOR INTERDISCIPLINARY RESEARCH

Discovering the causes of a disease requires the collaboration of researchers from many disciplines. However, those who have actually tried to engage in interdisciplinary research know how difficult and frustrating this experience can be. Researchers from different disciplines often use different methods and techniques, define terms differently, and have different research priorities and objectives. As a consequence, many investigators simply give up on interdisciplinary collaboration and opt instead for working with people who share their own research approach. While understandable, this withdrawal is unfortunate because it makes the search for the cause of disease more difficult.

The search for the causes of disease can be seen as taking place at several levels. At one level, we ask how specific disease agents act alone or together to produce disease in *one* individual. At another level, we ask why *one* person gets sick instead of *another*. At yet another level, we ask why *rates* of disease are higher in one group than in another.

One would think that the answer to a question at any one of these levels of inquiry would be useful in answering the questions posed at the other levels. Unfortunately, this often is not the case. For example, we have a very solid body of research information regarding the biological consequences that follow infection of the body by the cholera vibrio. This information is only of limited value in understanding why one person develops cholera while another does not. It is of even less use in shedding light on reasons for the distribution of cholera throughout the world.

The problem is not that there exists different levels of analysis in the search for the causes of disease. The problem is that researchers tend to focus their efforts at only one level so that, over time, scientific disciplines develop different techniques, methods and concepts that are particularly suitable to study at that level. This specialization tends to make difficult interdisciplinary communication and collaboration. This problem is not amenable to simple solution and it certainly cannot be resolved by well-meaning conferences in which researchers from different disciplines are urged to try hard to be cooperative and sharing.

Interdisciplinary cooperation might be enhanced if we could identify concepts that transcended various levels of research strategy. Control may be one of these concepts. If it were agreed that the concept of control is important, it might be easier to begin to specify and to more clearly visualize these differences in approach. This does not solve the problem but it narrows the range of disagreement and permits a specification of differences so that communication can proceed. In recent years, the concept of control has appeared more and more frequently to help explain variations in biological functioning in laboratory, clinical and population research. In this research, the term has of course been defined and measured differently, but enough common content seems included in this usage to suggest that a transcendent core may exist. Much of the material in the present volume is a demonstration of this. As can be seen, the concept of control—defined differently in virtually every instance—has been used effectively in research at several levels of inquiry; that these different approaches appear together in one collection provides a unique opportunity to examine the different meanings attributed to the concept and to begin the process of identifying common ground.

THE DEFINITION AND MEASUREMENT OF 'CONTROL'

It is perhaps not surprising that a concept as general and ill-defined as control should provide for integration among different research findings as well as across disciplinary boundaries. This vagueness may be the reason that the concept can encompass such a wide variety of heterogeneous ideas. Loss of control has been defined in terms of constraints on coping ability, diminished authority over decisions, threats to status and self-esteem, lessened opportunity to learn new skills and inappropriateness of coping. Question has been raised in the literature as to whether the concept refers to perceived control or to actual control. Some view controllability in terms of predictability, while others see it in terms of sense of coherence or sense of permanence. Control can be assessed as a property of individuals or of situations; it can reflect a quality of individuals as well as be a function of training and opportunities or of social and cultural circumstances. Control can be a positive or negative force depending on personality, cultural milieu and previous experiences. It can involve specific situations or all situations. People can be seen to desire control, need control or abhor control. The idea can refer to control over big things, little things or all things. Some think of control as a personal 'state of being' (of *being* in control) while others see it as a 'condition' (where *things* are under control).

In this circumstance, the temptation to move towards one common definition is strong. If we could agree on such a definition, we then could develop appropriate assessment methods and hopefully a coherent and comparable body of research evidence. While this is reasonable, there are some serious hazards in such an approach. In the first place, it is difficult to accomplish given our present state of knowledge. Each of the various conceptions of control currently in use have merit and it is not easy to see how one would choose the 'right' one. As noted earlier, with some ingenuity, substantial research evidence can be arranged to support any one of these approaches. In the end, the selection of the 'best' definition will depend on its usefulness in accounting for research observations.

In the second place, there is a hazard in prematurely moving toward one commonly agreed upon definition of such concepts. One need only review the recent history of research on type A behavior to see the damage that can follow from the decision to prematurely define terms and agree on measurement methods. Rosenman *et al.* (1975) had shown that, at least in their hands, a behavior type could be identified and measured so that it predicted coronary heart disease. Based on their one prospective study, investigators around the world tacitly accepted their definition of type A behavior and attempted to measure it by use of the structured interview and by questionnaires such as the Jenkins Activity Scale, the Bortner Scale or the Framingham Scale.

The results of this outpouring of research are so varied as to be uninterpretable. Many studies found a relationship between the behavior pattern but an approximately equal number have failed to do so. Several major conferences and workshops have been convened aimed at developing some consensus regarding these varied results, but these meetings have not achieved agreement (Ostfeld and Eaker, 1985). It is only in the last few years that new work by Williams *et al.* (1985), Scherwitz *et al.* (1983), Kobasa (1982) and others (Matthews and Haynes, 1986) is now providing some clarification in this area. This new work suggests that the concept of type A behavior was probably too vague a concept in the first place and that it was premature to try to capture it using one or another questionnaire or scale. The research now going on in this field is suggesting that the important element in type A behavior may really be a particular subcomponent that the global concept was reflecting but that now should be measured directly. Of course, these investigators have their own view of what that subcomponent is and few of them agree with one another about what it is. For example, one or another of these investigators has suggested that the important dimension of type A behavior is hostility, others that it is need for control, others that it is self-reference behavior, yet others that it is hardiness, and so on.

While we are still far from having a clear view of the meaning and importance of type A behavior, it is refreshing to see that research now under way is directed towards achieving an understanding of the concept rather than a more or less mindless and repetitive effort to replicate findings that emerged from one early study. This phenomenon is not limited to type A behavior. A more or less similar scenario can now be seen with reference to such other popular concepts as social support and stressful life events.

There are at least two alternatives to the 'consensus' movement. One, suggested by Cohen (1988), is to bring together in one place all of the various approaches and definitions of control so that a typology can be developed. This typology would help us to see what various definitions have in common and, at the same time, to see how they differ from one another. An important contribution of this approach would be to help in discerning underlying issues, themes and processes. A somewhat different approach is to think of control as a 'sensitizing' concept—a concept that raises consciousness about an issue and that directs thinking along certain lines but that does not provide specific guidance about definitions or assessment methods. This approach suffers from lack of rigor but it does encourage a very wide range of research perspectives so that the relative power of each can more easily be appreciated.

In either case, the issue of definitions is an empirical one, better settled by research than by argument and debate. As such, a major priority in this area of work is the initiation of research that specifically and systematically compares the usefulness of various definitions and approaches.

THE POTENTIAL FOR INTERVENTION

In the health field, the usefulness of a concept is enhanced if it can be used to help prevent disease: the concept of control seems clearly of potential value in this respect. The special and exciting potential of the concept of control, however, is that it is amenable to intervention and application not only at the individual level but also at the community and environmental level. This usefulness at the environmental level is worthy of note because we have had great difficulty in helping individuals to make changes in many behaviors that affect health. Many people who try to quit smoking fail (Syme and Alcalay, 1982). We have little success in getting people to lower the fat and salt content of their diet (Kirscht and Rosenstock, 1979), and the majority of people who try to lose weight and maintain losses do not succeed. Even in a specially designed program like the Multiple Risk Factor Intervention Trial (MRFIT) (1981, 1982), where optimal conditions existed for behavior change, many people were unable to follow recommendations for dietary change and smoking cessation. This occurred in spite of the fact that MRFIT included an informed and highly motivated group of participants, an excellent behavioral intervention plan, excellent and numerous staff, and enough time to work with each participant over a six-year period.

One major limitation of almost all intervention programs is that we have viewed high-risk behaviors almost exclusively as problems of the individual. When intervention programs focus exclusively on the individual and his behavior, they ignore the fact that these behaviors occur in a social and cultural context. By focusing on the individual's motivations and perceptions, we may be neglecting some of the most important influences on behavior such as social values, fashions and priorities (Leventhal and Cleary, 1980).

Even if we could induce people to change their behavior in one-to-one programs, the impact of such changes in the population would be modest. The reason for this is that new people continue to enter the 'at-risk' population even as high-risk people leave it since individually oriented programs do nothing to deal with the environmental factors that initiated the problem. In this circumstance, an environmental approach may be more useful than an individual one.

While control is a characteristic of individuals, it is also a product of the environment. Interventions to enhance control therefore can be directed both to the individual and to the environment. The work of Langer and Rodin (1976) and Rodin and Langer (1977) provides a classic example of the way in which control can be dealt with at the environmental level. These investigators provided arrangements whereby a group of elderly convalescent-home residents could make more choices about their living circumstance and have more control of day-to-day events. After 18 months of follow-up, these residents showed a significantly greater improvement in health than a comparable group of residents who were 'looked after' by the staff. Compared to a 25% mortality rate in the nursing home in the 18 months before intervention, only 15% of the subjects in the intervention group died. In the same time period, 30% in the control group died. Several other important interventions among elderly persons have yielded positive results (Rodin, 1986), as have interventions in other organizational contexts such as hospitals (Langer *et al.*, 1975; Taylor, 1979).

Another illustration of the power of environmental manipulations of control comes from the other end of the age spectrum. In this case, children 3 and 4 years of age from disadvantaged backgrounds during the 1960s in the United States were offered one or two years of special education prior to their enrollment in regular school. In 1977, the American Association for the Advancement of Science sponsored a symposium in which 100 longitudinal experiments on such early enrichment were evaluated. Over 90 of these studies reported long-term gains in social and emotional competence, intellectual and language development and 'meaningful parent involvement' (Brown, 1978). More interesting for our purposes, however, are the results reported from a 22-year follow-up of low-income children from Ypsilanti, Michigan. These children had been randomly assigned either to a Head Start program or to no program (Berrueta-Clement *et al.*, 1984). At age 19, those who had one or two years of early education were more likely than those in the control group to complete high school (67% versus 49%) and be employed (59% versus 32%) and were less likely to have been arrested (31% versus 51%), been on public assistance (18% versus 32%) and, for girls, were 50% less likely to have had a teenage pregnancy. Since these children were assigned at random to the Head Start program, these reported differences are probably attributable to the program itself and not to such other factors as motivated parents or differences in baseline intellectual level.

While these results come from only one study, other long-term follow-up studies have been done on Head Start children and it would be useful to collect and critically review data obtained in those studies. A new series of similar programs is now under way in England. If subsequent analyses support the findings from the Ypsilanti study, it will be important to explain how one or two years of early education could have such a profound impact on the quality of life many years later. Indeed, this type of analysis might be most useful in helping to identify crucial components of control.

Another illustration of interventions to enhance control comes from our work with San Francisco bus drivers. Several previous studies have noted that bus drivers, compared with workers in other occupations, have a higher prevalence of hypertension as well as diseases of the gastrointestinal tract and of the musculo-skeletal and respiratory systems. These results have been obtained from studies in different transit systems, under different conditions and in several countries (Berlinguer, 1962; Morris *et al.*, 1966; Garbe, 1980; Netterstrom and Laursen, 1981; Winkleby *et al.*, 1988). Based on these findings, it has been suggested that certain aspects of the bus-driving occupation may create an increased risk for disease among these workers.

In our study of drivers, we are monitoring such environmental factors as exposure to noise, vibration and carbon monoxide fumes, but we are paying particular attention to the drivers' social environment (Ragland *et al.*, 1987; Winkleby *et al.*, 1988). One of the most important aspects of that environment is that drivers must keep to a specific schedule that is arranged without realistic reference to actual road conditions and, in fact, cannot be met. From the instant drivers sit in the bus, they are behind schedule and are continually reprimanded for this.

In this circumstance, interventions to improve the work situation of drivers can be introduced not merely among bus drivers but directly on the schedule itself. For example, it may be that by changing the way in which schedules are arranged, the bus company will be able to earn more money than it loses because of reduced rates of absenteeism among drivers as well as lower rates of sickness, accidents and, in particular, turnover. It is possible that drivers could be invited to share in the schedule-making process: they probably have useful information to provide regarding important elements of the schedule. Even if the schedule itself is not changed much, however, drivers will at least have had a hand in creating it. It often is true that we can better tolerate bad situations if at least they are of our own choosing rather than imposed by others.

These examples illustrate the possibility of aiming interventions to ehance control not just at individuals but at the social environment. The modification of living arrangements in a nursing home is an institutional and organizational matter; the provision of early enrichment programs for children is a community issue; the opportunity for workers to participate in determining the factors that affect their working lives is a company issue. Without the availability of these structural resources, it is difficult for people, on their own, to enhance control over their lives. Clearly, we need both environmental support and individual initiatives. The concept of control is especially attractive because it is amenable to intervention at both levels.

CONCLUSION

One of the questions posed in the introduction to this chapter was whether or not there really is anything of value in the concept of control. Is it worth further study? My thoughts of this question are, of course, limited by my perspective and experience. In the work I know best, the concept clearly is of great interest because it provides a parsimonious approach to so many apparently unrelated ideas. Relying on the concept of control, loosely defined, I can better understand why higher rates of disease are found among people who have poor social support, who have been mobile, who have had stressful life events, who are in jobs with little latitude and little room for discretion, who are in lower socio-economic positions, and who exhibit type A behavior. So far, I have come across no findings in my field of knowledge that are consistent with the control hypothesis.

There are at least four reasons for this phenomenon. The first is that I have not covered all of the findings available and, if I had looked harder, I would certainly have found such contradictory evidence. The second is that I have been so ingenious that I have been able to fit almost anything into my pre-set schema. The third is that the concept is so vaguely and ambiguously defined that it can encompass virtually any idea simply because of that vagueness. The fourth is that it may really be a useful and parsimonious concept and that what we see is an accurate reflection of reality.

There probably is some validity to each of these possibilities and it ought to be a priority to see which have more weight. This volume contains an enormous range of research effort dealing in one way or another with the concept of control and, as such, it provides a rich resource for such comparative work. I come to this resource looking not for confirmation of my beliefs but for contradictions and negative evidence. Confirmatory evidence is reassuring but it does not help to clarify ideas. Negative evidence forces us to confront the inadequacy of our thinking and requires that we sharpen our concepts and assessment methods. One of the problems I face as a researcher, however, is my reluctance and/or inability to seek out such negative evidence and to recognize it when I see it. I tend to rationalize away such contradictory evidence with alarming ease so that the problem set before me rarely penetrates my conscious thought. This is one of the special advantages of inviting to a conference researchers from different fields with different perspectives and commitments in order to examine together one idea. In a conference setting, we still are able to talk past each other and avoid confronting unpleasant and contradictory data, but it is not as easy. To assemble the presented evidence from such a conference in one volume makes it more difficult to practice this type of avoidance and denial.

In answer to the questions 'Is there anything to the idea of control? Is it worth further study?' my answer is a firm 'yes', but I am concerned that my perspective is too narrow and specialized; examination of the evidence from other perspectives, therefore, would be great value.

The second and third questions posed in the introduction to this chapter dealt with the question of whether we could move toward a more precise definition of what is meant by the term control so that we can measure it reliably and validly. This is a difficult and controversial issue. One could argue with considerable justification that a clear and agreed-upon definition is necessary if we are to generate data that are comparable. My view is that this desirable goal is premature. Agreement on one definition means the exclusion of other definitions. While I have my own favorite definition, I doubt that others would agree with me. One way to deal with this problem is to develop a typology of control definitions by recognizing that seemingly dissimilar definitions of control in fact have themes in common. Another way to approach this issue is to encourage a variety of different definitions, to applaud rather than condemn negative and contradictory evidence, and to select from the resulting diversity of results those definitions that most usefully solve problems.

The fourth question posed in the introduction dealt with the steps that are needed next. The simple answer to this question is the time-honored one: more research is needed. The question remains 'What kind of research?' If the foregoing arguments make sense, we need a variety of research approaches among animals and humans, and in laboratory, clinic and population settings, aimed at answering questions such as why a person becomes ill, why one person becomes ill and not another, and why rates of illness are higher in one group than in another. But we can go further than this. One of the fascinating results from research on control is the diversity of outcomes that have been observed, ranging from physiological abnormalities to pychological distress to disease and death. In this work, a wide variety of organ systems and biological processes are seen to be affected by control or its absence.

That this one factor, control, is associated with higher rates of so many different diseases and conditions may at first glance seem biologically implausible. Two models come to mind that might account for this phenomenon. One model postulates that the concept of control includes so many diverse elements that each element separately influences the likelihood of different diseases and conditions. This often is the explanation offered to account for the higher rate of so many diseases and conditions associated with cigarette smoking. The second model suggests that stressors associated with the breakdown of control (however defined) act to depress the body's defense systems so that people affected are more vulnerable to a wide range of disease agents (Sklar and Anisman, 1979; Visintainer *et al.*, 1982; Laudenslager *et al.* 1983). In this model, the presence of such specific disease agents as viruses, bacteria, air pollutants or high blood pressure would not result in diseases unless the person was vulnerable to them. For this reason, the presence of breakdown in control would predict the likelihood of people getting sick, but not what disease they got. This model is attractive because it would account for the fact that (a) the concept of control is related to many different diseases involving many organ systems, and (b) most well-recognized disease-specific risk factors only sometimes result in disease.

If the second model seems reasonable, research on control should focus not only on specific diseases and conditions but also on compromised defense systems in general. In this way, the study of control—a concept that parsimoniously integrates a variety of seemingly unrelated *psychosocial* concepts—can lead to studies of immunological function—an approach that might parsimoniously integrate a variety of seemingly unrelated *disease* outcomes.

We are properly guarded about the introduction of trendy new ideas or of new words that merely provide a fresh package for old ideas. In the case of the concept of control, however, we may really be on to something important. In my view, the idea is worth serious study and consideration. This volume provides a wonderful opportunity to begin this process.

ACKNOWLEDGEMENTS

I am indebted to Sheldon Cohen, Meredith Minkler and Fiona North for comments and advice on an earlier draft of this chapter.

REFERENCES

Alfredsson, L., Karasek, R., and Theorell, T. (1982). Myocardial infarction risk and psychosocial work environment: An analysis of the male Swedish working force. *Social Science and Medicine*, **16**, 463–467.

Antonovsky, A. (1967). Social class, life expectancy and overall mortality. *Milbank Memorial Fund Quarterly*, **45**, 31–73.

Bandura, A. (1982). Self-efficacy mechanisms in human agency. *American Psychologist*, **37**, 122–147.

Bauman, K. E., and Udry, J. R. (1972). Powerlessness and regularity of contraception in an urban Negro male sample: A research note. *Journal of Marriage and the Family*, **34**, 112–114.

Berlinguer, G. (1962). *Maladies and Industrial Health of Public Transportation Workers* (Translation). Washington, DC: US Department of Transportation, UMTA-VA-06-0034-82-2.

Berrueta-Clement, J. R., Schweinhart, L. J., Barnett, W. S., Epstein, A. S., and Weikart, D. P. (1984). *Changed Lives: The Effects of the Perry Preschool Program on Youths Through Age 19*. Ypsilanti, Michigan: High/Scope Press.

Brown, B. (ed). (1978). *Found: Long-term Gains from Early Intervention*. American Association for the Advancement of Science Symposium. Boulder, Colorado: Westview Press.

Burger, J. (1985). Desire for control and achievement-related behaviors. *Journal of Personality and Social Psychology*, **48**, 1520–1533.

Cassel, J. (1974). Psychosocial processes and 'stress': Theoretical formulations. *International Journal of Health Services*, **4**, 471–482.

Cohen, S. (1980). Aftereffects of stress on human performance and social behavior. *Psychological Bulletin*, **88**, 82–108.

Cohen, S. (1988). Personal communication.

Garbe, C. (1980). *Health and Health Risks among City Bus Drivers in West Berlin* (Translation). Washington, DC: US Department of Transportation, UMTA-VA-06-0034-3.

Glass, D. C. (1977). *Behavior Patterns, Stress and Coronary Disease*. Hillsdale, New Jersey: Erlbaum.

Glass, D. C., and Singer, J. E. (1972). *Urban Stress: Experiments on Noise and Social Stressors*. New York: Academic Press.

Haan, M. N., and Aro, S. (1988). Job strain and ischemic heart disease: An epidemiologic study of metal workers. *Annals of Clinical Research*, **20**, 143–146.

House, J. S., Strecher, V., Metzner, H. L., and Robbins, C. A. (1986). Occupational stress and health among men and women in the Tecumseh Community Health Study. *Journal of Health and Social Behavior*, **27**, 62–77.

James, S. A., Hartnett, S. A., and Kalsbeek, W. D. (1983). John Henryism and blood pressure differences among black men. *Journal of Behavioral Medicine*, **6**, 259–278.

Karasek, R., Baker, D., Marxer, F., Ahlbom, A., and Theorell, T. (1981). Job decision latitude, job demands, and cardiovascular disease: A prospective study of Swedish men. *American Journal of Public Health*, **71**, 694–705.

Kirscht, J. P., and Rosenstock, I. M. (1979). Patients' problems in following recommendations of health experts. In: G. C. Stone, F. Cohen and N. E. Adler (eds), *Health Psychology: A Handbook*. San Francisco: Jossey-Bass.

Kitagawa, E. M., and Hauser, P. M. (1973). *Differential Mortality in the United States*. Cambridge: Harvard University Press.

Kobasa, S. C. (1982). The hardy personality: Toward a social psychology of stress and health. In: G. S. Sanders and J. Suls (eds), *Social Psychology of Health and Illness*. Hillsdale, New Jersey: Erlbaum.

Krantz, D., and Schulz, R. (1980). A model life crisis control and health outcomes: Cardiac rehabilitation and relocation of the elderly. In: A. Baum and J. E. Singer (eds), *Advances in Environmental Psychology, Vol. 3, Cardiovascular Disorders and Behavior*. Hillsdale, New Jersey: Erlbaum.

Langer, E. J. (1983). *The Psychology of Control*. Beverly Hills, California: Sage.

Langer, E. J., and Rodin, J. (1976). The effects of choice and enhanced personal responsibility for the aged: A field experiment in an institutional setting. *Journal of Personality and Social Psychology*, **34**, 191.

Langer, E. J., Janis, I. L., and Wolfer, J. A. (1975). Reduction of psychological stress in surgical patients. *Journal of Experimental and Social Psychology*, **11**, 155–165.

Laudenslager, M. L., Ryan, S. M., Drugan, R. C., Hyson, R. L., and Maier, S. F. (1983). Coping and immunosuppression: Inescapable but not escapable shock suppresses lymphocyte proliferation. *Science*, **221**, 568–571.

Leventhal, H., and Cleary, P. D. (1980). The smoking problem: A review of the research and theory in behavioral risk modification. *Psychological Bulletin*, **88**, 370–405.

Libassi, M. F., and Muluccio, A. (1986). Competence-centered social work: Prevention in action. *Journal of Primary Prevention*, **6**, 168–180.

Marmot, M. G., Rose, G., Shipley, M., and Hamilton, P. J. S. (1978). Employment grade and coronary heart disease in British civil servants. *Journal of Epidemiology and Community Health*, **3**, 244–249.

Matthews, K. A., and Haynes, S. G. (1986). Type A behavior pattern and coronary disease risk. *American Journal of Epidemiology*, **123**, 923–961.

Morris, J. N., Kagan, A., Pattison, D. C., Gardner, M. J., and Raffle, P. A. B. (1966). Incidence and prediction of ischemic heart disease in London busmen. *Lancet*, **1**, 533–559.

Multiple Risk Factor Intervention Trial Research Group (1981). The Multiple Risk Factor Intervention Trial. *Preventive Medicine*, **10**, 387–553.

Multiple Risk Factor Intervention Trial Research Group (1982). The Multiple Risk Factor Intervention Trial: Risk factor changes and mortality results. *Journal of the American Medical Association*, **248**, 1465–1476.

Netterstrom, B., and Laursen, P. (1981). Incidence and prevalence of ischemic heart disease among urban bus drivers in Copenhagen. *Scandinavian Journal of Social Medicine*, **2**, 75–79.

O'Leary, A. (1985). Self-efficacy and health. *Behavior Research and Therapy*, **23**, 437–451.

Ostfeld, A. M., and Eaker, E. D. (eds) (1985). *Measuring Psychosocial Variables in Epidemiologic Studies of Cardiovascular Disease: Proceedings of A Workshop*. Bethesda, Maryland: National Institutes of Health Publication No. 85-2270.

Pearlin, L. I., Menaghan, E. G., Leiberman, M. A., and Mullan, J. T. (1981). The stress process. *Journal of Health and Social Behavior*, **22**, 337–356.

Ragland, D. R., Winkleby, M. A., Schwalbe, J., Holman, B. L., Morse, L., Syme, S. L., and Fisher, J. M. (1987). Prevalence of hypertension in bus drivers. *International Journal of Epidemiology*, **16**, 208–213.

Rodin, J. (1986). Aging and health: Effects of the sense of control. *Science*, **233**, 1271–1276.

Rodin, J., and Langer, E. J. (1977). Long-term effects of a control-relevant intervention with the institutionalized aged. *Journal of Personality and Social Psychology*, **35**, 897–902.

Rosenman, R. H., Brand, R. J., Jenkins, C. D., Friedman, M., Straus, R., and Wurm, M. (1975). Coronary heart disease in the Western Collaborative Group Study: Final follow-up experience of $8\frac{1}{2}$ years. *Journal of the American Medical Association*, **233**, 872–877.

Rotter, J. B. (1975). Some problems and misconceptions related to the construct of internal versus external reinforcement. *Journal of Consulting and Clinical Psychology*, **43**, 56–67.

Scherwitz, L., McKelvain, R., Laman, C., Patterson, J., and Dutton, L. (1983). Type A behavior, self-involvement, and coronary atherosclerosis. *Psychosomatic Medicine*, **45**, 47–57.

Schulz, R. (1976). Effects of control and predictability on the physical and psychological well-being of the institutionalized aged. *Journal of Personality and Social Psychology*, **33**, 563–573.

Seeman, T. E., and Syme, S. L. (1987). Social networks and coronary artery disease: A comparison of the structure and function of social relations as predictors of disease. *Psychosomatic Medicine*, **49**, 341–354.

Seligman, M. E. P. (1975). *Helplessness: On Depression, Development, and Death.* San Francisco. Freeman.

Sherrod, D. R. (1974). Crowding, perceived control, and behavioral aftereffects. *Journal of Applied Social Psychology,* **4**, 171–186.

Sklar, L. S., and Anisman, H. (1979). Stress and coping factors influence tumor growth. *Science,* **205**, 513–515.

Susser, M. W., Watson, W., and Hopper, K. (1985). *Sociology in Medicine.* New York: Oxford University Press.

Syme, S. L. (1986). Social determinants of health and disease. In: J. M. Last (ed.), *Public Health and Preventive Medicine* (12th edn). Norwalk, Connecticut: Appleton-Century-Crofts.

Syme, S. L., and Alcalay, R. (1982). Control of cigarette smoking from a social perspective. *Annual Review of Public Health,* **3**, 179–199.

Syme, S. L., and Berkman, L.F. (1976). Social class, susceptibility and sickness. *American Journal of Epidemiology,* **104**, 1–8.

Taylor, S. E. (1979). Hospital patient behaviour: Reactance, helplessness or control? *Journal of Social Issues,* **35**, 156–184.

Theorell, T., Alfredsson, L., Knox, S., Persk, A., Svensson, J., and Waller, D. (1984). On the interplay between socioeconomic factors, personality and work environment in the pathogenesis of cardiovascular disease. *Scandinavian Journal of Work and Environmental Health,* **10**, 373–380.

Visintainer, M. A., Volpicelli, J. R., and Seligman, M. E. P. (1982). Tumor rejection in rats after inescapable shock. *Science,* **216**, 437–439.

Wallston, K. A., and Wallston, B. S. (1982). Who is responsible for your health? The construct of health locus of control. In: G. S. Sanders and J. Suls (eds), *Social Psychology of Health and Illness.* Hillsdale, New Jersey: Erlbaum.

Williams, R. B., Barefoot, J. C., and Shekelle, R. B. (1985). The health consequences of hostility. In: M. Chesney and R. Rosenman (eds), *Anger and Hostility and Cardiovascular and Behavioral Disorders.* Washington: Hemisphere Publishing.

Winkleby, M. A., Ragland, D. R., Fisher, J. M., and Syme, S. L. (1988). Excess risk of sickness and disease in bus drivers: A review and synthesis of epidemiologic studies. *International Journal of Epidemiology,* **17**, 255–262.

Winkleby, M. A., Ragland, D. R., and Syme, S. L. (1988). Self-reported stressors and hypertension: Evidence of an inverse relationship. *American Journal of Epidemiology,* **27**, 124–134.

Section I

Occupational aspects

CHAPTER 2

Personal control in an occupational context

KATHARINE R. PARKES
Department of Experimental Psychology, University of Oxford, UK

THE CONCEPT OF PERSONAL CONTROL IN THE WORK ENVIRONMENT

During recent years, the concept of control has been increasingly recognized as a topic of major importance in the context of research into work conditions and their impact on well-being and satisfaction. This importance is reflected not only in empirical studies (most recently, Adelmann, 1987; Bromet *et al.*, 1988; Karasek *et al.*, 1987; Pearson, 1987; Perrewe and Mizerski, 1987; Spector, 1987a; Tetrick and LaRocco, 1987), but also in several review articles which discuss the implications of control in occupational settings from individual, organizational and sociological perspectives (Ganster, 1989; Greenberger and Strasser, 1986; Jackson, 1989; Johnson, 1989; Sutton and Kahn, 1987).

It is clear from these articles that there is no single view of control common to all researchers in the areas of occupational and organizational psychology. Rather, interpretation of the control construct depends on the particular conceptual and methodological focus of the study concerned. Thus, in the psychological literature, it is possible to identify three approaches to defining personal control in the work environment: (1) control as an objective characteristic of the work situation, reflecting the extent to which the design of work tasks, and the work environment more generally, allow opportunities for control; (2) control as a subjective evaluation reflecting an individual's judgement about the extent to which his or her work situation is amenable to control; and (3) control as a generalized belief on the part of an individual about the extent to which

Stress, Personal Control and Health.   Edited by A. Steptoe and A. Appels.
Published by John Wiley & Sons Ltd.

important outcomes (including, but not limited to, occupational outcomes) are controllable. Most studies of control in work settings are concerned, by definition or implication, with one or more of these facets of control.

Control as an objective characteristic of the work situation

Sutton and Kahn (1987) provide a broad definition of control as an objective characteristic of the work situation. In their view, control is 'the exercise of effective influence over events, things and persons' (p. 276) in the work environment. This definition of control includes not only influence over specific work tasks, but also influence over people and over the organization as a whole. In contrast, other authors (e.g. Kahn, 1981) consider objective control in a more limited context, relating it specifically to control over immediate work tasks. Warr (1987) distinguishes between control at the level of individual jobs, and control at an organizational level. He refers to control over individual jobs as 'intrinsic' control, pointing out that jobs differ widely in the degree to which they allow control over work objectives, methods and scheduling. Karasek (1979) extends the concept of control to form a dimension of 'job decision latitude' which includes other work characteristics, such as variety, skill utilization, decision authority and opportunities for learning. Thus, this dimension incorporates job attributes which are conceptually distinct from, but often empirically correlated with, control over method and pacing of individual tasks.

Control at an organizational level (or, in Warr's terminology, 'extrinsic' control) refers to opportunities to influence other people in the work environment, and to bring about changes in the organization as a whole. For instance, employee-initiated changes in working methods to increase safety (Pasmore and Friedlander, 1982), and participation in decision-making (Jackson, 1983) and in setting performance goals (Pearson, 1987), are examples of ways in which the degree of control employees can exercise over people and activities in their work environment can be increased.

Control as a subjective construct

Some authors have argued that an individual's subjective perception of the extent to which he or she can control events and stimuli in the environment plays a more important role in influencing responses than the objective reality of the situation (Averill, 1973; Lazarus and Folkman, 1984; Lefcourt, 1973). Consistent with this view, control may be regarded as a subjective construct which reflects situational characteristics as appraised or evaluated in the light of the beliefs, attitudes and expectations of the individual concerned. Many published studies adopt this subjective interpretation, emphasizing self-reported perceptions of control rather than objective work characteristics. For instance, Spector (1986) defines control in terms of the extent to which an individual believes he or she can directly affect the work environment.

Greenberger and Strasser (1986) also take a subjective view of the concept of control; in their dynamic model, control is conceptualized as a cognitive construct, which is open to influence by the attitudes and behaviours of others. Hence, their formulation emphasizes that perceptions of control may not depend on 'absolute reality' and that, like other cognitions, perceptions of control may change over time. Similarly, Folkman (1984), writing from the viewpoint of transactional theories of stress and coping, conceptualizes one form of control as an appraisal made in relation to a particular stressful encounter, which is open to subsequent reappraisal during the coping process.

Control as a dimension of individual difference

The concept of control as a generalized belief on the part of an individual about the extent to which important outcomes are determined by internal factors such as ability and personal initiative, as opposed to fate, powerful others and similar external factors, derives originally from the work of Rotter (1966), and has subsequently been refined by other authors (e.g. Levenson, 1974; Paulhus, 1983). This dimension of individual difference, usually designated 'locus of control', has important implications for outcomes in work settings (O'Brien, 1984a; Spector, 1982); it impacts on each stage of the process by which objective control over work tasks influences psychological and physical well-being.

As discussed by Folkman (1984), generalized control beliefs tend to have the greatest effect on control perceptions when environmental characteristics are ambiguous or novel. On this basis, it would be predicted that locus of control would be less important in the context of highly structured and routine work, such as assembly tasks, than in relation to less clearly defined demands. Individual differences in preferences for, and expectations of, control may also be important in the work environment; although less widely studied than control beliefs, they are also relevant to work outcomes. For instance, Pryor (1987) identifies desire for control and freedom at work as one of three major dimensions of work preferences.

MODELS OF CONTROL

The three interpretations of control outlined above focus on different components of the process by which individual differences and objective situational character-istics jointly influence perceptions of control, and other responses to the work environment (see Figure 1). Thus, perceptions of control are seen as mediating relationships between objective aspects of job design which limit or facilitate control, and individual outcomes (including physical and mental health, and

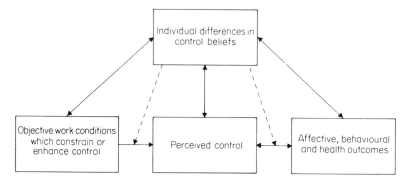

FIGURE 1. Components of control and their relationship to outcomes. Main effects shown by solid lines, interactive effects by dotted lines. Double-headed arrows indicate reciprocal relationships.

more specific work-related outcomes such as performance, absenteeism and turnover). However, causal direction between perceptions and outcomes is difficult to establish. Although a large body of empirical evidence links perceptions of control in the work setting to outcome measures, only rarely do studies allow inferences to be made about causal mechanisms. Consistent with cognitive theories of emotion, the direction of causation is usually assumed to be from work perceptions to short-term affective and behavioural responses, and to longer-term health-related outcomes. However, causal modelling suggests a 'post-cognitive, non-recursive' process in which objective conditions influence perceptions, perceptions influence affective responses, and these responses then further modify perceptions (James and Jones, 1980; James and Tetrick, 1986). Thus, the perceptions–outcomes relationship appears to be reciprocal rather than unidirectional.

At any stage in the process by which control affects outcomes, individual differences may influence the nature and magnitude of the relationships concerned. In the present context, locus of control is particularly relevant but other dimensions (for instance, type A behaviour) may also be important. As shown in Figure 1, the impact of locus of control can take the form of direct main effects on the variables concerned, or of interactive effects in which control beliefs influence relationships between objective control characteristics and subjective perceptions of these characteristics, or between perceptions and outcome variables. Again, reciprocal causation may occur; in this case, evidence suggests that there are long-term reciprocal relationships between individual control beliefs and objective job characteristics, work perceptions and outcome measures (Andrisani and Nestel, 1976; Kohn and Schooler, 1982, 1983; O'Brien, 1984b).

Individual differences in the abilities and skills required to exercise control may also act as moderators between control and outcome; laboratory findings suggest that the degree of congruence between the control opportunities provided by the environment and the individual's ability to make effective use of control is important in determining outcomes (Bazerman, 1982). Thus, consistent with person–environment fit models of work stress (French *et al.*, 1982; Harrison, 1978), increasing personal control in work settings may be detrimental if the individual does not have adequate skills and knowledge to use the control opportunities provided.

Similarly, an imbalance between the degree of control desired and the degree of control actually available may give rise to strain. The cognitive and behavioural mechanisms by which individuals attempt to reduce discrepancies between desired and perceived control at work are central to the model of personal control formulated by Greenberger and Strasser (1986). This model is not concerned with objective control; rather, it represents an attempt to explain and predict employees' reactions to situations in which perceived control is not congruent with desired control. The central hypothesis is that the ratio of perceived control to desired control determines individual reactions to the organizational environment, and that individuals seek to obtain a balance between perceived and desired levels. In particular, Greenberger and Strasser argue that, when perceived control is less than desired control, employees will persist in attempting to restore equilibrium in their control perceptions even when desired outcomes may not be attainable, and attempts to achieve them may require considerable expenditure of personal resources. If these attempts fail, 'learned helplessness' (Seligman, 1975) may result when a balance between perceived and desired control can only be restored by the employee ceasing to desire control. As yet this model of control in organizations remains a theoretical formulation; the concept of desired control has received less attention in the empirical literature than internal–external control beliefs.

Control as a component in general models of work stress

Although opportunities for personal control play an important role in influencing responses to the work environment, control is only one of a number of work characteristics that jointly determine individual outcomes. For instance, as reviewed by Warr (1987), adverse behavioural and affective responses to the work situation have been found to be associated with lack of variety, feedback and identity in tasks; with high levels of work demand and time pressure; with role conflict, overload and ambiguity; and with lack of support from colleagues. The possibility that lack of control acts not only as an independent source of stress but also combines with other work stressors to influence outcomes must therefore be considered. Two models of job stress in which the control plays a major part have been developed; both conceptualize control as a moderating factor which reduces the impact of other work stressors, and both view control as an objective characteristic of the environment, rather than a subjective construct.

The demand–control model of job strain

The more parsimonious of the two models is the 'demand–control' model
developed by Karasek (1979); this model conceptualizes job control (in the form
of decision latitude) and job demand as interactive predictors of strain; jobs
which combine low decision latitude with 'hectic work' and time pressure are
seen as producing an imbalance which is manifest as psychological strain, and
increased risk of mental and physical ill health. In contrast, 'active jobs' (high
demand and high control) promote growth and development. A recent extension
to the demand–control model incorporates social support as an additional
orthogonal dimension (Johnson and Hall, 1989). Cross-sectional and longitudinal findings reported by Karasek and his colleagues tend to support the
interactive demand–control model in relation to affective and behavioural
outcomes and, particularly, in relation to cardiovascular disease (Karasek, 1989).
Findings relating to Karasek's model are considered briefly later in this chapter,
and are reviewed in detail elsewhere in this volume.

'Prediction, understanding and control' as antidotes to work stress

A more general model conceptualizing control as an antidote to work stress has
recently been described by Sutton and Kahn (1987). In Sutton and Kahn's
formulation, control is seen as one of three factors—the other two being
'understanding' (knowledge about the causes of significant events in the workplace) and 'prediction' (the ability to predict the frequency, timing and duration
of events in the workplace)—which attenuate the effects of organizational
stressors on individual strain. As shown in Figure 2, the model incorporates both
main and moderating effects of prediction, understanding and control in relation
to work stress variables. In that it predicts that control will act to mitigate the

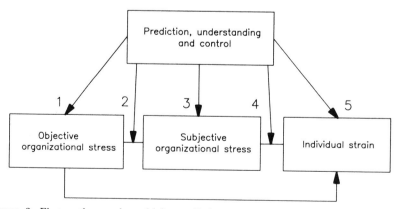

FIGURE 2. Five pathways by which prediction, understanding and control serve as
antidotes to organizational stress. (From Sutton and Kahn, 1987, reproduced with
permission, © Prentice Hall, Inc.)

effects of job demands, Sutton and Kahn's model incorporates the central idea of the demand–control model, although it is more wide-ranging in its overall formulation.

To date, only one published study has tested Sutton and Kahn's model; Tetrick and LaRocco (1987) used latent variable modelling to examine the effects of prediction, understanding and control on measures of perceived stress, and affective well-being, and their interrelationships. The results provided some support for the model, the control variable showing the most marked effects. However, individual differences in locus of control were not assessed in this study; in view of findings that locus of control and job attributes such as skill utilization, complexity and autonomy are reciprocally related (Kohn and Schooler, 1982; O'Brian, 1984b), it is unclear whether the effects found in Tetrick and LaRocco's study should be ascribed primarily to job characteristics or to individual differences in control beliefs. Extension of Sutton and Kahn's model to include individual differences as well as situational variables would more completely represent the moderating variables in the stress process (cf. the more general model of work stress described by House, 1981).

EMPIRICAL FINDINGS RELATING TO CONTROL AT WORK

A large number of empirical studies examine the role of personal control at work, and its implications for mental and physical well-being. These studies potentially contribute to the understanding of relationships between objective control over work tasks, perceptions of control, and individual control beliefs, and of the ways in which these variables jointly influence outcomes; more generally, empirical findings provide evidence of the extent to which control mitigates the effects of work stress.

In reviewing published work, a broad distinction can be made between studies based on 'objective' assessments of control, and those which conceptualize control in terms of 'subjective' or 'perceived' measures; studies which include measures of individual control beliefs form a further category. In practice, however, the distinction between objective and subjective interpretations of control is blurred in much of the literature. Thus, some authors use self-report methods to assess variables which they interpret as measures of 'objective' control, disregarding possible subjective bias. In other relevant studies, the issue of whether control is construed objectively or subjectively is not addressed.

In the material presented below, four types of studies are considered: (1) comparative studies carried out in specific job situations which differ objectively in the extent to which they limit or enhance personal control; (2) studies based on control ratings made independently of the job incumbent, i.e. by job analysts, supervisors or co-workers; (3) studies in which control is self-reported by job incumbents; and (4) studies which examine the role of individual control beliefs in relation to objective and perceived control over work tasks. Each of these approaches contributes in a different way to the empirical understanding of control at work.

The measures used to assess health-related outcomes (interpreting the term in its widest sense to include all aspects of physical and mental well-being, and working effectiveness) can also be classified as objective or subjective. Thus, diagnosed illnesses (e.g. cardiovascular disease, ulcers and psychiatric disorders); physiological responses (e.g. catecholamine excretion, cardiac responses and blood pressure changes); and behavioural measures (e.g. sickness absence, medical consultations and work performance), are all potentially amenable to objective assessment. In contrast, affective distress, somatic symptoms, mood state, sleep quality, turnover intention and other subjective aspects of well-being are normally assessed by self-report. Objective outcome measures involve more complex and costly data collection techniques than self-report measures; inevitably, therefore, subjective outcomes are more frequently reported. In particular, numerous correlational studies have been published in which both work attributes and individual outcomes are assessed by self-report. Limitations of these studies, particularly problems of methodology, psychometrics and interpretation, have been widely discussed (Algera, 1983; James and Tetrick, 1986; Spector, 1987b; Spector et al., 1988).

Comparisons of work conditions differing in objective control

In some work situations, similar tasks are carried out under two or more conditions differing in the extent to which they allow opportunities for personal control, e.g. machine-paced and manual letter-sorting. These different work conditions may co-exist as a normal part of the production situation; alternatively, naturally occurring or experimentally manipulated changes may be studied. Either way, conditions can be independently identified or manipulated for research purposes, and their effects on outcome measures evaluated. Comparisons are often made across groups exposed to different work situations (e.g. Clegg et al., 1987; LaRocco, 1985; Stellman et al., 1987), but this method has the disadvantage that the effects observed may be confounded by pre-existing differences between groups. Comparisons of the same individuals exposed successively to different conditions (e.g. Dunham et al., 1987; Jackson, 1983; Parkes, 1982; Wall et al., 1986) are methodologically stronger, but more difficult to implement in field settings.

Several specific areas of research can be identified in which direct comparisons are made between conditions differing in the extent to which they facilitate or constrain personal control at work: comparisons of machine-paced production work with equivalent tasks carried out under unpaced conditions; studies of computer-based office technology, as compared with traditional equipment; the effects of changes in opportunities for participation in work-related decision-making; and the introduction of flexible working hours. Findings relating to these four topics are outlined below. More generally, broadly based research, such as comparative studies of public and private organizations (Frantz, 1980; Solomon, 1986), and studies of worker ownership (Hammer *et al.*, 1981; Tannenbaum, 1983) may also throw light on the impact of control at an organizational level.

Paced versus unpaced work

The effects of machine-paced and unpaced tasks have been compared in both field and laboratory studies. The results demonstrate that constraints over the rate and method of work imposed by pacing are reflected in subjective perceptions of lack of control, and are associated with unfavourable physiological, somatic and affective outcomes. Thus, relative to comparable unpaced tasks, paced tasks are seen as low in skill utilization, job freedom and 'intrinsic rewards' (LaRocco, 1985; Wells, 1982), and as high in demand and low in decision latitude (Karasek, 1979).

Studies of physiological (e.g. Bohlin *et al.*, 1986; Frankenhaeuser and Gardell, 1976; Johansson, 1981; Jenner *et al.*, 1980) and psychological (e.g. Broadbent and Gath, 1979; Chamberlain and Jones, 1987; Clegg *et al.*, 1987; Hurrell, 1985; LaRocco, 1985; Stammerjohn and Wilkes, 1981) outcomes demonstrate the unfavourable effects of machine-pacing in a variety of different production tasks. In particular, paced work is associated with high levels of catecholamine excretion, and with work dissatisfaction, boredom, somatic and affective symptoms, and visual and muscular strain (for a review, see Smith, 1985). Collectively, the results do not imply that pacing is linked to specific types of distress, although it has been suggested that anxiety is the primary affective response to work demand, and the element of demand in pacing may act in a similar way (Broadbent, 1985; Hesketh and Shouksmith, 1986).

Office work: new technology compared with traditional methods

The development of computer-based visual display units (VDUs) for wordprocessing and other clerical tasks has had a marked impact on office work over the past decade. However, published studies suggest that the advantages of the new technology have not as yet resulted in increased well-being among clerical staff; indeed, much of the existing evidence points to adverse effects. Reported findings include unfavourable perceptions of VDU work as compared with conventional typing (Billette and Piche, 1987; Buchanan and Boddy, 1982; Stellman *et al.*, 1987); work dissatisfaction (Stellman *et al.*, 1987); physiological stress responses (Johansson, 1979); and musculoskeletal disorders (e.g. Evans, 1987; Smith *et al.*, 1981; Williams, 1985). In contrast, reports of favourable effects of office technology (e.g. Rafaeli and Sutton, 1986) are much less common.

Wordprocessors and other computer-based systems remove many of the repetitive and boring aspects of manual office work; hence, the question arises as to why research findings tend to demonstrate adverse, rather than positive, effects on well-being among office staff. Some physical health problems (e.g. musculo-skeletal disorders and visual strain) may be ascribed to poor ergonomic design of VDU systems (Grandjean, 1980). However, adverse psychological outcomes appear to reflect wider issues such as management styles, changes in the organization and structuring of office jobs, and equipment unreliability, rather than the use of computer-based systems *per se*. The extent to which new technology constrains the degree of personal control over work tasks is particu-larly relevant in the present context. Some evidence suggests that office techno-logy reduces both the variety of office work and its controllability, especially among women employees (Evans, 1987; Gattiker and Nelligan, 1988). Consistent with these findings, Gill (1985) points out that use of computer-based systems can result in 'de-skilling' of office work, in increased rigidity and structuring of jobs, and in reduction of personal control. A further problem is the possibility of close, and possibly intrusive, monitoring of performance by supervisors.

Gill notes that different consequences for work methods, people and organiza-tions will result from different techniques of designing and implementing computer-based systems. Clearly, much depends on whether VDUs are intro-duced in such a way as to enrich clerical jobs rather than to reduce their variety, controllability and skill levels. The negative findings dominating the existing literature suggest that there is a need for managers to become more aware of the personal, social and organizational implications of introducing new technology so that the potential benefits of such systems are more fully realized in the future, not only by organizations but also by individual employees.

Participation in decision-making and goal setting

Opportunities for personal control at work can potentially be enhanced by allowing employees more opportunities for participating in decision-making, both in relation to their own work tasks and in the organization as a whole. Several longitudinal field studies have investigated the effects of interventions intended to increase worker involvement in decision-making and goal-setting (Griffeth, 1985; Jackson, 1983, 1984; Pearson, 1987; Sarata, 1984; Wall *et al.*, 1986). Laboratory experiments provide further evidence (e.g. Breaugh and Becker, 1987; Vanderslice *et al.*, 1987). Taken together, these studies demonstrate that opportunities for participation in decision-making have favourable effects on perceptions of control and influence in the organization, on affective well-being, and on absenteeism, performance and turnover. Employee participation in decisions about work redesign may also lessen the disruptive effects of change and/or enhance the benefits obtained (Karasek, 1989; Latack and Foster, 1985). However, the nature of the tasks concerned may influence the extent to which participation is beneficial; tasks that are routine, highly structured or mechan-ized may show less favourable effects (House and Baetz, 1979). Empirical findings tend to support this view (Campbell and Gingrich, 1986). Organizational and cultural factors may also be important in influencing the effects of participation (Locke and Schweiger, 1979; Wilpert, 1984).

Flexible working hours and other aspects of work scheduling

At an organizational level, 'flexitime', and other innovative work-scheduling arrangements have implications for personal control in that they increase employees' autonomy in deciding which hours to work, and how work and non-work activities are combined. Pierce and Newstrom (1983) found that 'perceived time autonomy' mediated the effect of work schedules differing in flexibility on employee attitudes and symptoms of stress. More generally, non-standard work schedules enhance work satisfaction and reduce absence and sick leave, although the effects on other aspects of employee well-being are less consistent (Dunham *et al.*, 1987; Harrick *et al.*, 1986; Hurrell and Colligan, 1985; Kim and Campagna, 1981; McGuire and Liro, 1986; Ralston and Flanagan, 1985). Discrepancies between findings may be due to moderating effects of individual and social factors, particularly family commitments. In general, married women are found to benefit more than men from flexible hours (e.g. Krausz and Freibach, 1983; Staines and Pleck, 1986), although there may also be advantages for married men with children (Lee, 1983). Organizational factors, such as the extent to which resources are shared among many employees, may also influence the effects of flexible hours (Ralston *et al.*, 1985).

Other aspects of flexibility, for instance scheduling within the work period, have received less attention in the literature than flexitime. However, employees (e.g. bus drivers) who are required to maintain precise work schedules, while exposed to conditions which constrain their freedom to do so, experience both time pressure and lack of control. For instance, recent field studies of driving examiners in the UK and in the Netherlands have shown that a modest increase in the time allowed for each candidate brought about significant and favourable changes in perceptions of stress, in objective measures of alertness, and in affective and physiological responses (Meijman, personal communication, 1985; Parkes, unpublished data).

Comment

Two general conclusions can be drawn from the findings reviewed above: first, objective differences in work conditions are reflected in the employees' subjective perceptions of control; second, jobs which impose greater limitations on personal control are associated with less favourable responses. These findings are consistent across the four different areas of work considered, with particularly clear similarities between responses to paced work and to use of VDUs. However, from the point of view of providing evidence of relationships between objective control, perceived control and outcomes, there are two problems of interpretation which apply to much, although not all, of the work described above.

(1) Most of the studies do not allow evaluation of the extent to which affective, physiological and behavioural outcomes are specifically associated with objective control differences. For instance, control over speed and methods may not be the only difference between paced and unpaced work; other differences (e.g. in complexity, repetitiveness or opportunities for social interaction) may contribute to the observed outcomes. A further difficulty of interpretation in 'between-group' studies is that individuals who choose, and remain in, particular jobs may differ in pre-existing personality and mental health from those who choose to work under different conditions.

(2) Most of the studies outlined above measure either control perceptions or affective and behavioural responses to different work conditions, but not both perceptions and outcomes. Thus, inferences about the mediational role of control perceptions in predicting outcomes can only be made indirectly across studies. Few studies directly examine control perceptions as mediators of the effects of objective work conditions; however, mediational effects of this kind have been reported (Jackson, 1983, 1984; Parkes, 1982).

Studies based on independent ratings of control

The use of independent ratings of control made by job analysts, supervisors or co-workers of the job incumbent provides a means of assessing control in a wide range of jobs, while avoiding some of the problems inherent in self-report data. As described below, independent ratings have been used in two different ways in studies of job control.

Occupational ratings derived from population survey data

In Sweden, survey data have been used to produce ratings of job characteristics for each of 118 occupational codes (Alfredsson *et al.*, 1985), thus allowing epidemiological studies to be carried out by linking occupational data to census information and hospital records. Using this approach, Alfredsson *et al.* showed that several factors reflecting lack of control over work (e.g. low influence over working hours, over planning of work, and over co-workers) were associated with alcohol-related illness, but did not appear to play a major role in cardiovascular disease. However, in this study, and in other studies using occupational ratings (Alfredsson and Theorell, 1983; Alfredsson *et al.*, 1982), increased incidence of cardiovascular disease was found among men in monotonous jobs with 'few opportunities to learn new things'; the effects were more marked when job demand was high, but 'control over work tempo' did not appear to be important.

Shaw and Riskind (1983) used occupational ratings developed in the USA to analyse job characteristics in relation to outcomes derived from three separate studies. 'Performing controlled manual activities' was found to be significantly related to mortality from several different causes, including heart disease and ulcers, and to self-reports of affective distress. Adelmann (1987) also used archival data to provide independent ratings of job characteristics; in this study, self-report information about mental health outcomes was obtained from a large-scale survey. After taking into account age, education and income, job control ratings significantly predicted happiness and self-confidence in men, but only self-confidence in women.

Individual job ratings made by supervisors and co-workers

The studies reported above depend on ratings of occupations rather than individual jobs. To obtain independent assessments of individual job characteristics, supervisors' or co-workers' ratings can be used. Independent ratings of this kind have been analysed in relation to corresponding self-reports from job incumbents and/or in relation to self-reported outcomes (Algera, 1983; Birnbaum *et al.*, 1986; Kiggundu, 1980; Spector *et al.*, 1988). The Job Diagnostic Survey (JDS) (Hackman and Oldham, 1975) is most commonly used to assess job attributes, the 'autonomy' scale being closest to the concept of personal control. Results show that supervisors' and co-workers' ratings of autonomy are positively related to a variety of job incumbent outcomes including work satisfaction, low anxiety and good performance (Algera, 1983; Spector *et al.*, 1988; Birnbaum *et al.*, 1986), but not to more direct health measures such as minor symptoms and doctors' visits (Algera, 1983; Spector *et al.*, 1988). These relationships are smaller in magnitude than corresponding values obtained from self-reports of both job characteristics and outcomes (e.g. for correlations between autonomy and anxiety, comparative values from Spector *et al.* are $-.16$ and $-.34$, respectively). Thus, it appears that some inflation of correlations between job attributes and outcomes occurs when both variables are self-reported (e.g. due to similar response biases being reflected in both measures), but that the correlations remain significant when self-report artifacts are eliminated by the use of independent ratings.

Comment

The results outlined above demonstrate that lack of control over work tasks, as independently assessed, predicts increased risk of serious disease and affective distress among job incumbents. Thus, the adverse effects of lack of control are sufficiently robust to be apparent even when job ratings are obtained independently of the outcome data, and relate to classes of occupations rather than to individual jobs. The true effects of control are probably greater than those observed in analyses based on occupational category ratings, as such data do not take into account variations in actual exposure within each category. Failure to control statistically for differences in socio-economic status may inflate some reported results (e.g. Shaw and Riskind, 1983), but there is convincing evidence that control at work predicts health outcomes after taking socio-economic status into account (e.g. Alfredsson *et al.*, 1985; Adelmann, 1987).

Studies which include both self-reports and ratings by others potentially allow examination of the extent to which the job incumbents' own perceptions of control contribute to explained variance in well-being, over and above independent job ratings. At issue here is the role of individual perceptions as mediators of relationships between 'objective' work characteristics and outcomes; however, this question does not appear to have been examined in analyses of data relating to control at work (cf. Repetti's (1987) study of consensus and personal perceptions of social support at work as predictors of well-being).

Self-report studies of job control

Numerous studies have used self-report measures to examine relationships between job attributes and outcomes. In some work, outcomes are assessed independently but, more usually, outcome information is also self-reported. Although use of self-report methods has the advantage of allowing large data sets to be obtained with limited resources, it raises questions about the extent to which general response tendencies and other sources of bias act to inflate the observed correlations between job characteristics and outcomes. Thus, self-report studies are methodologically weaker than those that include independent measures, although recent findings suggest that, providing the measures are psychometrically adequate, the problem of common method variance may not be as serious as is often thought (Spector, 1987b).

Studies based on self-report data form the major part of the empirical literature on personal control at work, and help to establish the nature and magnitude of the relationships between control and a wide variety of outcome measures. Some researchers interpret self-report measures of control as assessing objective aspects of the work situation (e.g. Karasek, 1979; O'Brien, 1984b; Tetrick and LaRocco, 1987); they consider this interpretation to be justified by the factual nature of the questionnaire items, and observed correlations between self-reports and independent ratings. In other studies, self-report measures are treated as assessing subjective perceptions of control (e.g. Spector, 1987a). In general, self-reports of control in the work situation are most appropriately regarded as subjective measures although, if the items are of a clearly factual nature, interpretation in terms of objective control may be tenable.

A general overview of studies of perceived control is provided by Spector's (1986) meta-analysis of 88 studies of autonomy and participation at work, involving 102 samples. High levels of perceived control were found to be associated with high levels of job satisfaction, commitment, involvement, performance and motivation, and with low levels of somatic symptoms, emotional distress, role stress, absenteeism and turnover. Separate analyses of autonomy and participation yielded generally similar results, suggesting that perceived control is the common underlying factor. Although the data analysed by Spector do not allow causal interpretation, findings from several longitudinal studies suggest that increase in autonomy (for instance, resulting from organizational change or promotion) leads to increases in affective well-being, confidence and job satisfaction (Bhagat and Chassie, 1980; Kirjonen and Hanninen, 1986; Mortimer and Lorence, 1979; Wall and Clegg, 1981). Similarly, Gerhart (1987) found that, after control for previous job satisfaction, change in job complexity (a measure based on items from JDS dimensions, including autonomy) significantly predicted current satisfaction.

Although 'learned helplessness' theories (Seligman, 1975) suggest that prolonged exposure to 'uncontrollable' work conditions would lead primarily to depression rather than, say, anxiety or frustration, this specificity of affective response has not been demonstrated. Indeed, few researchers have considered this issue, although Broadbent (1985) examines specific responses to job demand (in which he includes pacing) and to social aspects of the work environment. Extending this idea, Hesketh and Shouksmith (1986) examined work characteristics reported by veterinary professionals as predictors of affective distress using 'residualized' scores, controlled for other dimensions of distress. The findings suggest that perceived lack of control over 'the speed at which things are done' was significantly related to the residualized scores for anxiety, but not to those for depression. However, neither of these studies should be interpreted as indicating that lack of control is specifically linked to anxiety; in both cases the evidence points more strongly to demand being associated with anxiety.

Perceived control has also been examined in relation to self-reports of physical health outcomes. For instance, Karasek *et al.* (1987) found that higher levels of perceived control at work were related to fewer physical symptoms and to less use of medication, but the method of analysis precluded tests of demand–control interactions. However, longitudinal data reported by Bromet *et al.* (1988) revealed significant interactions between job decision latitude and demand in predicting alcohol problems and symptom levels. This study provides good support for the demand–control model, particularly as the data were collected in face-to-face clinical interviews rather than by questionnaire, and pre-existing health problems and other work and personal factors were statistically controlled in the analysis.

Other studies in which the demand–control model has been tested using cross-sectional, self-report data have not provided convincing support. Findings include main effects for demand and control, but not the predicted interactions (Payne and Fletcher, 1983; Spector, 1987a); interactive effects too small to be of theoretical or practical importance (Beehr and Drexler, 1986); and, in a different interpretation of the model, little evidence of interaction between discretion and control over speed of work (Hesketh and Shouksmith, 1986). A recent laboratory study in which control and demand were objectively manipulated, and subjectively assessed, showed very little evidence of the predicted control–demand interaction, either for the objective or the perceived measures (Perrewe and Ganster, 1989). Thus, aside from the study by Bromet *et al.* (1988), evidence supporting the demand–control theory stems largely from the work of Karasek *et al.*

In his initial study, Karasek (1979) found that a number of adverse outcomes, including depression, dissatisfaction, use of sedative medication and days of sickness, were predicted by the demand–control interaction. Similarly, lack of control combined with high demand predicted cardiovascular risk in two case–control studies (Karasek *et al.*, 1981; Theorell *et al.*, 1987). In further work, Johnson and Hall (1989) found that control, social support and demand interacted as predictors of cardiovascular disease, greatest risk being associated with high demand, low support, and low control. However, findings from several other studies reviewed by Karasek (1989) suggest that 'monotony' and 'lack of opportunities to learn new things' (either independently or in interaction with demand) are more important predictors of cardiovascular risk than lack of control *per se*.

Comment

The studies outlined above demonstrate significant correlations between self-reports of control at work and a wide range of affective, behavioural and disease outcomes. However, there are a number of limitations of the work: in particular, few of the studies allow causal inferences; method variance may inflate observed correlations between self-reports of job characteristics and outcomes; and self-report scales do not clearly differentiate objective and perceived control, thus precluding consideration of the mediational effects of control perceptions. Several more specific issues also merit comment.

(1) Although the work reviewed clearly demonstrates that lack of control is associated with adverse outcomes, there are some discrepancies between different studies, particularly in which outcome measures show the most marked effects, and in whether control acts independently or in interaction with demand as implied by the demand–control model. A possible reason for these discrepancies is that in these studies control is assessed by a variety of different measures, ranging from single items to lengthy scales; from measures which focus exclusively on control over work pace and methods to more broadly based scales such as decision latitude; and from measures emphasizing factual job characteristics to those that are primarily evaluative in nature. Differences between subject groups (in particular, between general population samples and homogeneous occupational groups) may also underly differences in results obtained.

(2) From a psychometric viewpoint, identification and assessment of the separate components of control is important. In particular, a multidimensional measure would be valuable; Breaugh (1985) reports one attempt to develop such a scale. Ideally, a measure of control at work should have three parallel versions: one for the job incumbent to report factual job characteristics; one for a similar report by independent observers, e.g. supervisors; and one for the job incumbent to report perceived control, i.e. an evaluative rather than factual version. This threefold assessment would allow independent and self-report data to be obtained for the same job characteristics, and would also allow factual assessment to be separated from individual appraisals of the job situation, thus facilitating empirical clarification of the distinction between objective and perceived measures.

(3) There appears to be little evidence that lack of control is associated with specific affective outcomes. However, this issue has not been widely studied and would merit further investigation not only in relation to paced work but also in other contexts, e.g. participation in decision-making. The use of more sophisticated statistical techniques, such as latent variable models, would help to overcome some of the limitations of observed-score analyses of symptom checklist data (see, for instance, Parkes, 1987).

Locus of control, job attributes and outcomes

Individual differences in personal control beliefs have important implications for motivation, attitudes, adaptation and behaviour in many domains of life (Phares, 1976; Lefcourt, 1983). In relation to occupational settings, the balance of evidence suggests that, as compared with externals, internals seek work which allows greater use of skill; experience greater autonomy, satisfaction and well-being; and show higher occupational attainment and more effective leadership. O'Brien (1984a) and Spector (1982) review this literature; however, much of the earlier research in this area is of limited value. For instance, Spector describes the literature on job characteristics and locus of control as 'inconsistent and inconclusive' (p. 492). Both reviews draw attention to methodological weaknesses, the difficulties of determining causal direction, and the possibility of confounding factors in this research.

More recent studies have shown greater methodological sophistication. For instance, O'Brien (1984b), applying causal modelling to cross-sectional data, found that locus of control was reciprocally related to skill utilization for married men (but not for other subgroups in the overall sample), and income was causally related to locus of control. Similarly, Kohn and Schooler (1982) demonstrated reciprocal relationships between personality and job conditions in longitudinal data. In particular, 'self-directed orientation' (a dimension similar to locus of control), ideational flexibility (a measure of problem-solving ability) and occupational self-direction (lack of close supervision, and greater complexity of work), and were found to act as a 'mutually reinforcing triumvirate' (p. 153), each influencing the others over time. Also using longitudinal data, Andrisani and Nestel (1976) demonstrated that locus of control systematically influenced work success and, conversely, success at work enhanced internal control perceptions. Frantz (1980) reported similar findings for school-leavers entering private-sector employment, but in public-sector employment the opposite was true, career progress leading to increased externality.

The topic of 'congruency' between control beliefs and environmental conditions has also received attention in the recent literature. At issue here is the question of whether congruence between personal control beliefs and environmental control opportunities leads to more favourable outcomes than incongruence, as would be predicted by theories of person–environment fit (Caplan, 1987; French *et al.*, 1982). Warr (1987) suggests that congruency effects can be predicted *a priori*, but notes the lack of empirical evidence. Spector (1982) appears implicitly to accept a congruency model, advocating selection of internals for professional and managerial jobs, and externals for production line work, clerical tasks and unskilled labour; O'Brien (1984a) challenges this opinion as unjustified and discriminatory.

Some evidence of congruency in work situations has been reported. Marino and White (1985) found a significant interaction between locus of control and 'job specificity' (the extent to which work required rules and procedures to be closely followed). Under conditions of low specificity (i.e. high autonomy), externals reported more stress than internals, but the reverse was true under conditions of high specificity. A different type of congruence effect occurs in relation to coping behaviour; for instance, Parkes (1984) found that internals reported coping strategies congruent with their perceptions of control over work-related stressful episodes, whereas this was not true of externals.

Results consistent with a congruency model have also been found in laboratory studies (Brownell, 1982; Hrycenko and Minton, 1974). Brownell found that internal subjects performed a simulated management task better in conditions of high control, while external subjects performed better in the low control condition. In a more recent study, preference for high versus low job discretion was found to moderate the effects of work conditions differing in control (machine-paced versus self-paced work); cognitive performance measures and self-reported stress demonstrated significant effects associated with incongruency between preferred and actual conditions (Parkes *et al.*, 1988). Studies such as these, in which objective conditions are manipulated but perceived work characteristics are not assessed, reveal moderating effects on relationships between objective conditions and outcomes, but they do not indicate whether these moderating effects influence relationships between objective and perceived control, or those between perceived control and outcome. However, recent evidence suggests that locus of control may act in both ways (Perrewe, 1986; Perrewe and Mizerski, 1987), and may also moderate relationships between different outcomes measures, for instance performance and satisfaction (Norris and Niebuhr, 1984).

Comment

The results outlined above demonstrate that locus of control acts both independently and interactively with job characteristics, as a significant predictor of work-related outcomes. However, individual differences in locus of control usually account for only small amounts of explained variance. Possible reasons underlying these relatively weak findings are outlined below.

(1) Situational constraints inherent in work situations, particularly those which allow little objective control, may reduce opportunities for individual differences to exert an influence on outcomes. More attention needs to be given to identifying work situations which do, or do not, show moderating effects of locus of control on relationships between objective control, control perceptions and outcomes.

(2) Relationships between locus of control and outcomes may not be linear. Studies of life stress (e.g. Krause and Stryker, 1984) suggest that moderate control orientations may be more adaptive than extreme values. Similarly, O'Brien (1984a) suggests that extreme scorers on internal–external dimensions have distorted perceptions of social reality, as compared with an intermediate group of 'realists'. The idea that intermediate scores may reflect more effective adaptation suggests possible curvilinear relationships with outcomes, but the statistical tests required to demonstrate curvilinearity have not been reported in the work reviewed above. Thus, statistical weaknesses may contribute to the apparently small explanatory power of control beliefs.

(3) Rotter's (1966) scale has been widely used to assess locus of control in work settings, but more sophisticated measures of control beliefs are now available. For instance, the 'Spheres of Control' scale (Paulhus, 1983) assesses control in three behavioural domains (personal, interpersonal and sociopolitical), each of which is potentially important in relation to work outcomes. This scale was developed in the US, but data from a large sample of UK subjects have also been published (Parkes, 1988).

(4) Generalized control beliefs may not be sufficiently specific to predict responses to work settings. Spector (1988) has recently reported preliminary validation data from a new scale intended to provide greater specificity in assessing work-related locus of control. One difficulty in developing such a scale is the need to distinguish between an individual's perception of his or her current work situation, and general beliefs about control at work. If this problem is overcome, a work-specific control scale could prove to be a more sensitive predictor of work outcomes than more general measures.

Thus, more attention to psychometric and statistical issues in future research may help to clarify some unresolved questions about the role of control beliefs in adaptation to work environments. The issue of congruency is particularly important; more information is needed about the conditions under which externals respond unfavourably to work situations which allow high levels of control, about the outcome measures in which these effects are apparent, and about the mechanisms involved.

CONCLUSIONS

The material reviewed in this article reflects the range of research literature concerned with personal control in occupational settings, and the main empirical findings reported from several different types of studies. The diversity of the methods used, and the wide range of affective, behavioural and disease outcomes for which significant findings have been reported, strengthens the argument that opportunities for personal control in occupational settings have important implications for psychological and physiological functioning generally, and for specific work-related outcomes. In studies which show significant findings, greater control is almost always associated with more favourable outcomes; only when issues of congruency between environmental conditions and individual control beliefs or preferences are considered is there any empirical evidence to suggest that greater control may not always be beneficial to all individuals.

Although control over work tasks is almost always found to be associated with favourable outcomes, less is known about the underlying mechanisms by which these outcomes are manifest. The magnitude of the relationships reported, the methodological sophistication of the work, and the psychometric adequacy of the measures used, vary greatly from study to study. Furthermore, few of the studies conducted in field settings allow definite causal inferences to be drawn between lack of control and adverse outcomes, although laboratory studies in which control is experimentally manipulated do provide clearer evidence of causality. Thus, alongside what is currently known about the implications of control at work are many unresolved questions.

To make further progress in this research area, there is a need for research which combines the use of independent and self-reported measures of control and outcome to examine responses to work conditions differing objectively in control opportunities. In particular, greater use of independently diagnosed medical conditions as outcome variables would be desirable to increase understanding of the effects of control on physical and mental health. Ideally, locus of control and background variables (such as education, age, and pre-existing health problems) should be measured prior to the subject's entry to the work situation, and longitudinal data relating to perceived control and outcomes collected subsequently. Systematic field experiments such as that reported by Jackson (1983) potentially provide a strong basis for such work.

Applying statistical modelling techniques to such data would allow the causal relationships involved in objective control–perceived control–outcome relationships to be examined, together with the impact of control beliefs on this process. Within this framework, several other issues would merit further examination; e.g. gender differences in responses to the control characteristics of work situations; specificity in affective responses to lack of control; coping in relation to high and low levels of control; and further examination of interactive relationships between control and other aspects of the work environment. Studies of this kind, although difficult to undertake, would allow further clarification and integration of the present literature in this research area.

REFERENCES

Adelmann, P. K. (1987). Occupational complexity, control, and personal income: Their relation to psychological well-being in men and women. *Journal of Applied Psychology*, **72**, 529–537.

Alfredsson, L., and Theorell, T. (1983). Job characteristics of occupations and myocardial infarction risk: Effect of possible confounding factors. *Social Science and Medicine*, **20**, 1497–1503.

Alfredsson, L., Karasek, R. A., and Theorell, T. (1982). Myocardial infarction risk and the psychosocial work environment: An analysis of the male Swedish working force. *Social Science and Medicine*, **16**, 463–467.

Alfredsson, L., Spetz, C-L., and Theorell, T. (1985). Type of occupation and near-future hospitalization for myocardial infarction and some other diagnoses. *International Journal of Epidemiology*, **14**, 378–388.

Algera, J. A. (1983). 'Objective' and perceived task characteristics as a determinant of reactions by task performers. *Journal of Occupational Psychology*, **56**, 95–107.

Andrisani, P. J., and Nestel, G. (1976). Internal–external control as contributor to and outcome of work experience. *Journal of Applied Psychology*, **61**, 156–165.

Averill, J. R. (1973). Personal control over aversive stimuli and its relationship to stress. *Psychological Bulletin*, **80**, 286–303.

Bazerman, M. H. (1982). Impact of personal control on performance: Is added control always beneficial? *Journal of Applied Psychology*, **67**, 472–479.

Beehr, T. A., and Drexler, J. A. (1986). Social support, autonomy, and hierarchical level as moderators of the role characteristics–outcome relationship. *Journal of Occupational Behaviour*, **7**, 207–214.

Bhagat, R. S., and Chassie, M. B. (1980). Effects of changes in job characteristics on some theory-specific attitudinal outcomes: Results from a naturally occurring quasi-experiment. *Human Relations*, **33**, 297–313.

Billette, A., and Piche, J. (1987). Health problems of data entry clerks and related job stressors. *Journal of Occupational Medicine*, **29**, 942–948.

Birnbaum, P., Farh, J., and Wong, G. (1986). The job characteristics model in Hong Kong. *Journal of Applied Psychology*, **71**, 598–605.

Bohlin, G., Eliasson, K., Hjemdahl, P., Klein, K., Fredrikson, M., and Frankenhaeuser, M. (1986). Personal control over work pace: Circulatory, neuroendocrine and subjective responses in borderline hypertension. *Journal of Hypertension*, **4**, 295–305.

Breaugh, J. A. (1985). The measurement of work autonomy. *Human Relations*, **38**, 551–570.

Breaugh, J. A., and Becker, A. S. (1987). Further examination of the work autonomy scales: Three studies. *Human Relations*, **40**, 381–400.

Broadbent, D. E. (1985). The clinical impact of job design. *British Journal of Clinical Psychology*, **24**, 33–44.

Broadbent, D. E., and Gath, D. (1979). Chronic effects of repetitive and non-repetitive work. In: C. Mackay and T. Cox (eds), *Response to Stress: Occupational Aspects*. Guildford: IPC Science and Technology Press.

Bromet, E. J., Dew, M. A., Parkinson, D. K., and Schulberg, H. C. (1988). Predictive effects of occupational and marital stress on the mental health of a male workforce. *Journal of Organizational Behavior*, **9**, 1–13.

Brownell, P. (1982). The effects of personality–situation congruence in a managerial context: Locus of control and budgetary participation. *Journal of Personality and Social Psychology*, **42**, 753–763.

Buchanan, D. A., and Boddy, D. (1982). Advanced technology and the quality of working life: The effects of word processing on video typists. *Journal of Occupational Psychology*, **55**, 1–11.

Campbell, D. J., and Gingrich, K. F. (1986). The interactive effects of task complexity and participation on task performance: A field experiment. *Organizational Behavior and Human Decision Processes*, **38**, 162–180.

Caplan, R. D. (1987). Person–environment fit theory and organizations: Commensurate dimensions, time perspectives, and mechanisms. *Journal of Vocational Behavior*, **31**, 248–267.

Chamberlain, A. G., and Jones, D. M. (1987). Satisfactions and stresses in the sorting of mail. *Work and Stress*, **1**, 25–34.

Clegg, C., Wall T., and Kemp, N. (1987). Women on the assembly line: A comparison of the main and interactive explanations of job satisfaction, absence and mental health. *Journal of Occupational Psychology*, **60**, 273–287.

Dunham, R. B., Pierce, J. L., and Castaneda, M. B. (1987). Alternative work schedules: Two field quasi-experiments. *Personnel Psychology*, **40**, 215–242.

Evans, J. (1987). Women, men, VDU work and health: A questionnaire survey of British VDU operators. *Work and Stress*, **1**, 271–283.

Folkman, S. (1984). Personal control and stress and coping processes: A theoretical analysis. *Journal of Personality and Social Psychology*, **46**, 839–852.

Frankenhaeuser, M., and Gardell, B. (1976). Underload and overload in working life: Outline of a multidisciplinary approach. *Journal of Human Stress*, September, 35–46.

Frantz, R. S. (1980). The effect of early labor market experience upon internal–external locus of control among young male workers. *Journal of Youth and Adolescence*, **9**, 203–210.

French, J. R. P., Caplan, R. D., and Harrison, R.V. (1982). *The Mechanisms of Job Stress and Strain*. Chichester: Wiley.

Ganster, D. C. (1989). Worker control and well-being: A review of research in the workplace. In: S. L. Sauter, J. J. Hurrell and C. L. Cooper (eds), *Job Control and Worker Health*. New York: Wiley.

Gattiker, U. E., and Nelligan, T. W. (1988). Computerized offices in Canada and the United States: Investigating dispositional similarities and differences. *Journal of Organizational Behavior*, **9**, 77–96.

Gerhart, B. (1987). How important are dispositional factors as determinants of job satisfaction? Implications for job design and other personnel programs. *Journal of Applied Psychology*, **72**, 366–373.

Gill, C. (1985). *Work, Unemployment and the New Technology*. Cambridge: Polity Press.

Grandjean, E. (1980). Ergonomics of VDU's: Review of present knowledge. In: E.

Grandjean and E. Vigliani (eds), *Ergonomic Aspects of Visual Display Terminals.* London: Taylor & Francis.

Greenberger, D. B., and Strasser, S. (1986). Development and application of a model of personal control in organisations. *Academy of Management Review,* **11**, 164–177.

Griffeth, R. W. (1985). Moderation of the effects of job enrichment by participation: A longitudinal field experiment. *Organizational Behavior and Human Decision Processes,* **35**, 73–93.

Hackman, J. R., and Oldham, G. R. (1975). Development of the Job Diagnostic Survey. *Journal of Applied Psychology,* **60**, 159–170.

Hammer, T. H., Landau, J. C., and Stern, R. N. (1981). Absenteeism when workers have a voice: The case of employee ownership. *Journal of Applied Psychology,* **66**, 561–573.

Harrick, E. J., Vanek, G. R., and Michlitsch, J. F. (1986). Alternate work schedules, productivity, leave usage, and employee attitudes: A field study. *Public Personnel Management,* **15**, 159–169.

Harrison, R. V. (1978). Person–environment fit and job stress. In: C. L. Cooper and R. Payne (eds), *Stress at Work.* Chichester: Wiley.

Hesketh, B., and Shouksmith, G. (1986). Job and non-job activities, job satisfaction and mental health among veterinarians. *Journal of Occupational Behaviour,* **7**, 325–339.

House, J. S. (1981). *Work Stress and Social Support.* Reading, MA: Addison-Wesley.

House, R. J., and Baetz, M. L. (1979). Leadership: Some empirical generalizations and new research directions. In: B. M. Staw (ed.), *Research in Organizational Behaviour,* **1**, 341–423.

Hrycenko, I., and Minton, H. L. (1974). Internal–external control, power position and satisfaction in task-oriented groups. *Journal of Personality and Social Psychology,* **30**, 871–878.

Hurrell, J. J. (1985). Machine-paced work and the Type A behaviour pattern. *Journal of Occupational Psychology,* **58**, 15–25.

Hurrell, J. J., and Colligan, M. J. (1985). Alternative work schedules: Flextime and the compressed work week. In: C. L. Cooper and M. J. Smith (eds), *Job Stress and Blue Collar Work.* Chichester: Wiley.

Jackson, S. E. (1983). Participation in decision making as a strategy for reducing job-related strain. *Journal of Applied Psychology,* **68**, 3–19.

Jackson, S. E. (1984). Correction to 'Participation in decision making as a strategy for reducing job-related strain'. *Journal of Applied Psychology,* **69**, 546–547.

Jackson, S. E. (1989). Does job control control job stress? In: S. L. Sauter, J. J. Hurrell and C. L. Cooper (eds), *Job Control and Worker Health.* New York: Wiley.

James, L. R., and Jones, A. P. (1980). Perceived job characteristics and job satisfaction: An examination of reciprocal causation. *Personnel Psychology,* **33**, 97–135.

James, L. R., and Tetrick, L. E. (1986). Confirmatory analytic tests of three causal models relating job perceptions to job satisfaction. *Journal of Applied Psychology,* **71**, 77–82.

Jenner, D. A., Reynolds, V., and Harrison, G. A. (1980). Catecholamine excretion rates and occupation. *Ergonomics,* **23**, 237–246.

Johansson, G. (1979). Psychoneuroendocrine reactions to mechanized and computerized work routines. In: C. Mackay and T. Cox (eds), *Response to Stress: Occupational Aspect.* Guildford: IPC Science and Technology Press.

Johansson, G. (1981). Psychoneuroendocrine correlates of unpaced and paced perfor-mance. In: G. Salvendy and M. J. Smith (eds), *Machine Pacing and Occupational Stress.* London: Taylor & Francis.

Johnson, J. V. (1989). Control, collectivity and the psychosocial work environment. In: S. L. Sauter, J. J. Hurrell and C. L. Cooper (eds), *Job Control and Worker Health.* New York: Wiley.

Johnson, J. V., and Hall, E. M. (1988). Job strain, work place social support and cardiovascular disease. *American Journal of Public Health*, **78**, 1336–1341.

Kahn, R. L. (1981). *Work and Health*. New York: Wiley.

Karasek, R. A. (1979). Job demands, job decision latitude, and mental strain: Implications for job redesign. *Administrative Science Quarterly*, **24**, 285–308.

Karasek, R. (1989). Control in the workplace and its health related impacts. In: S. L. Sauter, J. J. Hurrell and C. L. Cooper (eds), *Job Control and Worker Health*. Wiley: New York.

Karasek, R., Baker, D., Marxer, F., Ahlbom, A., and Theorell, T. (1981). Job decision latitude, job demands, and cardiovascular disease: A prospective study of Swedish men. *American Journal of Public Health*, **71**, 694–705.

Karasek, R., Gardell, B., and Lindell, J. (1987). Work and non-work correlates of illness and behaviour in male and female Swedish white collar workers. *Journal of Occupational Behaviour*, **8**, 187–207.

Kiggundu, M. N. (1980). An empirical test of the theory of job design using multiple job ratings. *Human Relations*, **33**, 339–351.

Kim, J. S., and Compagna, A. F. (1981). Effects of flexitime on employee attendance and performance: A field experiment. *Academy of Management Journal*, **24**, 729–741.

Kirjonen, J., and Hanninen, V. (1986). Getting a better job: Antecedents and effects. *Human Relations*, **39**, 503–516.

Kohn, M. L., and Schooler, C. (1982). Job conditions and personality: A longitudinal assessment of their reciprocal effects. *American Journal of Sociology*, **87**, 1257–1286.

Kohn, M. L., and Schooler, C. (1983). *Work and Personality: An Inquiry into the Impact of Social Stratification*. Norwood, NJ: Ablex.

Krause, N., and Stryker, S. (1984). Stress and well-being: The buffering role of locus of control beliefs. *Social Science and Medicine*, **18**, 783–790.

Krausz, M., and Freibach, N. (1983). Effects of flexible working time for employed women upon satisfaction, strains, and absenteeism. *Journal of Occupational Psychology*, **56**, 155–159.

LaRocco, J. M. (1985). Effects of job conditions on worker perceptions: Ambient stimuli vs. group influence. *Journal of Applied Social Psychology*, **15**, 735–757.

Latack, J. C., and Foster, L. W. (1985). Implementation of compressed work schedules: Participation and job redesign as critical factors for employee acceptance. *Personnel Psychology*, **38**, 75–92.

Lazarus, R. S., and Folkman, S. (1984). *Stress, Appraisal, and Coping*. New York: Springer.

Lee, R. A. (1983). Flextime and conjugal roles. *Journal of Occupational Behaviour*, **4**, 297–315.

Lefcourt, H. M. (1973). The function of the illusions of control and freedom. *American Psychologist*, **28**, 417–425.

Lefcourt, H. M. (ed.) (1983). *Research with the Locus of Control Construct. Vol. 2. Developments and Social Problems*. New York: Academic Press.

Levenson, H. (1974). Activism and powerful others: Distinction within the concept of internal–external control. *Journal of Personality Assessment*, **38**, 377–383.

Locke, E. A., and Schweiger, D. M. (1979). Participation in decision-making: One more look. In: B. M. Staw (ed.), *Research in Organizational Behaviour*, Vol. 1. Greenwich, DT: JAI Press.

Marino, K. E., and White, S. E. (1985). Departmental structure, locus of control, and job stress: The effect of a moderator. *Journal of Applied Psychology*, **70**, 782–784.

McGuire, J. B., and Liro, J. R. (1986). Flexible work schedules, work attitudes, and perceptions of productivity. *Public Personnel Management*, **15**, 65–73.

Mortimer, J. T., and Lorence, J. (1979). Occupational experience and the self-concept: A longitudinal study. *Social Psychology Quarterly*, **42**, 307–323.

Norris, D. R., and Niebuhr, R. E. (1984). Attributional influences on the job performance–job satisfaction relationship. *Academy of Management Journal*, **27**, 424–431.

O'Brien, G. E. (1984a). Locus of control, work, and retirement. In: H. M. Lefcourt (ed.), *Research with the Locus of Control Construct. Vol. 3. Extensions and Limitations*. Orlando, FL: Academic Press.

O'Brien, G. E. (1984b). Reciprocal effects between locus of control and job attributes. *Australian Journal of Psychology*, **36**, 57–74.

Parkes, K. R. (1982). Occupational stress among student nurses: A natural experiment. *Journal of Applied Psychology*, **67**, 784–796.

Parkes, K. R. (1984). Locus of control, cognitive appraisal, and coping in stressful episodes. *Journal of Personality and Social Psychology*, **46**, 655–668.

Parkes, K. R. (1987). Field dependence and the differentiation of neurotic syndromes. In: P. Cuttance and R. Ecob (eds), *Structural Modeling by Example: Applications in Educational, Behavioral, and Social Research*. New York: Cambridge University Press.

Parkes, K. R. (1988). Locus of control in three behavioural domains: Factor structure and correlates of the 'Spheres of Control' scale. *Personality and Individual Differences*, **9**, 631–643.

Parkes, K. R., Styles, E. A., and Broadbent, D. E. (1988). Work preferences as moderators of the effects of paced and unpaced work on mood and cognitive performance (under review).

Pasmore, W., and Friedlander, F. (1982). An action research program for increasing employee involvement in problem-solving. *Administrative Science Quarterly*, **27**, 343–362.

Paulhus, D. (1983). Sphere-specific measures of perceived control. *Journal of Personality and Social Psychology*, **44**, 1253–1265.

Payne, R., and Fletcher, B. C. (1983). Job demands, supports, and constraints as predictors of psychological strain among schoolteachers. *Journal of Vocational Behavior*, **22**, 136–147.

Pearson, C. A. L. (1987). Participative goal-setting as a strategy for improving performance and job satisfaction: A longitudinal evaluation with railway track maintenance gangs. *Human Relations*, **40**, 473–488.

Perrewe, P. L. (1986). Locus of control and activity level as moderators in the quantitative job demands–satisfaction/psychological anxiety relationship: An experimental analysis. *Journal of Applied Social Psychology*, **16**, 620–632.

Perrewe, P. L., and Ganster, D. C. (1989). The impact of job demands and behavioral control on experienced job stress. *Journal of Organizational Behavior* (in press).

Perrewe, P. L., and Mizerski, R. W. (1987). Locus of control and task complexity in perceptions of job dimensions. *Psychological Reports*, **61**, 43–49.

Phares, E. J. (1976). *Locus of Control in Personality*. Morristown, NJ: General Learning Press.

Pierce, J. L., and Newstrom, J. W. (1983). The design of flexible work schedules and employee responses: Relationships and processes. *Journal of Occupational Behaviour*, **4**, 247–262.

Pryor, R. G. L. (1987). Differences among differences: In search of general work preference dimensions. *Journal of Applied Psychology*, **72**, 426–433.

Rafaeli, A., and Sutton, R. I. (1986). Word processing technology and perceptions of control among clerical workers. *Behaviour and Information Technology*, **5**, 31–37.

Ralston, D. A., and Flanagan, M. F. (1985). The effect of flextime on absenteeism and turnover for male and female employees. *Journal of Vocational Behavior*, **26**, 206–217.

Ralston, D. A., Antony, W. P., and Gustafson, D. J. (1985). Employees may love flextime, but what does it do to the organization's productivity? *Journal of Applied Psychology*, **70**, 272–279.

Repetti, R. (1987). Individual and common components of the social environment at work and psychological well-being. *Journal of Personality and Social Psychology*, **52**, 710–720.

Rotter, J. B. (1966). Generalized expectancies for internal versus external control of reinforcement. *Psychological Monographs*, **80**, (1, whole No. 609).

Sarata, B. P. (1984). Changes in staff satisfactions after increases in pay, autonomy and participation. *American Journal of Community Psychology*, **12**, 431–444.

Seligman, M. E. P. (1975). *Helplessness: On Depression, Development and Death*. San Francisco: Freeman.

Shaw, J. B., and Riskind, J. H. (1983). Predicting job stress using data from the Position Analysis Questionnaire. *Journal of Applied Psychology*, **68**, 253–261.

Smith, M. J. (1985). Machine-paced work and stress. In: C. L. Cooper and M. J. Smith (eds), *Job Stress and Blue Collar Work*. Chichester: Wiley.

Smith, M. J., Cohen, B. G. F., Stammerjohn, L. W., and Happ, A. (1981). An investigation of health complaints and job stress in video display operators. *Human Factors*, **23**, 387–400.

Solomon, E. E. (1986). Private and public sector managers: An empirical investigation of job characteristics and organizational climate. *Journal of Applied Psychology*, **71**, 247–259.

Spector, P. E. (1982). Behavior in organizations as a function of employee's locus of control. *Psychological Bulletin*, **91**, 482–497.

Spector, P. E. (1986). Perceived control by employees: A meta-analysis of studies concerning autonomy and participation at work. *Human Relations*, **39**, 1005–1016.

Spector, P. E. (1987a). Interactive effects of perceived control and job stressors on affective reactions and health outcomes for clerical workers. *Work and Stress*, **1**, 155–162.

Spector, P. E. (1987b). Method variance as an artifact in self-reported affect and perceptions at work: Myth or significant problem? *Journal of Applied Psychology*, **72**, 438–443.

Spector, P. E. (1988). Development of the Work Locus of Control Scale. *Journal of Occupational Psychology*, **61**, 335–340.

Spector, P. E., Dwyer, D. J., and Jex, S. M. (1988). Relation of job stressors to affective, health, and performance outcomes: A comparison of multiple data sources. *Journal of Applied Psychology*, **73**, 11–19.

Staines, G. L., and Pleck, J. H. (1986). Work schedule flexibility and family life. *Journal of Occupational Behaviour*, **7**, 147–153.

Stammerjohn, L. W., and Wilkes, B. (1981). Stress/strain and linespeed in paced work. In: G. Salvendy and M. J. Smith (eds), *Machine Pacing and Occupational Stress*. London: Taylor & Francis.

Stellman, J. M., Klitzman, S., Gordon, G. C., and Snow, B. R. (1987). Work environment and the well-being of clerical and VDT workers. *Journal of Occupational Behaviour*, **8**, 95–114.

Sutton, R. I., and Kahn, R. L. (1987). Prediction, understanding, and control as antidotes to organizational stress. In: J. Lorsch (ed.), *Handbook of Organizational Behavior*. Englewood Cliffs, NJ: Prentice-Hall.

Tannenbaum, A. S. (1983). Employee-owned companies. In: L. L. Cummings and B. M. Staw (eds), *Research in Organizational Behavior*, Vol. 5. Greenwich, CT: JAI Press.

Tetrick, L. E., and LaRocco, J. M. (1987). Understanding, prediction, and control as moderators of the relationships between perceived stress, satisfaction, and psychological well-being. *Journal of Applied Psychology*, **72**, 538–543.

Theorell, T., Hamsten, A., de Faire, U., Orth-Gomer, K., and Perski, A. (1987). Psychosocial work conditions before myocardial infarction in young men. *International Journal of Cardiology*, **15**, 33–46.

Vanderslice, V. J., Rice, R. W., and Julian, J. W. (1987). The effects of participation in decision-making on worker satisfaction and productivity: An organizational simulation. *Journal of Applied Social Psychology*, **17**, 158–170.

Wall, T. D., and Clegg, C. W. (1981). A longitudinal field study of group work redesign. *Journal of Occupational Behaviour*, **2**, 31–49.

Wall, T. D., Kemp, N. J., Jackson, P. R., and Clegg, C. W. (1986). Outcomes of autonomous workgroups: A long-term field experiment. *Academy of Management Journal*, **29**, 280–304.

Warr, P. (1987). *Work, Unemployment and Mental Health*. Oxford Science Publications. Oxford: Oxford University Press.

Wells, J. A. (1982). Objective job conditions, social support and perceived stress among blue collar workers. *Journal of Occupational Behaviour*, **3**, 79–94.

Williams, T. A. (1985). Visual display technology, worker disablement and work organisation. *Human Relations*, **38**, 1065–1084.

Wilpert, B. (1984). Participation in organizations: Evidence from international comparative research. *International Social Science Journal*, **36**, 355–366.

CHAPTER 3

Personal control at work and health: a review of epidemiological studies in Sweden

Töres Theorell
National Institute for Psychosocial Factors and Health, Stockholm, Sweden

JOB CHARACTERISTICS AND PERSONAL CONTROL

To have personal control at work can be defined as a feeling that *most situations that could occur in the near or distant future at work could be anticipated and dealt with*. This chapter concentrates on the characteristics of jobs that may affect sense of personal control.

Two dimensions relevant to control

Authority over decisions

The most direct feature of jobs that promote personal control is that they allow the worker to influence decisions regarding his or her job. These decisions could relate to work content (*what* is produced and what is the goal?) as well as to ways of production (*how* is it produced?). The dimension '*authority over decisions*' arose out of a long sociological tradition (Kohn, 1976). In Karasek's factor analysis of the American Quality of Employment Surveys in 1968, 1974 and 1977, the factor corresponding to this dimension consisted of two questions, namely (1977 version):

'I have freedom to decide what I do on the job'
'My responsibility is to decide how much work gets done'

For each item four fixed response categories were used (from 1 = strongly disagree to 4 = strongly agree).

Stress, Personal Control and Health.   Edited by A. Steptoe and A. Appels.
Published by John Wiley & Sons Ltd.
© ECSC–EEC–EAEC, Brussels–Luxembourg, 1989

50   *Töres Theorell*

These questions were slightly modified (the second items states . . . . to decide *how* to get work done . . .), translated into Swedish, and were used in a study of six widely different occupations, namely physicians, air traffic controllers, symphony musicians, baggage carriers in an airport, aeroplane mechanics and waiters. Figure 1 shows the mean age-adjusted scores of the participants' sense of authority over decisions in the six occupational groups. It can be seen that there is a highly significant difference between the groups (age-adjusted one-way analysis of variance). Symphony musicians have the lowest mean score. This might have been expected, since a symphony orchestra functions as a large school class with more than one hundred pupils. The company board decides *what* the orchestra should play, and the conductor makes practically all the decisions—even about minute details—about *how* to play. Other groups with low mean scores in this study are air traffic controllers and waiters. Air traffic is regulated in minute detail by laws of practice, and the individual air traffic controller's opportunity to make spontaneous decisions is small. Waiters have to follow the customers' wishes. A frequent complaint stated in group interviews in our study was that customers often abuse this position, and the waiter is put in many humiliating situations.

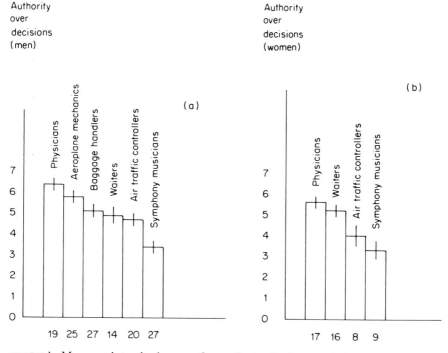

FIGURE 1. Means and standard errors of mean for 'authority over decisions': (a) men; (b) women.

Skill discretion

This dimension is related to personal control *in the future*. It consists of questions relating to utilization of workers' skills, their opportunities to learn new things at work and variety of tasks. The assumption is that workers who feel that their capabilities and ideas are used, that they constantly develop new skills and that their tasks vary, will develop a sense of mastery—whatever happens in the future they will be able to handle the situation.

In Karasek's factor analysis of the American Quality of Employment Surveys, the 1977 version of the *skill discretion* dimension consisted of four questions (Karasek *et al.*, 1988):

'My job requires that I be creative'
'My job requires that I do things over and over' (reverse scoring)
'My job requires that I learn new things'
'My job requires a high level of skill'

These questions were translated into Swedish and used in the study of six occupations. Figure 2 shows the average age-adjusted scores among participants in the six occupations. The difference between the groups is highly significant (one-way analysis of variance). In this case the baggage carriers have the lowest scores. This is also consistent with their statements in group interviews in the study. During these they claimed that their work was monotonous and boring and that they had to seek compensation for this.

'Authority over decisions' and 'skill discretion' are strongly correlated (Karasek *et al.*, 1988). Despite this, there are striking exceptions to this rule in the study of six occupations. Despite the low mean score for skill discretion in baggage carriers, men in this group do *not* claim that they have low 'authority over decisions' (see Figure 1a). In group interviews they commented on this: 'Whenever a crisis occurs—such as too many pieces of baggage in one place—we can always use our internal communication system and ask the supervisors to send more men.' Thus, there was frequently a feeling of good authority over decisions. Symphony musicians, on the other hand, claim that skill discretion is good although 'authority over decisions' is low (see Figures 1 and 2). Skill utilization has been regarded as an important dimension in work psychology by many research groups. For instance, German researchers (Volpert, 1975) have developed a theory of skill development including manual as well as intellectual components.

In the study of six occupations (Theorell et al., 1987b), 118 men had one to four measurements from self-administered questionnaires of both 'authority over decisions' and 'skill utilization'. Table 1 shows the *inter-subject* correlations between each one of these two dimensions and each one of a number of health-related variables. Blood pressure was measured by the subjects themselves by means of Cardiocare 2000 instruments. The subject was asked to sit down once

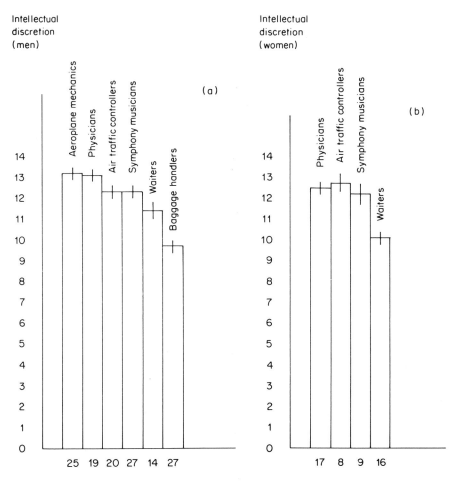

FIGURE 2. Means and standard errors of mean for 'skill discretion': (a) men; (b) women.

every hour or as close to once an hour as possible and measure blood pressure
without previous rest. In a sample of healthy subjects, the correlations between
blood pressure measured on the same occasion by conventional means and self-
measured blood pressure was 0.85 for systolic and 0.73 for diastolic. Average
blood pressure at work and during leisure was calculated for each subject. The
means were based upon an average of 7 measurements at work and 7 measurements during leisure during 1–4 ordinary work-days. Table 1 shows that men
with a low level of self-reported skill discretion are much more overweight than
other men—as reflected in the striking negative age-adjusted correlation between
skill discretion and body mass index. There is also a similar significant negative
relationship between average systolic blood pressure during leisure hours and

TABLE 1. Age-adjusted correlation between health indicators and 'skill discretion' and 'authority over decisions' indices, 118 men aged 40–60 in six occupations

	Skill discretion	Authority over decisions
Mean systolic blood pressure[a] during work hours	−0.15	−0.05
Mean distolic blood pressure[a] during work hours	−0.12	−0.09
Mean systolic blood pressure[a] during leisure hours	−0.19*	−0.06
Mean diastolic blood pressure[a] during leisure hours	−0.12	−0.09
Average rating of sadness in diaries	−0.16[0]	−0.04
Log. γ-glutamyltransferase in blood (liver enzyme sensitive to long-lasting, excessive alcohol consumption)	−0.11	−0.10
Body mass index (kg body weight/square of m height)	−0.43***	−0.06
Gastrointestinal symptom index	−0.06	−0.09
Muscle tension index	0.00	−0.28**

[a] Measurements approximately once an hour by means of self-triggered apparatus, one to four working days.
[0] $p < 0.10$.
* $p < 0.05$.
** $p < 0.01$.
*** $p < 0.001$.

skill discretion—the lower skill discretion the higher systolic blood pressure. During work hours skill discretion is also negatively related to systolic blood pressure, but in this case the relationship is not significant. There tends to be a relationship between a high average level of self-reported sadness in diaries and skill discretion—the higher skill discretion the lower sadness level ($p < 0.10$).

'Authority over decisions', on the other hand, shows no significant relationship with the health outcome variables, with one important exception. Men who report a low level of 'authority over decisions' also report a much higher level of muscle tension than other men. Thus, the two components of decision latitude are associated with health variables in different ways.

In summary, the two dimensions 'authority over decisions' and 'skill discretion' may not always be correlated, and they may also have different consequences for health. Despite this, they have mostly been combined into the 'decision latitude' concept proposed by Karasek (1979). Factor analyses have indicated that it is meaningful to combine them (see Karasek *et al.*, 1988; Johnson, 1986). However, when we interpret data from analyses of decision latitude we should bear in mind that the two dimensions could have separate effects.

In Swedish epidemiological studies an occupational classification system has been used that was constructed on the basis of national surveys of random Swedes of working age (Alfredsson *et al.*, 1982). Each one of a number of questions describing the job were explored. What proportion of workers in a given occupation describe their job as monotonous, for instance? Three questions that are close to the 'decision latitude' concept have been used, namely:

'Is your work monotonous?'
'Do you learn anything new in your job?'
'Do you have influence over your work tempo?'

The prevalence of 'monotony', 'not learning anything new' and 'no influence over work tempo' was described in more than a hundred occupations (male and female separately and age below and above 40 separately). In two different studies, occupation classification (three-digit codes) based upon this knowledge were used in order to test whether 'monotonous' occupations have a higher myocardial infarction incidence than other occupations. The same test was made for 'not learning anything new' and 'no influence over work tempo'. In this procedure the upper half of the distribution was compared with the lower half—for instance, occupations with a percentage of workers reporting 'monotony' *above* the median being compared with occupations *below* the median. In the first study all men living in one region of greater Stockholm who had suffered a myocardial infarction between the ages of 40 and 64 in the years 1975 and 1976 were identified. These men were compared with regard to occupation characteristics to a sample of similarly aged men living in the same geographical area. Potential confounders were explored using the Mantel–Haenszel test. Confidence intervals were calculated using the technique introduced by Miettinen (1976). Occupational title was identified mainly in the census in 1970, and cases were identified in the official death and hospitalization registers.

In this first study, which included about 300 cases of myocardial infarction and about 800 non-cases, all three questions were significantly associated with myocardial infarction risk. Significant confounding was observed, however. For instance, the variable 'monotony' was confounded by educational level and by 'heavy lifting'. Thus, part of the association between 'monotony' and risk could be explained by these other variables—those in 'monotonous' occupations who had increased risk were partly the same subjects as those in occupations with a low average level of education in which heavy lifting was common. A previous study by our group showed that concrete work was associated with a higher risk of developing myocardial infarction than other kinds of construction work. Concrete work is associated with excessive physical static loads (Theorell *et al.*, 1977).

In the next study, the 'Five Counties Study' (Alfredsson *et al.*, 1985), a much larger sample was studied, almost one million working men and women in five counties in Sweden. In this case, the follow-up period was shorter (occupational title identified in 1975 and case in 1976), and deaths outside hospitals were not included. The age span was also larger—20–64 years. Only those associations that remained significant throughout a series of confounding tests were reported. In this study 'monotony' was significantly associated with myocardial infarction risk for both men and women. 'Not learning' showed a strong association with risk for men but not for women. 'Influence over work tempo' did not have any significant association with risk either for women or men.

In both these epidemiological studies, we also tested the hypothesis that the combination of lack of personal control (as reflected in 'monotony', 'not learning' and 'lack of influence over tempo') and quantitative demands (as reflected in percentage of workers reporting 'hectic work') would be particularly dangerous. In this respect both studies yielded the same result: for men, in particular for men below the age of 55, a combination of 'not learning' and 'hectic' in an occupation is the most powerful psychosocial predictor of risk. For women, the variable 'not learning' was not a predictor either alone or in combination with 'hectic', but as in the case of men the combination of 'monotony' and 'hectic' was a strong predictor of risk. Both for men and for women, 'hectic' *per se* did not have any predictive value, but in combination with 'monotony' and 'not learning' it turned out to be important.

There was information available for each one of the participants in the follow-up that enabled analyses of possible confounders to be carried out. Except for age (which was adjusted for in all the analyses), several social factors were explored such as geographical region, type of residence, income, part-time or full-time job and type of employment, and two factors that were based upon the occupational classification—percentage reporting heavy lifting and the percentage who were cigarette smokers. Confounding was not a problem in this association. When 'percentage of cigarette smokers' was adjusted for, the association was actually strengthened.

Non-cardiovascular illness in the 'Five Counties Study'

Hospitalization for other illnesses except myocardial infarction could also be explored in the 'Five Counties study'. Table 2 shows the relative risks associated with 'monotony' and 'not learning' for hospitalization due to several illnesses, both for men and women. All the associations that are presented with relative risk values are significant (using two-tailed tests and a p-value of 5% as cut-off point) even after adjusting for the potential confounding factors mentioned above. A striking observation is that 'monotony' is a significant predictor both for men and women for general ill health in the near future. 'Not learning' is also a very general predictor of ill health but only for men, not for women. We have no explanation of the gender difference in the importance of 'not learning'—maybe this simply reflects a difference in male and female language; the way in which men and women describe the same conditions at work may be different.

TABLE 2. Aggregated occupation analyses of psychosocial characteristics in relation to relative age-adjusted risk of hospitalization for different illness categories. Five counties, one-year follow-up of all working men and women

	Myocardial infarction			Alcohol-related illness		Psychiatric illness		Gastrointestinal illness		Traffic accident	
	Men 20–54	Men 20–64	Women 20–64	Men 20–64	Women 20–64	Men 20–64	Women 20–64	Men 20–64	Women 20–64	Men 20–64	Women 20–64
Few possibilities to learn new things	1.1	1.4	ns	2.6	ns	2.8	ns	1.7	ns	1.5	ns
Monotony	ns	1.4	1.3	2.3	1.9	2.1	1.5	1.6	1.6	1.5	ns
Hectic	ns	ns	ns	0.5	1.2	0.6	ns	ns	ns	0.7	ns
Hectic and few possibilities to learn new things	1.3	1.6	ns	1.4	1.3	1.4	ns	1.5	ns	ns	ns
Hectic and monotonous	1.2	1.5	1.6	ns	3.1	ns	1.6	ns	2.2	ns	ns

ns = not significant.

An important observation is that, among men, 'hectic' occupations have *lower* relative risks for hospitalizations due to alcohol-related illness, psychiatric illness or traffic accidents. This finding is hard to interpret. It could be due either to a psychiatric 'salutogenic' effect of having an important job (that is frequently associated with a hectic tempo) or to a 'downward drift' social phenomenon —when somebody starts drinking excessively there is increasing likelihood that he or she will be put in a less 'hectic' job. Alcoholism increases the risk of traffic accidents and psychiatric problems.

Other studies in Sweden separating 'authority over decisions' and 'skill utilization' as possible predictors of ill health

A cardiovascular symptom indicator was defined in the Swedish Survey of Level of Living in 1968–1974 by Karasek *et al.* (1981). Using this indicator as a health end-point, defining cases as those 1600 men who were asymptomatic or had one mild symptom in 1968 and then had developed at least one serious symptom in 1974, a prospective study was carried out. Two different factors related to the individual's sense of personal control at work were identified in 1968 from questionnaires by means of factor analysis, namely:

Skill discretion
   'Is your work monotonous?'
   'Does your work require more than mandatory education?'
Influence over decisions
   'Can you receive a visitor for at least half an hour during working hours?'
   'Can you get away from work for private business for at least half an hour during working hours?'
   'Can you make a private telephone call during working hours?'

These two factors were analysed as predictors of cardiovascular symptom development during the years 1968–1974, along with an indicator of 'psychological demands' composed by two questions ('Is your work hectic?'; 'Is your work psychologically demanding?'), age, cigarette-smoking and self-reported overweight. Age, skill discretion and psychological demands were the only independent predictors in multiple logistic regression analysis.

In a study of young (below age 45) male victims of myocardial infarction in the greater Stockholm area, those who had survived acute illness for three months were subjected to a clinical examination and an interview regarding the psychosocial work conditions before illness onset (Theorell *et al.*, 1987a). One index relating to 'demands' (the same as in the previous study) and one relating to 'authority over decisions' (the same as in the previous study) and finally two indices relating to 'skill discretion', namely 'variety' and 'skill discretion', were used. The latter two were assessed as follows:

Variety
'Is your work monotonous?'
The responses were graded from 1 = 'Yes, very much' to 4 = 'Not at all'.
Intellectual discretion
'Does your work provide you with good opportunities to learn new things?'
The responses were simply 'Yes' = 2 and 'No' = 1.

All four indices were used along with several clinical predictors (education, type A behaviour, smoking habits, history of hypertension, serum lipoproteins, family history of myocardial infarction) in a multiple logistic regression analysis in order to find independent characteristics of cases of myocardial infarction (MI) in young age ($n = 72$) as opposed to non-cases in the same ages living in the same areas ($n = 117$). In this analysis, 'lack of variety' was observed to be a statistically independent characteristic of the occupations of MI cases. The statistical strength of the association was of almost the same magnitude as cigarette-smoking, and of the same magnitude as 'family history of myocardial infarction'.

When the index of 'psychological demands' was divided by each one of the indices in 'skill discretion' and 'authority of decisions', two of the ratios had significant independent statistical power in separating the cases from the non-cases, even after having taken all the clinical risk factors into account; namely, demands divided by 'variety' and demands divided by 'influence over work' (see Table 3).

TABLE 3. Variables significantly correlated with myocardial infarction by multiple logistic regression analysis in a case–control study of medical and psychosocial risk factors among men below age 45 in greater Stockholm (cases, $n = 72$; controls, $n = 116$)

Term	Coefficient/ standard error	*P*-value*
LDL/HDL cholesterol ratio	4.382	0.0000
Cumulative tobacco consumption	3.455	0.0010
High demand in relation to variety at work	3.356	0.0014
High demands in relation to influence over work	2.266	0.0292
Alcohol consumption	−2.241	0.0311

* Approximation for *F* to remove.

STUDIES COMBINING 'AUTHORITY OVER DECISIONS' AND 'SKILL DISCRETION'

Johnson (1986) has performed studies of the illness-predictive power of three psychosocial job dimensions, namely 'psychological demands', 'control' and 'social support'. The 'control' dimension was a combination of 'skill discretion' and 'authority over decisions' based upon factor analysis. The 'control' dimension included the following eleven items:

Influence over the planning of work
Influence over the setting of the workplace
Influence over how time is used in work
The planning of work breaks
The planning of vacations
Flexible working hours
Freedom to receive a phone call during working hours
Freedom to receive a private visitor during working hours
Varied task content
Varied work procedures
Possibilities for ongoing education as part of the job

Each item was graded from $0 = $ 'Never' to $2 = $ 'Often'. The analysis was based upon 13 779 subjects, 52% men and 48% women. All three dimensions were independently associated with self-reported symptoms of heart disease, low back pain and gastrointestinal disease. Statistically significant interactions were observed between all three (control–demands, support–demands and support–control as well as control–demands–support). The multiplied standardized combination formed the 'iso-strain' factor. All three scores were transformed into z-scores, and a constant was added in order to transform them into positive scores. In this way, the scores for lack of control, demands and lack of support became mathematically equal. Subsequently they were multiplied with each other. The $8\frac{1}{2}$-year incidence of cardiovascular mortality was then related, by use of a logistic analysis of age trends for cardiovascular mortality, with age in three groups—upper and lower quintiles or 'iso-strain' as well as an intermediate group (three middle quintiles). This is shown in Figure 3. There is a strong relationship—those who initially reported low iso-strain died from cardiovascular disease at a later age than those who reported high or intermediate iso-strain. There was, however, no difference between the intermediate and high iso-strain groups. These data point at a protective 'salutogenic' effect of a good job. Similar, albeit weaker, findings were observed among women (Johnson *et al.*, 1989).

An important finding was that the general model seems to fit white-collar workers considerably less well than blue-collar workers. One reason for the

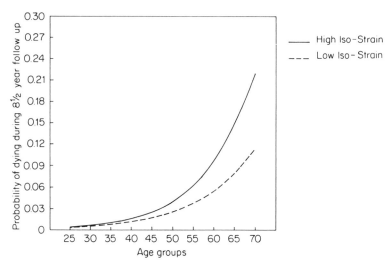

FIGURE 3. Iso-strain and cardiovascular mortality. Logistic estimates based on $8\frac{1}{2}$-year follow-up. Male Swedish working population, $n = 7299$. (From Johnson *et al.*, 1989.)

difference between upper and lower classes is that higher executives may not perceive lack of control or intellectual discretion as a problem. For instance, in the study of six occupations described earlier, physicians (both male and female) were the only group who reported 'too much complexity' to be a problem. This should be the subject of future research. However, regardless of kind of illness, age and social group, those who experienced a high level of personal control and support as well as a low level of psychological demands reported, on average, fewer illness symptoms of all kinds than others.

In conclusion, epidemiological studies have shown that 'decision latitude' (a combination of possibilities to influence decisions and to develop new skills at work) is correlated with health—the more decision latitude, the better health. Cross-sectional as well as prospective studies point in the same direction. In those studies in which relevant individual characteristics have been taken into account, such factors have not been able to 'explain away' all of the association. The results are similar when people themselves describe work (individual studies) and when all members of a group describe it (aggregated studies). This speaks in favour of the interpretation that work structures, not only personal characteristics, are important in generating a sense of personal control at work. The influence of 'decision latitude' is strengthened when 'demands' are taken into account—when decision latitude is low, high demands are particularly damaging. High demands and low decision latitude probably creates a pronounced feeling of lack of personal control.

In studies which have separated 'skill discretion' and 'authority over decisions', the former factor has been of greater importance than the latter one. This may indicate that the long-term perspective is more important to health than the short-term one in 'personal control at work'—development of new skills may be associated with development of a sense of mastery over unexpected difficulties in the future.

In most of the studies which have adjusted for social class or similar variables such as education and income, it has been observed that measures of decision latitude provide more precise information and more predictive value than these conventional social class variables.

SPONTANEOUS VARIATIONS IN THE RATIO BETWEEN DEMANDS AND DECISION LATITUDE

Since a sense of personal control is probably to a great extent dependent on the relationship between psychological demands and possibilities for action, a study was undertaken in which intra-subject variations in the self-reported ratio between demands and decision latitude (authority over decisions plus skill utilization) were studied. Seventy-three working men and women in six different occupations (described above) were assessed on four different occasions (Theorell *et al.*, 1988). For each subject, the occasions were ordered from the least favourable ratio (worst 'strain') to the most favourable one (least 'strain'). These occasions were unrelated to season and whether they were the first, second, third or fourth measurement, and thus probably mainly reflect true variations in the work situation. Figure 4 shows how these four levels of work strain relate to a number of health-relevant variables. It should be mentioned that the variations in work strain showed no significant association with smoking habits, liver enzymes (reflecting excessive alcohol abuse) or body weight. The figures show that increasing strain has effects on several outcome variables, namely sleep disturbance, gastrointestinal symptoms and systolic blood pressure during working hours. In male participants blood testosterone levels decreased (Theorell *et al.*, 1989). Blood prolactin levels decreased, but this was only shown in men who reported at least once during the study that they felt depressed or sad.

This means that increasing strain at work (which may mean decreasing sense of personal control) is associated with a number of physiological changes. We know from experimental studies that this may indeed be the case. Studies of unemployment processes (Brenner and Levi, 1987) and the bereavement process (Parkes *et al.*, 1969) have shown that catastrophic losses of personal control may have profound physiological effects. Karasek (1989), studying a large group of clerks in Sweden longitudinally, found that those clerks who claimed that they had a lower level of decision latitude at follow-up than initially reported significantly more deterioration of their health than did others. Aronsson and Barklöv (1981), studying bus drivers, were also able to show that demands

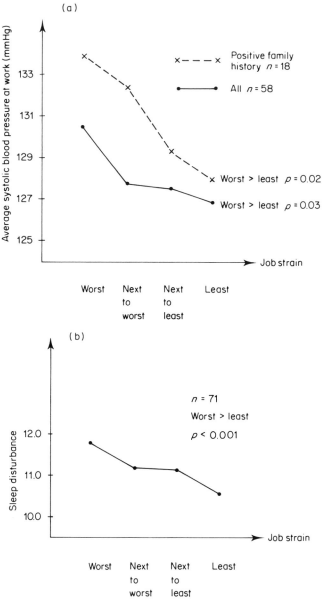

FIGURE 4. (a) Average systolic blood pressure during work hours in 58 working men and women in relation to reported job strain (demand/decision latitude). Observations ranked according to worst–least job strain. Subgroup ($n = 18$) with family history of hypertension. (From Theorell, 1989) (b) Sleep disturbance index in 71 working men and women in relation to reported job strain (demand/decision latitude). Observations rated according to worst–least job strain.

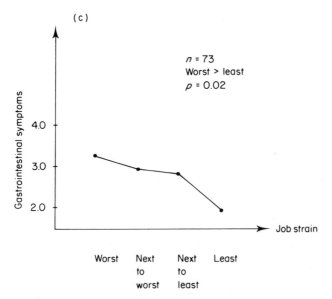

FIGURE 4. (c) Gastrointestinal symptom index in 71 working men and women in relation to reported job strain (demand/decision latitude). Observations rated according to worst–least job strain.

'exceeding resources' were associated with deteriorated health and physiological reactions.

In conclusion, it seems to be possible to identify work situations that facilitate a sense of control. Such jobs promote the development of good health.

REFERENCES

Alfredsson, L., Karasek, R. A., and Theorell, T. (1982). Myocardial infarction risk and psychosocial work environment: An analysis of the male Swedish working force. *Social Science and Medicine*, **16**, 463–467.

Alfredsson, L., Spetz, C.-L., and Theorell, T. (1985). Type of occupation and near-future hospitalization for myocardial infarction and some other diagnoses. *International Journal of Epidemiology*, **14**, 378.

Aronsson, G., and Barklöv, K. (1981). *The work environment of the public transportation personnel in Stockholm* (in Swedish). Work Environment Fund, Stockholm.

Brenner, S. O., and Levi, L. (1987). Long-term unemployment among women in Sweden. *Social Science and Medicine*, **25**, 153–161.

Johnson, J. (1986). *The impact of workplace and social support, job demands and work control upon cardiovascular disease in Sweden*. Doctoral thesis, Department of Psychology, University of Stockholm, ISSN 0283-3670.

Johnson, J. V., Hall, E., and Theorell, T. (1989). The combined effects of job strain and social isolation on the prevalence and mortality incidence of cardiovascular disease in a random sample of the Swedish working population. *Scandinavian Journal of Work. Environment and Health* (in press).

Karasek, R. A. (1979). Job demands, job decision latitude and mental strain: Implications for job design. *Administrative Science Quarterly*, **24**, 285–308.

Karasek, R. A. (1989). Reduced health risk with increased job control among white collar workers. *Journal of Occupational Behaviour* (in press).

Karasek, R. A., Baker, D., Ahlbom, A., and Theorell, T. (1981). Job decision latitude, job demands and cardiovascular disease: A prospective study of Swedish working men. *American Journal of Public Health*, **71**, 694–705.

Karasek, R., Theorell, T., Schwartz, J., Schnall, P., Pieper, C., and Michela, J. (1988). Job characteristics in relation to prevalence of myocardial infarction in the U.S. HES and HANES. *American Journal of Public Health*, **78**, 910–918.

Kohn, M. L. (1976). Occupational structure and alienation. *American Journal of Sociology*, **82**, 111–130.

Miettinen, O. (1976). Estimability and estimation in case-referent studies. *American Journal of Epidemiology*, **103**, 226–235.

Parkes, C. M., Benjamin, B., and Fitzgerald, R. G. (1969). Broken heart. A statistical study of increased mortality among widowers. *British Medical Journal*, **1**, 740.

Theorell, T. (1989). Spontaneously occurring stressors. In: H. Weiner, I. Florin, R. Murison and D. Hellhammer (eds), *Neuronal Control of Bodily Function: Basic and Clinical Aspects (Frontiers of Stress Research)*. Stuttgart: Hans Huber.

Theorell, T., Olsson, A., and Engholm, G. (1977). Concrete work and myocardial infarction. *Scandinavian Journal of Work, Environment and Health*, **3**, 144–153.

Theorell, T., Hamsten, A., de Faire, U., Orth-Gomér, K., and Perski, A. (1987a). Psychosocial work conditions before myocardial infarction in young men. *International Journal of Cardiology*, **15**, 33–46.

Theorell, T., Ahlberg-Hultén, G., Berggren, T., Perski, A., Sigala, F., Svensson, J., and Wallin, B.-M. (1987b). Work environment, personal habits and heart disease risk (in Swedish). *Stress Research Reports No. 195*, National Institute for Psychosocial Factors and Health and the Department of Stress Research, Karolinska Institute, Sweden.

Theorell, T., Perski, A., Åkerstedt, T., Sigala, F., Ahlberg-Hultén, G., Svensson, J., and Eneroth, P. (1988). Changes in job strain in relation to changes in physiological states: A longitudinal study. *Scandinavian Journal of Work Environment and Health*, **19**, 189–196.

Theorell, T., Karasek, R. A., and Eneroth, P. (1989). Job strain variations in relation to plasma testosterone fluctuations in working men: A longitudinal study. *Journal of Internal Medicine* (submitted).

Volpert, W. (1975). Die Lohnarbeitswissenschaft und die Psychologie der Arbeitstitägkeit. In: P. Groskurth and W. Volpert (eds), *Lohnarbeitspsychologie*. Frankfurt: Fischer.

CHAPTER 4

Restricted status control and cardiovascular risk

JOHANNES SIEGRIST AND HERBERT MATSCHINGER
Department of Medical Sociology, Medical School, University of Marburg, FRG

INTRODUCTION

Cardiovascular health and disease are prominent topics in sociomedical research owing to their substantial role in preventing or promoting premature illness and death in advanced societies at large. In scientific terms, cardiovascular diseases offer an opportunity to develop and to test pathogenic concepts of interaction between genetic, behavioural and socio-emotional factors. This opportunity has stimulated an impressive amount of innovative transdisciplinary research. Knowledge based on this approach has contributed to a broadening of medical intervention in terms of preventive public health, and of new types of professional cooperation including behavioural and microsocial intervention.

The present chapter focuses on the role of chronic socio-emotional distress in the development of two important cardiovascular (and especially coronary) risk factors: hypercholesterolaemia and systemic hypertension in middle adulthood (Kannel *et al.*, 1984; Castelli and Anderson, 1986). The first part develops a theoretical model of socio-emotional influences on cardiovascular health which stresses the mismatch between demand-related efforts and rewards in occupational life. In the second part, the chapter presents empirical findings from an ongoing prospective study on cardiovascular risk factors in male blue-collar workers.

Theoretical modelling of associations between socio-emotional distress and cardiovascular disease is difficult owing to the complexity and variety of potential stressors, the modulating action of individual and social coping resources, the

Stress, Personal Control and Health.   Edited by A. Steptoe and A. Appels.
Published by John Wiley & Sons Ltd.
© ECSC–EEC–EAEC, Brussels–Luxembourg, 1989

time course of assumed interactions, and the multidisciplinary approach needed to integrate sociological, psychological and biological information into patho-physiologically meaningful concepts. In view of these problems, it would seem difficult to advance cumulative knowledge in the field. Yet, over the past two decades, a substantial body of evidence on the impact of socio-emotional distress on cardiovascular health and disease has been developed (for overviews, see Ballieux *et al.*, 1984; Beamish *et al.*, 1985; Steptoe *et al.*, 1985; Matthews *et al.*, 1986; Schmidt *et al.*, 1986). This evidence needs further theoretical clarification and specification at different levels of scientific analysis. The model developed below represents but one such attempt at theoretical clarification and specification.

A MODEL OF RESTRICTED STATUS CONTROL AND CARDIOVASCULAR RISK

Every theoretical model is selective in terms of predicting variables, and this selection normally is not self-evident. The following statements explain the reasons for our emphasis on a mismatch between effort and reward in occupational life, and they define the relevant associations of components in the model.

(1) Clinical, epidemiological and experimental evidence suggests that cardiovascular risk and disease are associated with conditions of excessive catabolic, energy-mobilizing and effort-related activities of an organism (Schneiderman, 1983). Whatever additional specifications may be necessary in terms of environmental stressors, in terms of neuronal and neurohormonal response sustained activation of the sympatho-adrenomedullary system seems a potent source of cardiovascular risk.

(2) Sustained activation of the sympathoadrenergic system is likely to occur under conditions of low control or low reward in effort-related activities (Henry and Stephens, 1977; Frankenhaeuser, 1979; Karasek *et al.*, 1982). It usually involves additional systems, causing hormonal imbalance and changed patterns of hormonal release with long-term implications for cardiovascular health (Axelrod and Reisine, 1984).

(3) In human beings, demand, effort, control and reward are cognitively appraised phenomena. Appraisal means cognitive evaluation of the significance of a person's transaction with the environment for his or her well-being (Lazarus and Folkman, 1984). Therefore, perception of a mismatch between demand/effort and control/reward triggers emotional states of distress. It is important, however, to note that affective processing sometimes bypasses conscious neocortical evaluation (LeDoux, 1987). In addition, experienced emotional distress may not be admitted at a cognitive level. For these reasons, the association between sustained activation and perceived emo-

tional distress is difficult to evaluate, and inference from the first to the second phenomenon remains a critical assumption in human research.

(4) We suggest that within an individual's hierarchy of appraisal, fulfilment and continuity of crucial social roles are of primary importance (Siegrist *et al.*, 1986). In adult life, one of the crucial social roles is defined by occupational demands. Discrepancies between demand/effort and control/reward in occupational life provide powerful triggers of sustained activation and of related emotional distress.

(5) The most relevant components of high occupational demand and of related effort are quantitative workload (e.g time pressure), qualitative workload (e.g. responsibility) and structural role conflicts (Caplan *et al.*, 1975). The most relevant components of low occupational control and reward are poor incentives at work (low payment, rigid time schedule, low degree of self-direction in work), as well as conditions conducive to relative deprivation and to restricted status control (Kohn and Schooler, 1983; Pearlin *et al.*, 1981). Relative deprivation refers to those occupational characteristics which provoke unfavourable social comparison (e.g. 'dirty' work, work with low prestige). Restricted status control defines limitations and threats to occupational biography such as job instability (including unemployment, downward mobility and forced change), lack of promotion and low position in hierarchy (Siegrist *et al.*, 1986).

(6) Although discrepancies between components of high demand and of low control/reward may cause emotional distress in general, adaptation and routine are thought to reduce the amount of perceived emotional distress in the long run. To some extent, this also holds true for poor incentives and relative deprivation. However, adjustment to restricted status control is particularly difficult, since this condition threatens the continuity of a crucial social role in adult life. More generally speaking, adjustment to stressors which threaten a basic dimension in a person's hierarchy of appraisal is most difficult to achieve. Therefore, discrepancies between high demand in work and restricted status control are assumed to trigger chronic emotional distress and—most importantly—to modify its effects on cardiovascular risk (see Figure 1). The reasons for assuming an inconsistent association between the amount of high demand/low reward and the amount of perceived distress (as expressed by a dotted line in the model) have been explained above (see point 3): cognitive misperception to some extent may operate as a bias.

(7) In addition to the direct effect of high demand and low control/reward on the amount of perceived emotional distress, this latter depends on resources of coping with the demands of occupational life. It has been shown that interpersonal resources in terms of valuable social support operate as buffering mechanisms (House, 1981). In addition, intrapersonal patterns of coping have been identified which may enhance or reduce the amount of perceived emotional distress. We have shown elsewhere that a distinct

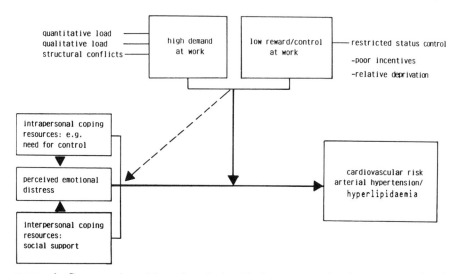

FIGURE 1. Conceptual model on the relationship between restricted status control and cardiovascular risk.

intrapersonal pattern of coping with demands termed 'need for control' increases the amount of perceived emotional distress and contributes to the explanation of cardiovascular risk (Matschinger *et al.*, 1986). Therefore, social support and need for control are designed as variables with conditional effects on cardiovascular risk in our model (see Figure 1).

As an analytical model, Figure 1 describes an oversimplified reality. Its emphasis is exclusively on occupational demand and control/reward. Additional stressful conditions for an individual, such as chronic difficulties in one's personal life or negative life events, are not considered explicitly. Even within the model, feedback loops between variables are not defined. On the other hand, the validity of this model can be tested empirically in terms of linear structural equation models, in terms of log-linear models and, with restrictions, in terms of analysis of variance and covariance (see below). Distinct from current psychological models of stress and disease, this model postulates a hierarchical (conditional) structure of effects: the variables measuring perceived emotional distress, social support and individual pattern of coping with demand exert significant effects on indicators of cardiovascular risk only under conditions of high demand and low control/reward in occupational settings.

METHODS AND STUDY SAMPLE

Measurement of the model

The model outlined above combines three different sources of information: first, descriptive social and individual facts with face validity (as collected by observational data, or, as a proxy measure, interviewer-based data); second, subjective attitudes (as measured by a questionnaire using scales or by in-depth interview); and third, biological data measuring cardiovascular risk.

Components of high demand and low control/reward are measured by techniques providing descriptive information, whereas variables measuring emotional distress, need for control and evaluation of social support rely on scales. In some parts, our methodology is specified with respect to the characteristic population under study. For instance, this chapter summarizes results of a prospective study on cardiovascular risk in male blue-collar workers (see below). Components of demand and control/reward are measured with special reference to this occupational group. Other parts of the methodology can be applied to a variety of populations under study (e.g. the scale: need for control, several indicators of emotional distress). The following lines provide an overview of the most relevant measures of the model.

High demands

Several alternative measures have been used defining subgroups of blue-collar workers who are exposed to at least one of these conditions:

- workplace under shift-work schedule (two-shift scheme, changing from 6 a.m. to 2 p.m. to 2 p.m. to 10 p.m.);
- workplace defined by piece-work;
- workplace with exposure to heavy noise and/or to overwork (workers' information on level of noise being validated by independent measurement);
- workplace with conflicting demands (foremen only).

Low control

Again a set of alternative measures has been used, defining subgroups of blue-collar workers who are exposed at least to one of these conditions:

Restricted status control:
- unstable occupation, defined by membership to a plant which cut down their personnel by 20% during the observation period;
- occupational downward mobility, defined by a discrepancy between level of training and/or former position and current job status;
- low-status job (unskilled or semiskilled workers).

Relative deprivation—poor incentives:
- low level of wage (within company and in relation to other companies);
- low self-direction in work (routine production versus individual production, group work versus individual work).

Owing to considerable overlap of subgroups defined by specific components of high demand *and* of low control/reward, our analysis basically focuses on four indicators of a mismatch between high demand and restricted status control:

(1) 'Forced piece-work': workers who for years were forced by economic pressure to do piece-work although they preferred easier jobs.
(2) 'Chronic shift-work': men who for years worked under shift-work without an opportunity to change their workplace.
(3) 'Low occupational position': unskilled or semiskilled workers who were exposed to heavy work (noise, overwork) to a large extent.
(4) 'Occupational instability': workers belonging to a plant which reduced their personnel by 20% during the observation period, compensating for this reduction by increase of workload.

Five tests of the model are presented in the Results section, below. Two of the three linear structural equation models (LISREL) are performed using forced piece-work as an indicator of a mismatch between high demand and restricted status control, and one using low occupational position. The two analyses of variance (ANOVA) are based on chronic shift-work and occupational instability as indicators of a mismatch between high demand and restricted status control.

Need for control

A scale containing 45 dichotomous items measures the following subscales of the construct: (1) need for approval, coping with success and failure; (2) competitiveness, independence and latent hostility; (3) work commitment, hard driving; (4) perfectionism, need for making plans; (5) impatience and disproportionate irritability; (6) inability to withdraw from work obligations. Unidimensionality of each subscale was tested by the dichotomous probabilistic test model developed by Rasch (1960). By means of a confirmatory factor analysis, two latent factors were found which are moderately correlated: the subscales 3 and 4 load on the factor labelled 'vigor', the other subscales on the second latent factor, labelled 'immersion'. Information on criterion validity and reliability of the scale can be found elsewhere (Matschinger *et al.*, 1986).

Social support

Amount of support received at work from superiors and from colleagues (index based on the following two LIKERT scale items):

(1) In the event of difficulties at work, how much support do you get from your colleagues (5 answers from 'not at all', to 'very strong')?
(2) In the event of difficulties at work, how much support do you get from your superior (5 answers from 'not at all' to 'very strong')? (Siegrist, 1986).

Emotional distress

A set of indicators has been developed which focus either on characteristics of work perceived as subjectively stressful or on aspects of the person's own behaviour reflecting emotional distress: perceived workload; perceived job insecurity; perceived anger/irritation; perceived helplessness; perceived sleep disturbances. Most indicators are based on LIKERT scale items (for detail see Siegrist *et al.*, 1987).

Cardiovascular risk

Hyperlipidemia

Total serum cholesterol and trigycerides were determined enzymatically (Cremer *et al.*, 1985). Lipoproteins were measured by a quantitative lipoprotein electro-phoresis (Wieland and Seidel, 1983). In addition to lipoprotein quantification, the main protein components of high- and low-density lipoproteins, i.e. apo-A1 and apo-B, were assessed by kinetic nephelometry. All analyses of blood samples were performed blind by an external institution, the Department of Clinical Chemistry at the University of Göttingen. The help of Dr P. Cremer and Dr D. Seidel is gratefully acknowledged here again. On the basis of current understanding of the pathophysiological aspects of lipoprotein metabolism and athero-genesis, the atherogenic index was defined as the ratio between low-density lipoprotein (LDL) and high-density lipoprotein (HDL) cholesterol (Lewis, 1982). This ratio has been shown to be predictive of future cases of overt coronary heart disease (Castelli *et al.*, 1983; Kannel *et al.*, 1984).

Arterial hypertension

Blood pressure readings were performed by sphygmomanometry according to WHO criteria at standardized diurnal time.

Confounding variables

Information on body weight and height was obtained by screening data. Information on age, cigarette-smoking, individual and family history of disease, physical exercise and recreational activities was collected by interview.

Statistical analysis

As mentioned above, the three predominant techniques used in our analysis are linear structural equation models (LISREL), log-linear models and analysis of variance and covariance (ANOVA). Each approach has its specific strengths and limitations, especially so with regard to an appropriate representation of the hierarchical structure of our theoretical approach.

LISREL (Jöreskog and Sörbom, 1979) represents a statistical program for analyses which combines factor analysis (for latent variables such as vigour and immersion) and path analysis. It allows a test of the assumption of a confirmatory factor analysis in one or more populations and a simultaneous analysis of the relations between such factors. Furthermore, one can test the model fit under certain restrictions for model parameters such as the restriction of invariance of parameters between different groups of observation.

In our LISREL analyses, indicators of restricted status control and high demand are used to define homogeneous subgroups for which identical models are estimated. By doing so, the hierarchical concept can be tested to some extent; effects of exogenous and endogenous variables on the criterion (blood pressure) are postulated to be much more pronounced in subgroups defined by a stressful occupational context. Results on three models testing this hypothesis will be briefly summarized below.

Log-linear models are appropriate if predictors consist of categorical data and if the criterion is not normally distributed (this latter condition is present with regard to atherogenic lipoproteins). On the other hand, restricted sample size limits the application of this type of model in the present data set.

ANOVAs allow for a test of interactive and separate effects of predictors on a criterion as well as for a simultaneous adjustment for effects of confounders (covariates). The hierarchical nature of the model can be tested in part by referring to non-symmetrical hypotheses: the subgroup characterized by restricted status control *and* by perceived emotional distress is expected to exhibit a significantly increased level of cardiovascular risk. No linear trend is assumed for the total group.

For an estimate of parameters of ANOVA in unbalanced designs, the program 2V of BMDP was used (Dixon *et al.*, 1983). The 'regression approach' used in this program is the most appropriate method for an estimation of the main and interactional effects in unbalanced designs (Winer, 1971). All ANOVAs were preceded by log-linear analysis confirming the stochastic independence of descriptive and attitudinal indicators of occupational stress. In one case, however, a dependence was observed: for obvious reasons occupational instability and job insecurity were significantly interrelated.

The study sample

A prospective study on cardiovascular risk factors in 416 middle-aged male (25–55 years, mean: 40.8 ± 9.6) blue-collar workers was performed to test relevant parts of the model. The initial study population was recruited from three industrial steel and metal plants owned by a West German company. The three plants were comparable in terms of size, type of production and composition of labour-force. However, in one plant, an economic crisis occurred during the observation period. This plant was forced to cut down its personnel by 20%. The total male blue-collar labour-force of the appropriate age group ($n = 735$) of all three plants was invited to participate in the study; 60% of all workers underwent initial screening, and after excluding workers with documented coronary events (as established by ECG) 416 men were included into follow-up. The sample was representative of the total labour-force, with the exception of a slight under-representation of unskilled workers.

Three screenings took place in 1982, 1983 and 1985. Medical data included blood pressure readings at all three occasions, height, weight and resting ECG at the beginning and at the end, and blood samples during second and third screening. The final sample size was 310 (75%). Compared to the initial group, the final sample was biased with respect to two out of 34 relevant characteristics: workers with high blood pressure and workers with high job instability were more likely to withdraw from follow-up. Therefore, an estimate of effects of occupational stress on indicators of cardiovascular risk based on final sample size is considered a conservative test of the research hypotheses.

RESULTS

This section is divided into two parts. The first part presents findings of different LISREL analyses entering blood pressure (hypertension as cardiovascular risk factor) as the most endogenous criterion. Results of the first two models have been published elsewhere (Matschinger *et al.*, 1986), therefore they are summarized here. A third model, unpublished so far, is discussed in more detail.

The index of atherogenic lipoproteins (LDL/HDL ratio) is the relevant criterion of coronary risk in a series of ANOVAs presented in the second part of this section.

LISREL models

Two structural equation models were tested, dividing the total population into two groups: forced piece-work (yes or no) and low occupational position (yes or no). In both models, the latent factors 'vigour' and 'immersion' (which are underlying dimensions of 'need for control'), social support at work and two indicators of emotional distress (perceived workload, anger and hopelessness) were included, as well as the confounding variables age, body weight and cigarette-smoking. The degree of model fit, the relative size of beta and gamma coefficients, and the total amount of blood pressure variation explained by the respective model were analysed.

In both cases the model fit was acceptable, and in both cases significant direct and indirect beta and gamma coefficients were observed. Most interestingly, a significant direct positive effect of the latent factor vigour on blood pressure was present in the subgroup characterized by high demand and restricted status control but not in the remaining group. The amount of explained variance of systolic blood pressure in the group of workers suffering from forced piece-work was 44% compared with 14% in the remaining group, and it was as high as 54% in the low occupational status group and 27% in the less-distressed higher-status group (Matschinger *et al.*, 1986).

A third linear structural model was tested for two groups defined by forced piece-work (yes or no), including variables of emotional distress, of social support and of coping with demands. The most endogenous criteria, however, were systolic blood pressure at first measurement *and* change of blood pressure between first and second measurement. For both subgroups, an identical structure of effects and invariant measurement models are assumed. In Figure 2, the structure of effects for the two subgroups indicating significant unstandardized beta and gamma coefficients is demonstrated, where the upper coefficients refer to the group characterized by forced piece-work and the lower coefficients (in parentheses) refer to the group without piece-work.

As can be seen, several hypothesized effects are significant and are much higher in the group of piece-workers as compared to the less distressed group. For instance, a direct positive effect of the latent factor 'vigour' on blood pressure is

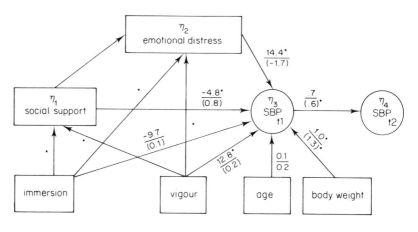

FIGURE 2. LISREL model on the effects of psychosocial variables on systolic blood pressure (SBP, two screenings within two years) in a group with and in a group without forced piece-work, indicating the most important unstandardized beta and gamma coefficients in the stressed (underlined) and in the non-stressed (in parentheses) group (for further discussion see text).

observed (12.8* v. 0.24). Also, a direct positive effect of perceived emotional distress on blood pressure is present in the group characterized by heavy occupational load, but not in the group without heavy load (14.4* v. −1.7). In addition, a direct negative effect of social support on blood pressure is evident in the high-stressed group, indicating a buffering mechanism, but no such effect can be found in a group exposed to less severe occupational demands (−4.8* v. 0.8). The buffering effect of social support is diminished to some extent by direct effects of 'vigour' and 'immersion' on blood pressure.

Results so far show important differences in the strength of effects of psychosocial variables on an indicator of cardiovascular risk, according to the presence or absence of a stressful social context. However, with reference to Figure 1, the theoretical model is not perfectly met by empirical results: indirect as opposed to direct effects of coping resources on blood pressure are rather weak.

One interesting finding needs further comment: as can be seen from Figure 2, a negative effect of the latent factor 'immersion' on blood pressure is present in the highly distressed group (−9.7* v. 0.1). As this latter finding is replicated in several other analyses (Matschinger *et al.*, 1986), we hypothesize that high need for control involves some kind of cognitive misperception of demand-related efforts: men who score high on scales measuring vigour tend to underestimate occupational efforts and to overestimate their own coping resources. Therefore they are more likely to disregard the behavioural and emotional consequences of their excessive efforts. Those who score high on vigour are likely to score low on immersion, at least for a certain period in their coping career (see below). The negative effect of immersion on blood pressure may indicate the presence of chronic sustained activation which 'bypasses' perceived distress and associated attenuating mechanisms.

In addition to the effects described in Figure 2, analogous direct effects of vigour and immersion on blood pressure at t_2 are observed, which do not reach statistical significance. However, in the group characterized by forced piece-work, substantially more variance in change of blood pressure between first and second measurement is explained by psychosocial factors than is the case in the less-distressed group.

ANOVAs

In Figure 3 results of two ANOVAs with separate and interactional effects of occupational instability and perceived emotional distress (job insecurity) (left panel) and of chronic shift-work and emotional distress (perceived workload) (right panel) on the LDL–HDL ratio are shown, adjusted for body weight, age and cigarette-smoking as covariates. In both cases, significant interaction effects of indicators of high demand/restricted status control and of emotional distress are observed: The subgroup of workers (D, left side) suffering from both objectively unstable occupation and subjectively perceived job insecurity exhibits

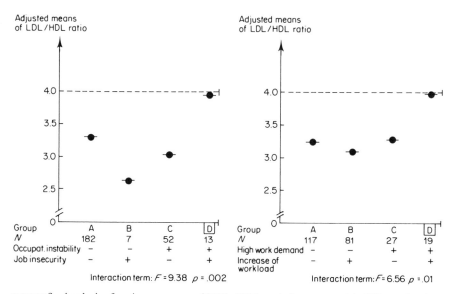

FIGURE 3. Analysis of variance: mean of LDL–HDL ratio in groups with different levels of occupational stress, adjusted for age, body weight and cigarette-smoking ($N = 254$, resp. 244). (Reproduced from Siegrist *et al.*, 1988, by permission of Elsevier Science Publishers B.V.)

a mean LDL–HDL ratio close to 4.0, and the same holds true for the subgroup of workers (D, right side) who were exposed to chronic shift-work and who experienced a steady increase of workload during the last years. An LDL–HDL ratio of 4.0 and above indicates a high risk of extended coronary atherosclerosis as documented by coronary angiography (Castelli *et al.*, 1983). As Figure 3 indicates, the association is not strictly linear, but the highly distressed subgroups D exhibit consistently elevated lipid levels (non-symmetric hypothesis).

In both analyses, significant effects of all three covariates are observed in addition to the interaction effects postulated by theory. Again, this finding points to the truly multifactorial nature of hyperlipidaemia, including genetic, nutritional, behavioural and socio-emotional factors (for detailed presentation and discussion of results see Siegrist *et al.*, 1988).

The two ANOVAs presented were replicated using LDL, HDL, apo-A1 and apo-B as dependent variables. This procedure was performed in order to improve the validity of reported results. It was shown that the LDL–HDL ratio provides the strongest findings, although similar results were obvious with the other dependent variables as well. In this respect apo-A1 is of special interest as the apo-A1 gene is viewed at present as the strongest genetic marker reported for coronary artery disease (Galton, 1987). Table 1 presents results of an ANOVA with separate and interactional effects of chronic shift-work and of perceived

TABLE 1. Analysis of variance: effects of chronic shift-work and perceived increase of workload on apo-A1 lipoprotein as indicator of atherogenic risk, with body weight, age and cigarette-smoking as covariates ($n = 244$ male blue-collar workers)

	F	P	b	
Chronic shift-work	0.07	0.79		
Perceived increase of workload	6.78	0.01		
Interaction shiftwork × increase of workload	8.97	0.003		
Body weight	23.67	0.000	−0.69	
Age	0.29	0.59	0.09	
Cigarette-smoking	3.51	0.06	0.27	
Adjusted means[a]				
apo-A1				
Shift-work	Absent	Absent	Present	*Present*
Increase of workload	Absent	Present	Absent	*Present*
mg/dl	133.80	135.41	145.25	121.73
N	117	81	27	19

[a] Results are presented as arithmetic means between first and second measurement as there is no emphasis on change over time in this analysis. For the same reason, F and P values for repetition were omitted in this table.

workload on adjusted means of apo-A1 level, with the covariates of body weight, age and smoking.

As can be seen, the interaction term (chronic shift-work × perceived workload) exerts a highly significant effect on adjusted level of apo-A1 which is even stronger than the effects of the covariates (age and smoking). Only body weight, a well-documented risk factor of hyperlipidaemia, exceeds the statistical influence of a relevant indicator of occupational stress on apo-A1. This result may be seen as a starting point for further analyses which elaborate more closely on a highly suggestive interaction between environmental (especially socio-emotional) and genetic influences on atherogenic risk.

The analysis reported here has shown interactive effects of indicators of high demand/restricted status control and of emotional distress on the mean level of atherogenic lipoprotein. However, additional ANOVAs were performed with similar results. For example, a highly significant interaction effect between low occupational position and perceived job insecurity on the LDL–HDL ratio was found ($F = 12.45$; $P = 0.001$). Another interaction effect was observed between chronic shift-work and perceived job insecurity ($F = 4.93$; $P = 0.03$).

If change of mean level of atherogenic lipoprotein over time is analysed, an interaction term of occupational instability with increase of workload on change of adjusted mean LDL over time becomes apparent ($F = 4.27$; $P = 0.04$).

A similar although statistically not significant effect is observed with the LDL–HDL ratio as dependent variable.

DISCUSSION

A summary of results on the influence of high demand/restricted status control in occupational life and of perceived emotional distress on high blood pressure, as well as on atherogenic hyperlipidaemia, was presented above, based on linear structural equation models and on analysis of variance and covariance. The findings have shown that unfavourable occupational conditions such as forced piece-work, job instability, low-status job and chronic shift-work systematically modify effects of indicators of perceived emotional distress and of related coping resources on high blood pressure and on high atherogenic lipoproteins. Perceived emotional distress *per se* does not produce consistent significant effects on cardiovascular risk. These effects become significant and consistent only in the presence of an occupational context characterized by high demand and low reward in terms of status control. It is evident that adjustment to this type of situation is difficult to achieve and that recurrent intense arousal in terms of a sympatho-adrenergic activation may occur, especially so as a basic dimension in a person's hierarchy of appraisal is involved.

In theoretical terms, the findings have several implications. First, they argue in favour of an interactional approach towards studying human stress. Although such an approach is verbally acknowledged in much of the current literature on human stress, many studies in fact concentrate on indicators of individual coping and of subjective strain without specifying associations between external stressors and subjective strain in terms of measurement and in terms of statistical analysis. This failure may produce bias and spurious relationships in respective empirical results. Despite the fact that sources of error involved in a measurement approach which does not specify environmental characteristics and individual coping characteristics have been convincingly demonstrated by sociologist George W. Brown (1974), the majority of studies still follow a research tradition which might be labelled 'from stressors to strains' (van Dijkhuizen, 1980). ANOVAs and LISRELs may not provide the best statistical approaches towards an appropriate modelling of conditional effects, and better methods may exist of separating contextual from individual characteristics. Yet, results presented in this chapter argue for a new emphasis on explicitly interactive concepts of stressor–strain relationships in research on personal control and health.

A second theoretical implication relates to the role of cognitive misperception. In our data, we have found inconsistent associations between the amount of demand/reward and the amount of perceived emotional distress (dotted line in Figure 1), and we have found a negative effect of immersion on blood pressure. Both findings point to cognitive misperception, at least in the subgroup of workers who are characterized by high need for control. Further studies are needed to clarify under what conditions misperception is likely to occur. Elsewhere we have argued that the probability of misperception decreases as a function of the chronicity and severity of experienced social stressors in an individual's coping career (Matschinger *et al.*, 1986). The more an individual becomes exhausted as a result of unsuccessful coping efforts, the more likely is the occurrence of symptoms of adaptive breakdown which are difficult to misperceive or to deny (Appels, 1983). At the same time, we suggest that conscious evaluation of emotional responses to demanding and threatening stimuli occurs more often than usual and that the burden of negative feelings itself may contribute to adaptive breakdown. This vicious circle may explain the high frequency of signs of disproportionate irritation and of exaggerated emotional outbursts observed in individuals who are subjected to severe chronic stress. In terms of LeDoux's model of emotion, the amygdaloid–cortical circuits of affective information-processing are permanently activated during this critical stage, with recurrent negative input from reward-sensitive areas in the orbitofrontal cortex and its connections to the amygdala (LeDoux, 1987).

The present chapter does not provide enough space to discuss the convergences and divergences of our conceptual approach with other research traditions in the field of sociobehavioural factors in cardiovascular disease. It is evident that our emphasis on high demand at work is derived from important previous studies, especially those provided by the Michigan group (e.g. Caplan *et al.*, 1975; House, 1981), from the important work on job decision latitude and job discretion (Theorell *et al.*, 1987), and from Kornitzer's studies on job stress and coronary disease (Kornitzer *et al.*, 1981). However, by stressing the dimension of restricted status control, our approach relates the issue of control in terms of characteristics of the workplace to control and reward in terms of occupational biography and role continuity. It would be desirable to design further studies in a way which permits a test of the relative contribution of either dimension of control to explaining cardiovascular risk under conditions of high demand.

The same holds true for further specification of individual coping characteristics. Our approach so far has focused on high need for control and its latent factors, vigour and immersion. Other coping patterns, not necessarily focusing on cognitive and motivational aspects, might be included. One such pattern, 'suppressed anger', has been found to be predictive of hypertension, if combined with occupational stress, and especially with future job ambiguity (Cottington *et al.*, 1986). Again, testing the relation between these concepts in terms of predictive validity might be an interesting step.

A prominent topic for further discussion is the question of mechanisms which link sustained activation to increased cardiovascular risk. Whereas the issue of neurogenic hypertension has been discussed at substantial length (e.g. Weiner, 1979), neurogenic regulation of lipid metabolism has been investigated less vigorously so far. New information on hypothalamic modulation of atherogenesis

(Gutstein, 1988), on stress-induced progression of atherosclerosis (Clarkson *et al.*, 1987) and on influence of stress hormones on blood lipids (e.g. Atkinson and Milsum, 1983) point to a promising area of further research.

Finally, the practical implications of the research results presented in this chapter need to be emphasized. According to recent data from the Framingham study, there is a powerful interaction between hypertension and increased level of blood lipids in the production of coronary heart disease (Castelli and Anderson, 1986). Our data show that the probability of experiencing high atherogenic lipoproteins and/or high blood pressure partly depends on exposure to and coping with specific occupational characteristics and that this association holds true after adjusting for relevant confounders. Given a high prevalence of hypertension and of hyperlipidaemia in working adults, preventive efforts should be redirected at improving occupational life and individual coping through comprehensive programmes of intervention.

ACKNOWLEDGEMENTS

The authors thank Dr Jere A. Wysong (visiting professor at the Department of Medical Sociology, University of Marburg), Dr Thomas Abel, Dr Astrid Junge, Siegfried Geyer, Achim Hättich, Richard Peter, Birgit Reime and Rolf Völckel (as members of a research seminar at the department) for fruitful discussion. We also thank Professor Dieter Seidel and Dr Peter Cremer (Department of Clinical Chemistry, Univeristy of Göttingen) for their cooperation in providing analysis of blood lipids.

REFERENCES

Appels, A. (1983). The year before myocardial infarction. In: T. M. Dembroski, T. H. Schmidt and G. Blümchen (eds), *Biobehavioral Bases of Coronary Heart Disease*. Basel: Karger.

Atkinson, C., and Milsum, J. H. (1983). A system model of the metabolic response to stress. *Behavioral Science*, **28**, 268–274.

Axelrod, J., and Reisine, T. D. (1984). Stress hormones: Their interaction and regulation. *Science*, **224**, 452–459.

Ballieux, R. E., Cullen, J., Fielding, J. F., L'Abbate, A., Siegrist, J., and Wegman, H. M. (eds) (1984). *Breakdown in Human Adaptation to 'Stress'* (2 vols). The Hague: Nijhoff.

Beamish, R. E., Singal, P. K., and Dhalla, N. S. (eds) (1985). *Stress and Heart Disease*. Boston, MA: Nijhoff.

Brown, G. W. (1974). Meaning, measurement and stress of life events. In: B.S. Dohrenwend and B. P. Dohrenwend (eds), *Stressful Life Events: Their Nature and Effects*. New York: Wiley.

Caplan, R. D., Cobb, S., French, J. R. P., Harrison, R. V., and Pinneau, S. R. (1975). *Job Demands and Worker Health*. Washington: US Government Printing Office.

Castelli, W. P., and Anderson, K. (1986). A population at risk. *American Journal of Medicine,* **80** (Suppl. 2A), 23–32.

Castelli, W. P., Abbot, R. D., and McNamara, P. M. (1983). Summary estimates of cholesterol used to predict coronary heart disease. *Circulation,* **67**, 730–736.

Clarkson, P. B., Weingand, K.W., Kaplan, J. R., and Adams, M.R. (1987). Mechanisms of atherogenesis. *Circulation,* **76** (Suppl. I), 120–128.

Cottington, E. M., Matthews, K. A., Talbott, E., and Kuller, L. H. (1986). Occupational stress, suppressed anger, and hypertension. *Psychosomatic Medicine,* **48**, 249–261.

Cremer, P., Seidel, D., and Wieland, H. (1985). Quantitative Lipoproteinelektrophorese. *Laboratoriums Medizin,* **9**, 39–44.

Dixon, W. J., Brown, M. B., Engelman, L., Frane, J. W., Hill, M. A., Jenrich, R. I., and Toporek, J. D. (1983). *BMDP Statistical Software.* Berkeley, CA: University of California Press.

Frankenhaeuser, M. (1979). Psychoneuroendocrine approaches to the study of emotions related to stress and coping. In: D. Howe (ed.), *Nebraska Symposium on Motivation.* Lincoln, NB: University of Nebraska Press.

Galton, D. J. (1987). DNA polymorphisms for genetic analysis of atherosclerosis. In: G. Schlierf and H. Moerl (eds), *Expanding Horizons in Atherosclerosis Research.* Berlin: Springer.

Gutstein, W. H. (1988). The central nervous system and atherogenesis: Endothelial injury. *Atherosclerosis,* **70**, 145–154.

Henry, J. P., and Stephens, P. M. (1977). *Stress, Health and the Social Environment.* Berlin: Springer.

House, J. S. (1981). *Work Stress and Social Support.* Reading, MA: Addison-Wesley.

Jöreskog, K. G., and Sorbom, D. (1979). *Advances in Factor Analysis and Structural Equation Models.* Cambridge, MA: Abt Books.

Kannel, W. B., Doyle, J. B., Ostfeld, A. M., Jenkins, C. D., Culler, L., Podell, R. N., and Stamler, J. (1984). Optimal resources for primary prevention of atherosclerotic diseases. *Circulation,* **29**, 157A–205A.

Karasek, R., Russel, S., and Theorell, T. (1982). Physiology of stress and regeneration in job-related cardiovascular illness. *Journal of Human Stress,* **8**, 29–38.

Kohn, M. L., and Schooler, C. (1983). *Work and Personality.* Norwood, NJ: Ablex.

Kornitzer, M., Kittel, F., Debacker, G., Dramaix, M., Sobolski, J., and Degre, S. (1981). Work load and coronary heart disease. In: J. Siegrist and M. J. Halhuber (eds), *Myocardial Infarction and Psychosocial Risks.* Berlin: Springer.

Lazarus, R. S., and Folkman, S. (1984). *Stress, Appraisal and Coping.* New York: Springer.

LeDoux, J. E. (1987). Emotion. In: F. Plum (ed.), *Handbook of Physiology V: The Nervous System.* Washington, DC: American Physiological Society.

Lewis, B. (1982). The lipoproteins: Predictors, protectors, pathogens. *British Medical Journal,* **278**, 1161–1164.

Matschinger, H., Siegrist, J., Siegrist, K., and Dittmann, K. (1986). Type A as a coping career: Towards a conceptual and methodological redefinition. In: T. H. Schmidt, T. M. Dembroski and G. Blümchen (eds), *Biological and Psychological Factors in Cardiovascular Disease.* Heidelberg: Springer.

Matthews, K. A., Weiss, S. M., Detre, T., Dembroski, T. M., Falkner, B., Manuck, S. B., and Williams, R. B. (eds) (1986). *Handbook of Stress. Reactivity, and Cardiovascular Disease.* New York, Wiley.

Pearlin, L. J., Menaghan, E. G., Lieberman, M. A., and Mullan, J. T. (1981). The stress process. *Journal of Health and Social Behaviour,* **22**, 337–356.

Rasch, G. (1960). *Probabilistic Models for Some Intelligence and Attainment Tests.* Copenhagen: Nielsen & Lydiche.

Schmidt, T. H., Dembroski, T. M., and Blümchen, G. (eds) (1986). *Biological and Psychological Factors in Cardiovascular Disease*. Berlin: Springer.

Schneiderman, N. (1983). Behavior, autonomic function and animal models of cardiovascular pathology. In: T. M. Dembroski, T. H. Schmidt and G. Blümchen (eds), *Biobehavioral Bases of Coronary Heart Disease*. Basel: Karger.

Siegrist, J., Siegrist, K., and Weber, I. (1986). Sociological concepts in the etiology of chronic disease: The case of ischemic heart disease. *Social Science and Medicine*, **22**, 247–253.

Siegrist, J., Matschinger, H., and Peter, R. (1987). *Der Einfluß sozialer Belastungen und ihrer Verarbeitung auf die Entwicklung kardiovaskulärer Risiken*. Marburg: unpublished research report.

Siegrist, J., Matschinger, H., Cremer, P., and Seidel, D. (1988). Atherogenic risk in men suffering from occupational stress. *Atherosclerosis*, **69**, 211–218.

Siegrist, K. (1986). *Sozialer Rückhalt und kardiovaskuläres Risiko*. München: Minerva.

Steptoe, A., Rüddel, H., and Neus, H. (eds) (1985). *Clinical and Methodological Issues in Cardiovascular Psychophysiology*. Heidelberg: Springer.

Theorell, T., Hamsten, A., de Faire, U., Orth-Gomer, K., and Perski, A. (1987). Psychosocial work conditions before myocardial infarction in young men. *International Journal of Cardiology*, **15**, 33–46.

van Dijkhuizen, N. (1980). *From Stressors to Strains*. Lisse: Swets & Zeitlinger.

Weiner, H. (1979). *The Psychobiology of Essential Hypertension*. New York: Elsevier.

Wieland, H., and Seidel, D. (1983). A simple and specific technique for precipitation of low-density lipoproteins. *Journal of Lipid Research*, **24** 904–909.

Winer, B. J. (1971). *Statistical Principles in Experimental Design*, 2nd edn. New York: McGraw-Hill.

Section II

The clinical perspective

CHAPTER 5

Assessment of control in health-care settings

KENNETH A. WALLSTON
Vanderbilt University, Nashville, Tennessee, USA

INTRODUCTION

The focus of this chapter is on the various ways in which control can be assessed in health-care settings. In illustrating these methods, I draw heavily on the work my colleagues, students, and I have done over the past 15 years as we wrestled with how best to assess this construct in our own research. This will be a 'how to do it' (or 'how not to do it') chapter, focusing more on methodological considerations than on a review of substantive findings.

Because the other chapters of this book deal explicitly with why it is important to assess control in the context of the relationship between stress and health, it is not necessary to go into great detail here about the role that control plays in contributing to, moderating, or mediating that relationship. For the reader of *only* this chapter, however, I offer a number of possible theoretical linkages: (a) a lack of control can act as a stressor and have a direct, negative effect upon one's health status; (b) providing a sense of control to a person experiencing a stressor may buffer the deleterious effects of the stressor; or (c) a sense of control might increase the likelihood that the individual would engage in one or more health behaviors, thus having a direct, positive effect on his or her health status.

Control is a multifaceted construct. It is especially important, for assessment purposes, to be clear about which aspect of control one wishes to measure and why one wishes to do so. Most often, in health-related research, 'control' means 'perceived control' as opposed to veridical or 'actual control'. Perceived control is 'the "belief" that one can determine one's own internal states and behavior, influence one's environment, and/or bring about desired outcomes' (Wallston *et*

Stress, Personal Control and Health.   Edited by A. Steptoe and A. Appels.
Published by John Wiley & Sons Ltd.
© ECSC–EEC–EAEC, Brussels–Luxembourg, 1989

al., 1987). Defining perceived control as a belief indicates that it is an individual difference construct; something which, when assessed, varies among individuals and within the same individual over time. In contrast, veridical or actual control is conceived of as a property of the situation and setting. Although it, too, may vary over time, in assessing veridical control one looks for low inter-observer variability in judging how much control is present at a given point in time.

Because we have done no research assessing veridical control, the majority of this chapter will concentrate on measures of perceived control. The targets of these measures varied from perceived control over one's health status (typically assessed by a measure of health 'locus of control'), over one's health behavior (using measures of 'self-efficacy' beliefs), or over one's health-care situation (using a combination of measures described below). In addition to perceived control, this chapter will describe our assessment of a related but different individual difference construct, 'desire for control' over one's health-care situation. 'Desire for control of health care is a preference for behaviors that (a) allow direct influence on the process of health care, (b) provide relevant information about the health care situation, or (c) do both' (Smith *et al.*, 1984, p. 416).

A theme running throughout the entire chapter is the issue of the optimum level of specificity at which to measure control. Is it better to design or tailor instruments to fit each researcher's unique situation or should one sacrifice 'goodness-of-fit' and utilize a more general scale—one whose psychometric properties are well-established and the use of which would more easily allow cross-study or cross-situational comparisons?

PERCEIVED CONTROL OVER THE HEALTH-CARE SETTING

A few years ago, under the auspices of a grant from the National Center for Health Services Research, my colleagues and I carried out a series of three field experiments in which we attempted to manipulate patients' perceived control over their health-care situation. We based this work on the findings of social psychologists who had demonstrated the positive health benefits of small-scale control-enhancing interventions such as: (a) letting blood donors choose from which arm the blood should be drawn (Mills and Krantz, 1979); (b) giving nursing-home residents a plant to take care of and letting them choose which night to attend a movie (Rodin and Langer, 1977); or (c) allowing nursing-home residents to select the frequency and timing of a visit from a college student volunteer (Schulz, 1976). Our research was designed to manipulate perceived control by giving certain patients predictability information about and choice over selected aspects of their health-care regimen.

Although not all of the studies upon which we based our work reported assessing perceived control, we felt it was essential to do so. One reason was as a manipulation check. An assessment of perceived control following the manipulation would inform us if our manipulation had been successful. Secondly, by assessing perceived control part way through our study, we would be able to correlate this measure of the hypothesized 'intervening variable' with the various assessments of physical and psychological well-being which constituted the dependent variables. The following are three case studies of how the best of intentions do not always pan out like they are supposed to.

Study one

In our first experiment in this series (Wallston, B. S. *et al.*, 1987), the stressor was having to prepare for a barium enema on an out-patient basis. Having a barium enema is, in and of itself, a highly stressful experience for any patient. The unpleasantness of the situation, however, is compounded by having to follow a strict bowel-cleansing regimen at home or at work for 24–48 hours prior to the radiological examination. (The standard regimen at that time involved a combination of a liquid diet, ingesting an evil-tasting, caster-oil-like preparation, and taking laxatives in order to ensure that one's bowels and intestines would be empty before being given the barium enema.) Our proposed means of 'improving' the situation was to develop two other alternative regimens, each of which had equal efficacy. One-third of our patient–subjects were allowed to choose from among the three regimes after we carefully described what each experience would involve. We hypothesized that patients randomly assigned to this 'choice' condition would perceive the greatest amount of control and, subsequently, would have the most favorable outcomes (e.g. be less distressed and most likely to follow the regimen).

To complete the design of this randomized clinical trial, another third of the patients were given one of the regimens along with the complete description of what it would involve—including the sensations they would experience. These patients constituted the 'predictability' condition. We were not sure how much perceived control to hypothesize for these subjects, since Schulz (1976) had found that his 'predictability alone' subjects fared as well as those given choice. The remaining patients were given neither choice nor enhanced sensory information about the regimen assigned them. We hypothesized that these latter subjects would have the least perceived control.

In this study we assessed perceived control in two ways. Because we were already using a 'multiple affect adjective checklist' (MAACL) to assess anxiety, depression and hostility, we modified that MAACL by adding three items: helpless, in control, and powerless. Then we constructed a Helpless score (or an assessment of feeling 'out of control') by giving one point each time the subject checked 'helpless' or 'powerless' or did not check 'in control'. The second method was an 11-item Likert scale which we termed PCON (for 'perceived control'). The instructions and items for PCON, which had an alpha reliability of 0.81, can be found in Table 1.

Unfortunately, we did not find condition main effects for PCON or Helpless (measured 30 minutes or so before the barium enema was to take place), even though other manipulation checks indicated that patients in the 'choice' condition did, indeed, perceive that they were given a choice over their mode of preparation. Elsewhere I have referred to our manipulation of control in this study as 'choose your poison'. Perhaps patients in this condition looked at our options as a sham choice, and reacted against having to select from among three unappealing alternatives.

One alternative explanation for these null results is that the measures of the constructs are invalid. In this study we had some evidence that this might be the case, but we also had some results which were less pessimistic. On the side of invalidity was the finding of no relationship ($r = -0.10$) between PCON and Helpless, our two purported measures of perceived control. This lack of concurrent validity could mean that either one or both of the indicators was not tapping the construct. On the other hand, both measures correlated significantly ($r = 0.20$, $p < 0.05$) with anxiety as assessed by the MAACL, thus providing some indication of the construct validity of both. Also, in a separate study, we found that the mean PCON score of our out-patient subjects was significantly ($p <$

TABLE 1. The perceived control (PCON) scale as utilized in the barium enema study (Wallston, B. S. *et al.*, 1987)

Instructions: Mark the degree to which you agree or disagree (using a six-point LIKERT scale) with the following statements:

The other day in clinic, when I was being told about preparation for today's barium enema I felt ...

1. That I was unable to influence the type of preparation I received.
2. That I was in control of the situation.
3. That I was just told what to do.
4. That I could get all of my questions answered.
5. That I was allowed to play an active role in my health care.
6. That what I did or said made no difference.

During the past few days, while I was getting ready for today's barium enema examination, I felt ...

7. Very much 'on top' of the situation.
8. Totally out of control.
9. At a loss to know what I would be experiencing.
10. If I wanted to, I could change the way I got ready for the barium enema.
11. I knew what the preparation would do to me.

0.04) higher than PCON for a sample of hospitalized in-patients awaiting a barium enema. This, too, provided some indication of construct validity.

Our strongest correlational findings ($r = 0.81$, $p < 0.01$) was between PCON and a six-item Likert scale measure of patients' satisfaction with how they had been treated (e.g. 'I was very satisfied with the manner in which I was told to get 'ready for my barium enema.'). Although this correlation was in the hypothesized direction, we felt it was *too* high. When two measures of theoretically distinct constructs correlate ≫ 0.70, it is probably due to shared method variance and/or a lack of discriminant validity. In this instance we knew there was too much shared method variance (the satisfaction measure was filled out immediately after PCON and used a similar six-point Likert response scale). We suspected that we should not make too much of the finding that the more control patients perceived they had, the more satisfied they were.

Study two

In this study the stressor was receiving chemotherapy for cancer and its attendant side effects, especially nausea and vomiting. We used a two-group experimental design. Half of the patients were randomly assigned to the 'choice' condition where they were given information about three distinctly different antiemetic treatments, each purportedly equivalent in reducing the noxious side effects of the chemotherapy treatments. The other group of cancer patients were assigned an antiemetic treatment, rather than being given a choice, but were provided the same sensory and procedure information as those in the 'choice' condition. (For ethical reasons, we did not feel comfortable in utilizing a no-information 'control' group in this study.) The patients, all of whom were just beginning chemotherapy or resuming chemotherapy after at least a year's time, were studied for four consecutive sessions.

Perceived control was assessed in a similar fashion as in study one, except that PCON was shortened to five items. In this study, PCON assessed the degree of agreement/disagreement with statements such as 'Since I began this treatment for nausea and vomiting, I felt very much "on top" of the situation.' This Likert scale, which had a low alpha reliability (0.49), was administered at the beginning of the second and fourth sessions. The test–retest stability of PCON across these two sessions ($r = 0.15$) was also low. The MAACL, containing the Helpless subscale, was given at the beginning of the third and fourth sessions. The test–retest stability of the Helpless index was 0.77. Once again, the two ways of measuring perceived control were not highly correlated with one another ($r = 0.00$ to -0.36).

As in study one, there were no differences between experimental groups on PCON at either session 2 or 4. On the Helpless index, however, there were condition main effects at both session 3 ($p = 0.06$) and session 4 ($p < 0.04$). In both instances, the patients in the choice condition checked fewer helpless adjectives than those in the no-choice condition.

Study three

In the final study in this series the health care stressor was the postoperative period in the hospital following major surgery. Patients were studied for five days post-surgery (or after being released from the surgical intensive care unit). Typically, patients feel dreadful for a day or two post-surgery, then they begin to recover. By five to seven days post-surgery, if complications have not occurred, they are usually well enough to be discharged. In the immediate postoperative period, when one is not feeling well, being 'in control' is probably not highly salient for most patients. However, as they begin to recover, many patients become distressed at being in a situation characterized by some (e.g. Taylor, 1979) as lacking in opportunities for patients to have any control. We reasoned that this would especially be the case for those aspects of the patients' lives that they would normally control if they were at home instead of being in the hospital (such as if and when to take a bath or to receive visitors).

In the hypothesized high perceived control condition, one of our research nurses visited the patient–subject on four consecutive postoperative days to offer a 'menu' of choices in a number of areas: sleeping aids; bathing; diet; visitors; telephone calls. The patient was free to make as many, or as few, choices off the 'menu' as desired, and could change the selections on a daily basis. In contrast, those randomly assigned to the 'predictability-only' condition were not given choices but were, instead, given enhanced predictability information (e.g. they would/would not receive a back rub that evening, or a half bath in the morning). Finally, those assigned to the 'standard operating procedure' condition received only the routine nursing care available to all patients on those post-surgical units.

A modification of the PCON scale was administered on the afternoon of the third and fifth postoperative days. This seven-item, seven-point Likert scale asked the patient to agree or disagree with such statements as 'Since my operation, I was given as much control over my activities in the hospital as I have at home', and 'I was unable to have a say in what my daily routine was during this hospital stay'. The alpha reliabilities of this scale were 0.67 on day 3 and 0.64 on day 5, and the test–retest reliability over two days was 0.58. We did not use the MAACL in this study, so we did not have an alternative measure of perceived control.

Once again, as in the other two studies, we found no condition main effects for PCON on either of the two postoperative days. We did, however, have one intriguing finding involving our final assessment of perceived control. We had kept track of the number of choices off the menu selected by patients in the choice condition over the four days during which they were offered choices. When we correlated this 'number of environmental changes' with PCON measured on day 5, we found a significant 'negative' relationship ($r = -0.34$, $p = 0.02$). When given an option, the more that patients said 'No thanks' to a change in routine, the more control they reported they had!

Discussion

In all three of our field experiments in which we attempted to increase patients' sense of perceived control over their health-care setting, our assessments of perceived control generally told us that we had failed to accomplish our objective. Assuming that our PCON scales were valid, what do these null results tell us? It might mean we were poor experimenters, unable to manipulate perceived control by the particular methods we selected to do so. While that is possible, it is not likely. In each of the three studies, we had some results on other outcome variables which were interpretable in light of a hypothesized interaction between patient's desire for control and the experimental conditions (see below).

We prefer to think that our Likert scale measure of perceived control, although probably valid, was insensitive to the subtle differences between groups in the settings in which we conducted these investigations. In other words, in order to have the situational control necessary to carry out these complex field experiments, we worked in settings (e.g. a university medical center) where all patients experienced a fair degree of control. This was even the case in study three, where the level of nursing care on the post-surgical units was excellent.

Another factor mitigating against significant condition differences in perceived control is the fact that all patient–subjects had given their informed consent to participate in our studies. The knowledge that, as volunteers, they could end their participation whenever they wished in and of itself could have contributed to their overall high perception of control over the health-care settings we studied. Finally, it is also possible that the subjects in the no-choice conditions experienced an 'illusion of control' (see Langer, 1975) and indicated experiencing more control than the situation offered them. This argument is bolstered by the fact that the mean PCON score for all subjects in all three studies was above the hypothetical midpoint, suggesting that, on the whole, patients felt in control no matter what we did to them. All of these factors taken together make it extremely difficult to assess significant condition differences in perceived control in this type of experimental study.

DESIRE FOR CONTROL OVER THE HEALTH-CARE SETTING

In each of the three experiments described above, we measured, at the outset, how much control each patient wanted in the particular health-care setting. Our theoretical prediction was that the outcome variables (e.g. psychological well-being, compliance) would be determined by an interaction between this individual difference variable, desire for control, and the experimental conditions (in which we felt we would be differentially manipulating perceived control). When we first began these studies, we hypothesized that patients high in desire for control would respond very favorably to our choice conditions and negatively to being assigned to the standard operating procedure conditions. Conversely, we felt that those low in desire for control would do all right if left alone, but might even become somewhat stressed if 'forced' to make choices (i.e. exercise decisional control) or if presented with sensory and procedural information (i.e. heightened informational control). We soon learned how naive we were in making those predictions. We were correct in looking for an interaction, but the form of the interaction surprised us.

Based upon a series of pilot studies (described in detail in Smith *et al.*, 1984), we measured desire for control by combining two seven-item scales: the Information subscale (K–I) from the Health Opinion Survey (Krantz *et al.*, 1980), and a shortened version of our own DCON scale (Smith *et al.*, 1984). The K–I scale, consisting of items such as 'I usually wait for the doctor or nurse to tell me about the results of a medical exam rather than asking them immediately', assessed persons' preference for health-care-related information in a variety of health-care settings. The DCON scale, on the other hand, was designed to be tailored for specific health-care settings. For example, in the barium enema study, when patients filled out the DCON scale, they were instructed to respond with what they wanted 'as a patient in this particular clinic'. By combining K–I and DCON, the two measures which showed the greatest discriminant validity in our pilot studies (Smith *et al.*, 1984), we had a measure of desire for control which was somewhere between highly and moderately situation-specific.

In analyzing the data for study one, while attempting to test the hypothesized interaction between desire for control and the experimental conditions, we soon realized that we had many more 'significant' findings if we did a three-way rather than a two-way split on desire for control. This decision to trichotomize rather than dichotomize our individual difference variable proved fortunate; indeed, by doing so we established a pattern of findings which we replicated over the next two studies. If we had stuck by our initial decision to simply separate patients into high v. low desire for control (or if we had adopted a regression rather than an ANOVA approach to the analysis), we probably would have missed the most important findings. Briefly, what we found in all three of these studies was that the *only* patients who profited by our 'enhanced control' manipulation were those who were *moderate* in desire for control. Contrary to prediction, those high in desire for control who were given choices did poorly (e.g. became upset, were non-compliant), while those low in desire for control who were given choices did fine, but not as well as those moderate in desire for control (Wallston, B. S. *et al.*, 1987; Wallston, K. A. *et al.*, 1987).

In study three, one of my graduate students, Marc Zylstra, examined for his master's thesis whether patients' desire for control scores changed from the pre-surgical assessment to five days post-surgery. The mean scores on K–I and DCON remained constant over time regardless of experimental condition. This null finding suggests that desire for control over health-care settings might be more stable than measures of perceived control over health-care settings.

Discussion

What did we learn from these findings? We learned that, for these particular settings, we could not give a sufficient amount of control to the high desire for control patients to meet their needs. For patients with a high desire (or need) for control, the kinds of choices we were able to give were not enough to satisfy them. We may, in fact, have raised their expectations by dangling choices in front of them, and then dashed their hopes when the choices did not lead to the control they desired. Perhaps certain patients can only feel in control by seizing it. Control which is 'given'to them does not meet their needs.

We also learned that health-care providers will not do any harm by offering enhanced choices and/or information to patients who do not want control. Across all three studies, our low desire for control patients did fine no matter which condition they were in. Theoretically, there are two ways one could be low in desire for control. One could actively 'not want' control or one could be indifferent to it. Apparently our subjects were more of the latter type. Because 'being in control' was not a salient issue for them, they were able to 'go with the flow' and were not affected by whether or not they had choices or predictability information. In examining the demographic correlates of desire for control, two variables—age and educational level—consistently showed significant negative relationships with desire for control scores. When controlling for educational level, we still found significant age effects for both K–I and DCON. Persons aged 60 or older professed less of a desire to control their health-care setting than younger adults (Smith *et al.*, 1988). Given our finding that elderly patients are more apt to be lower in desire for control than younger patients, it is reassuring, but not surprising, that those low in desire for control were not adversely affected by our interventions.

Most importantly, we learned that providing opportunities for taking control had a positive benefit for at least some patients—those with moderate desire for control. Although their perceived control scores were no different than any other subjects, the moderate desire for control patients who were given choices did significantly better on many of the other dependent variables than other patients given choices or moderate desire for control patients in other conditions. Too often, when assessing control, we assume that linearity prevails; the more control perceived or desired, the better. As will be pointed out again below, this assumption of straightforward linearity may mask the true role that individual differences in control play in helping us explain variance in health outcomes.

PERCEIVED CONTROL OVER ONE'S HEALTH STATUS

By far, the most typical means of assessing control in health-care settings is the use of some measure of locus of control beliefs. 'Locus' means 'place', and the logic behind the use of locus of control measures is that a person perceives more control when the locus of that control is 'internal'—i.e. dependent upon the person's own behavior—than when the locus is 'external'—i.e. dependent upon the actions of other persons, or a matter of fate, luck or chance. This assumption that internality is more related to perceived control than externality is debatable in the context of certain health-care situations.

Rotter put forth the locus of control construct as one generalized expectancy within his version of social learning theory (Rotter, 1954, 1982). The target of control was 'valued reinforcements'. His widely adopted I–E Scale (Rotter, 1966) assesses the extent to which individuals typically believe that important outcomes occur as a function of what they do or who they are (an internal locus of control orientation). If individuals cannot endorse these internal beliefs, the 'forced-choice' nature of the I–E Scale leads them to endorse externally worded items, statements which reflect control being in the hands of powerful other people or random happenings. Because these beliefs are cross-situational and are learned over a lifetime of experiences, they are considered to be relatively stable. In fact, most researchers (see Lefcourt, 1976; Phares, 1976) typically accord generalized locus of control orientation the status of a personality variable, an enduring trait not easily amenable to change.

In social learning theory (Rotter, 1954), the principal function of expectancy measures is to aid in the prediction of behavior. The major formula in the theory states that the potential for a given behavior to occur in a given psychological situation is a function of the expectancy that the behavior will lead to a particular reinforcement and the value of that reinforcement to the individual in that situation. Generalized expectancies, such as locus of control, operate predominantly in novel situations in which the individual has not had enough experience to develop specific expectancies. According to Rotter (1979), 'Measurement in a specific area is enhanced by devising tests limited to that specific area, particularly if the specific area is one in which the individual has a great deal of experience' (p. 265). For many people, especially adults, health is one specific domain where experience is plentiful.

The Multidimensional Health Locus of Control Scale

While the I–E Scale and other, similar, generalized locus of control measures have been and continue to be used to assess perceived control in health-related research (see Strickland, 1978; Wallston and Wallston, 1978 for reviews of this work), many health researchers over the past 10–12 years have chosen to use more situation-specific, health-related locus of control measures in their investigations. The most widely used instrument of this sort is the Multidimensional Health Locus of Control (MHLC) Scale developed by this author and his colleagues (Wallston *et al.*, 1978). The MHLC Scale consists of two alternative forms (A and B), each of which contain 18 items. Each form, in turn, contains three six-item Likert scales which, in 'normal, healthy' populations, are uncorrelated, or only slightly correlated, with one another (Wallston and Wallston, 1981). The Internal Health Locus of Control (IHLC) dimension assesses the degree to which one believes one's health status (a valued outcome or reinforcer) is influenced by one's own behavior. People who score high on the IHLC are said to have a sense of responsibility for their own health (Wallston and Wallston, 1982). PHLC measures the belief that powerful other people—one's family, friends or health-care providers—control one's health. Lastly, CHLC assesses perceived *non*-control of health, or the belief that one's health status is determined by fate, luck or chance.

Discussion

Both PHLC and CHLC are external dimensions; however, scoring high on the PHLC dimension does not necessarily indicate low perceived control. In many health-care situations, particularly if one is acutely or chronically ill, it is realistic to believe that other people's actions can influence one's health status. It may also be beneficial to hold these beliefs, particularly if the 'powerful other' people are expert practitioners who have only one's best interests at heart. Scoring high on the CHLC dimension usually does mean low perceived control (except if one truly believes one can control random events); however, moderately high CHLC beliefs may be advantageous in certain circumstances when, in fact, there is little one could actually do to change one's health status (e.g. Burish *et al.*, 1984). Finally, a high score on the internal health dimension (IHLC) does not necessarily signify that one thinks one is in control of one's health; agreement with IHLC items could indicate perceived responsibility for one's poor health status but not one's good health.

Some consumers of the MHLC Scale have mistakenly tried to compute a total health locus of control score by, for example, subtracting the two external dimensions (PHLC and CHLC) from IHLC, and treating the resultant score as a measure of perceived control. This is fallacious, owing to the ambiguous nature of PHLC, and is rarely, if ever, justified. On the other hand, particularly if one wishes to use the MHLC scores to predict an index of health behaviors in 'normal, healthy' individuals, it is all right to subtract CHLC from IHLC and to use the difference score in place of the two raw scores. This has the added advantage of eliminating response set bias, since people's tendency to agree or disagree with items regardless of their content will be cancelled out in the difference score. In those analyses, PHLC scores can be treated separately, or even ignored (since they are less relevant to the prediction of health behavior in healthy samples).

Currently, the MHLC Scale still predominates in the literature as the preferred means of assessing control in health-related settings. Although this measure is well used, it is not always used well or wisely. Some suffer from what I call the 'silver bullet complex'—the belief that a single measure of a single construct will somehow magically help explain a significant amount of the variance in health behavior or health status. They mistakenly assume that 'locus' of control is the only aspect of control that there is to measure, and that an often-cited instrument (such as the I–E Scale of the MHLC Scale) is the best brand of silver bullet available.

Hardly any researcher who has used the MHLC Scale has examined the individual dimensions in a non-linear fashion—for example, investigating whether it was 'better' to be moderately high on the IHLC dimension (e.g. a score of 26–30) than very high (a score of 31–36). The discussion above, about the value of a three-way split on desire for control, would indicate that it is at least worth while to explore the possibility with internality that 'too much of a good thing is no good'. It might also be the case that failing to perceive (or denying) the true role that chance plays in determining many aspects of our health can be as detrimental as placing too high a belief in random occurrences.

Although examining the non-linearity of locus of control scores remains a fertile area left to be explored, examining the joint actions of two or three of the dimensions at once is being done with increasing frequency. Much of this work is based on a multidimensional typology in which median splits on the three dimensions are crossed in a $2 \times 2 \times 2$ fashion to create eight hypothetical types (see Wallston and Wallston, 1982). One of the more interesting types to emerge is the 'believers in control', those persons who score above the median on both IHLC and PHLC but below the median on CHLC. These are people for whom the issue of 'locus of control' is irrelevant, as long as health status is determined by something other than luck. Roskam (1986), for example, found that patients with rheumatoid arthritis who were classified as 'believers in control' on the basis of their MHLC scores were 'inoculated' against increases in depression when their arthritis flared up. In fact, this type of rheumatoid arthritis patient actually became less depressed over time, while other MHLC types became more depressed if their condition worsened.

A caution must be given to those considering using a typology approach such as the one described above. The MHLC scales are not meant to be assessments of relatively enduring beliefs. They are more state-like than trait-like measures of expectancies. People's health beliefs should change as a function of their direct or vicarious experience. Thus, typologies of individuals determined by MHLC scores should not be accorded the status of 'personality' types. The typologies are not necessarily stable. From our longitudinal investigation of patients with rheumatoid arthritis, we have found that only about two-thirds will be classified in exactly the same manner based on MHLC scores obtained a year later.

As mentioned above, the easiest way to classify a person into one of the eight MHLC types is to do median splits on each dimension. However, Rock *et al.* (1987) have recently shown that cluster analysis can be used to assign persons to types. Their method of cluster analysis came up with six groupings of persons, exactly mapping six of the eight MHLC types posited by Wallston and Wallston (1982). We are currently working on other analytical approaches, such as creating interaction terms by multiplying two or more MHLC subscales together, which approximate the information obtained in the typologies. These interaction terms can then be used more efficiently in regression analyses than having to dummy code each of the separate MHLC types. Again, however, it must be remembered that all of these approaches suffer from linear rather than non-linear thinking. If the 'best' profile is to be moderately high on the IHLC, moderate on the PHLC and moderately low on the CHLC, none of these approaches will discover it.

Other measures

Within the last year, we have developed and tested a new form of the MHLC Scale—tentatively labeled Form C—which is designed to be used with persons who already have an existing medical condition (such as cancer, diabetes, AIDS, arthritis, pneumonia, headache). Form C was developed for two reasons: (1) many investigators who attempted to use the MHLC Scale with persons with a chronic disease discovered that some patients had difficulty in knowing how to respond to items which referred to their 'health' when, in reality, what was most salient to them was their disease; and (2) there began to appear in the literature a proliferation of new measures, modelled after the MHLC, assessing such constructs as 'cancer locus of control', 'diabetes locus of control' and 'pain locus of control'. Each of these new scales used a different set of items; thus, results on those scales were not comparable across studies. Furthermore, scale development is not an easy process and it was terribly inefficient for each investigator to have to construct a new measure to suit his or her unique purpose.

Form C is a generic instrument, useful for assessing locus of control beliefs about any health condition. In its current form, it consists of 24 items, 8 for each of the 3 dimensions: internality, powerful others and chance. (It is our intention, after sufficient preliminary work has been done, to shorten Form C to 18 items to make it comparable to forms A and B.) Each of the 24 items contain the word 'condition'. All a researcher has to do to use Form C is to substitute a specific entity (e.g. 'diabetes') for 'condition' in each item. We have tested Form C in our longitudinal investigation of patients with rheumatoid arthritis (by changing 'condition' to 'arthritis') and the preliminary results look very promising. The alpha reliabilities of the subscales and the intercorrelations of the Form C subscales with their counterparts on Form B are presented in Table 2.

A different approach toward assessing perceived control over one's chronic condition was developed by Clare Bradley and her colleagues in the UK (Bradley et al., 1984a). They based their assessment of perceived control of diabetes on the attribution style questionnaire (ASQ) developed by Seligman and his associates (Peterson et al., 1982), but embellished it with the health locus of control dimensions from our work and some wrinkles of their own. Their measure presents the diabetic patient with six hypothetical diabetes-related events, three 'positive' and three 'negative', and asks the patient to indicate what the most likely cause of each event might be. Patients are then asked to rate each of the likely causes on a series of seven dimensions: internality; treatment; powerful others and chance externality; personal control; medical control; and foreseeability. These scales have been found to be useful in understanding patients' choice of treatment regimen, individual differences in the efficacy of treatment and the occurrence of the life-threatening complication of diabetic ketoacidosis (Bradley et al., 1984b; Bradley et al., 1986)

We have adapted the Bradley et al. (1984a) attributional approach for use in our study of rheumatoid arthritis patients, dropping the medical control and forseeability dimensions and adding stability and globality. These dimensions, which are included on the ASQ but were not included by Bradley et al. (1984a), tap the longevity of the cause and the generalizability of the cause to many aspects of one's life. In our work with these dimensions, we only assessed attributions of causes of negative events, such as arthritic symptoms. The alpha reliabilities of our seven dimensions (across three items) ranged from 0.60 to 0.73. The internal dimension (the cause is totally due to me v. not at all due to me) is uncorrelated with the personal control dimension (I have control over the cause v. I have no control over the cause) or, for that matter, any of the other five dimensions. The personal control dimension, which is a purer measure of

TABLE 2. Alpha reliabilities and intercorrelations of the subscales of forms C and B of the MHLC Scale

	Form C Arthritis—specific			Form B Health—general		
	I	P	C	I	P	C
Arthritis—internality	(0.85)					
Arthritis—powerful others	0.12	(0.75)				
Arthritis—chance	−0.04	0.17	(0.72)			
Health—internality	0.60	−0.05	−0.16	(0.59)		
Health—powerful others	0.06	0.67	0.08	0.10	(0.67)	
Health—chance	−0.09	0.18	0.71	−0.15	0.19	(0.54)

Note: (N = 266). Numbers in parentheses are alpha reliabilities. The Form C subscales have eight items each, compared to six items each for the Form B subscales.

perceived control than the locus dimensions, is correlated with stability and globality, the two attributional dimensions which are most related to feelings of helplessness. One of my students, Carolyn Dobbins, is investigating whether these attributional measures of perceived control moderate the relationship between stress due to arthritis symptomatology and psychological well-being.

Discussion

The trend toward an ever-increasing variety of instruments, many tailored to highly specific situations, is a mixed blessing. While a larger selection of tools can be helpful to investigators, it makes it more difficult to compare results across studies. Also, the proliferation of measures does not address the theoretical shortcomings of many of these investigations. As an example, Rotter's social learning theory states that behavior is a joint function of expectancies and reinforcement value, yet many investigators try to predict health behavior from an expectancy measure alone (usually a locus of control measure). Even some researchers who include a measure of health value do so in an additive rather than multiplicative fashion. In other words, they fail to test the critical theoretical proposition that one's behavior is determined by one's values moderated by one's expectancies.

A discussion of the assessment of health value is worth a chapter in its own right. In our research, we use a modification of Rokeach's (1973) value survey in which subjects are asked to rank order 'health (physical and mental well-being)' against other highly desirable end states of existence (e.g. 'a comfortable life'; 'an exciting life'; 'inner harmony'). One recent improvement in our use of that technique comes from the work of Kristiansen (1986), who developed the idea of 'relative health value'. Relative health value is computed by subtracting the value of 'an exciting life' from the value of 'health'. People who value health as an outcome more than they value an exciting life will engage in recommended health behaviors providing that they perceive that those behaviors will get them what they value. This latter expectancy is only partially tapped by the construct, locus of control. As will be discussed below, locus of control might be the least important of all the aspects of control one could measure.

PERCEIVED CONTROL OVER ONE'S BEHAVIOR

There is nothing inherent in the definition of locus of control which speaks to the person's expectancies that they *can actually perform* the behavior necessary in order to get the reinforcement. Rotter's followers simply assumed that having an internal orientation meant that one was competent. Bandura (1977), another social learning theorist, refers to locus of control as an outcome expectancy—a belief about one's control over one's outcomes, and uses the term 'self-efficacy' for a behavioral expectancy. Self-efficacy, according to Bandura (1977, 1982, 1986), is the belief that one *can do* a particular behavior in a particular situation. One cannot, logically, be self-efficacious without being somewhat internal, but one can easily be internal without being self-efficacious (see Strecher *et al.*, 1986, for an excellent discussion of the distinction between self-efficacy and locus of control expectancies).

Many health researchers have begun to assess self-efficacy beliefs as a means of determining a person's perceived control over their behavior. If one is persuaded by Bandura's assertion that there is no such thing as a generalized behavioral expectancy, and that the construct only has value when it refers to specific behaviors in specific situations, one must use or develop unique measures for each individual health behavior. Kaplan *et al.* (1984), for example, needed to assess how efficacious their patients with chronic obstructive pulmonary disease (COPD) felt in regard to a series of six exercise behaviors taught as part of their intervention. They adapted a technique whereby the subject was presented with a series of progressively more difficult performance requirements within a specific exercise type (e.g. 'walk one block—approximately 5 minutes' up to 'walk 3 miles—approximately 90 minutes'). The patients indicated whether they could perform each of the behaviors and also the degree of certainty of their expectations that they would perform the activity. If other researchers studied exactly the same set of behaviors in a similar situation, they could use the measures developed by Kaplan *et al.*, or they could make up their own. In some areas, such as smoking cessation, a number of behavior-specific self-efficacy measures have been developed (e.g. Condiotte and Lichtenstein, 1982) which are available for use by those studying smoking cessation.

Behavior-specific self-efficacy measures make a great deal of sense if one is investigating a limited number of behaviors. Many investigators, however, are interested in predicting a wide range of behaviors—such as an index of preventive health behaviors—or wish to use a measure of perceived control over one's behavior as an indicator of cognitive helplessness. For these purposes, a generalized expectancy approach as advocated by Rotter would be preferable to the highly specific approach discussed by Bandura. For our research with arthritis patients, we use a scale which we call 'perceived competence' (or 'behavioral ineffectiveness', depending on which direction we score it). Each item (e.g. 'I'm generally able to accomplish my goals') assesses the belief that the person *can do* whatever is necessary in order to get what the person wants. The perceived competence scale has a high degree of internal consistency (alpha = 0.83), and correlates significantly and meaningfully with almost every other variable we have assessed in our arthritis study. In Bandura's (1986) terms, our perceived competence scale is an 'omnibus test' which assesses a global disposition to perceive oneself as capable across a number of domains.

One of my students, Shelton Smith, has recently converted an eight-item version of the perceived competence scale to a measure she calls 'health self-efficacy' (HSE) by rewording the items to be relevant to health behaviors. In a pilot test with students in a health promotion course, the internal consistency of the HSE Scale was > 0.80. Data from this pilot study demonstrated that HSE scores moderated the relationship between relative health value and a composite index of preventive health behaviors ($r = 0.38$; $N = 80$; $p < 0.001$). The HSE measure comes closer to what Bandura (1986) means by a 'domain-linked' scale, much in the same way that the health locus of control scales are 'domain-linked'. Shelton Smith's dissertation research, currently in progress, will help add to the validity evidence for the HSE Scale.

Discussion

As with assessments of locus of control, or perceived control over outcomes, the literature contains more and more examples of measures of perceived control over health behaviors. Again, careful scale development takes a considerable amount of time and effort, and there are an awful lot of health behaviors which people wish to investigate. Nevertheless, as more of these scales get developed and put into the literature, the need for developing new behavior-specific measures should subside.

Over the past several years, I have been trying to bring about a rapprochement between the two social learning theories of Rotter and Bandura. I have concluded from the evidence in the literature that, in general, measures of self-efficacy are much stronger predictors of behavior than measures of locus of control beliefs (assuming, of course, that reinforcement value is sufficiently high in the sample). However, in my 'newly revised', modified social learning theory, the effect of self-efficacy beliefs on behavior potential is modified by one's locus of control orientation. Only for 'internals' do self-efficacy beliefs predict behavior; if someone does not believe that their behavior influences their outcomes, then it is irrelevant whether the person believes he or she can do the behavior. Initial evidence for this theory can be found in the Kaplan *et al.* (1984) study with COPD patients. One of my students, Keith Peterson, and I have recently conceptually replicated this finding with a sample of newly diagnosed cardiovascular patients involved in a smoking-cessation project. Thus, it is the interaction of perceived control over behavior and perceived control over outcomes which best predicts behavior, not either one alone.

Our perceived competence scale is more than simply a self-efficacy measure. Because it combines a behavioral expectancy with an outcome expectancy it captures the full range of the expectancy construct described in social learning theory. One problem, however, with a 'generalized self-efficacy' construct such as this is that it is difficult to distinguish it, both theoretically and psychometrically, from a similar construct, self-esteem. In fact, a colleague gave the eight-item version of our perceived competence measure along with the Rosenberg Self-Esteem Scale (Rosenberg, 1965) to a sample of college students and found that the two measures were very highly correlated (R. F. DeVellis, personal communication, August 1985). The fact that perceived competence highly correlates with self-esteem may not be a problem to many investigators; after all, perceived competence is a large determinant of one's sense of self-worth. Showing that measures of the two constructs correlate is a demonstration of construct validity, but such a high correlation raises questions about discriminant validity. It is likely, however, that our new 'health self-efficacy' scale will be less highly correlated with measures of self-esteem than the more omnibus-perceived competence scale, because one's overall sense of esteem is not totally dependent on one's perceived capability in any one specific domain.

PERCEIVED CONTROL AS A COMPONENT OF HARDINESS

Personality hardiness (Kobasa, 1979, 1982) is an individual difference variable which has been shown to moderate the relationship between stress and negative health outcomes. Over the past nine years there have been a myriad of studies in the literature showing that 'hardy' individuals do not break down and become ill in the face of stressors, as do non-hardy individuals. Based upon an existential theory of personality (Kobasa and Maddi, 1977), personality hardiness is believed to be a combination of three constructs: perceived control, commitment, and challenge. Perceived control, defined as the tendency to believe and act as if one can influence the course of events, has been a major, if not *the* major, component of hardiness in almost every analysis which has looked at the components separately.

The assessment of personality hardiness has been problematical from the onset, although the challenge component has had more difficulties than either control or commitment (Hull *et al.*, 1987). In the original version of the hardiness scale, perceived control was assessed by a combination of Rotter's I–E Scale and the Powerlessness and Nihilism scales of the Alienation Test (Maddi *et al.*, 1979). In the latest 50-item version (distributed by the Hardiness Institute in Chicago), the perceived control items read more like self-efficacy (or perceived competence) than locus of control items. Interestingly, the latest version of perceived control in the hardiness scale only correlates 0.24 ($p = $ NS) with the previous assessment of perceived control (S. Kahn, personal communication, August 1987).

Pollock (1986) developed a health-related hardiness scale (HRHS) in which the MHLC Scale constituted the perceived control dimension. Pollock originally computed a total control score by subtracting IHLC from the sum of PHLC and CHLC, but subsequent analyses of her data from a sample of diabetic patients and our data from our sample of rheumatoid arthritis patients have shown that eliminating the PHLC items from the control dimension increases the scale's internal consistency. One of my students, Deborah Abraham, and I have recently developed a completely new HRHS in which we assess control through a combination of IHLC, CHLC and HSE (health self-efficacy) items. We are in the process of testing the concurrent and discriminant validity of our new HRHS against the 50-item personality hardiness measure.

Discussion

I am convinced that, once the measurement problems have been resolved, the construct of choice for researchers examining the role of individual differences as moderators of the stress–health status relationship will be hardiness. Hardy individuals are apparently healthier to begin with and are more resistant to stressors if and when they occur. The jury is still out on whether the measurement of hardiness should be at the more general, personality level or via a health-specific assessment such as the HRHS. It is also not clear whether a composite hardiness score should be calculated by simply adding together the component subscores, as is currently the case, or by some multiplicative function, which is more consistent with hardiness theory (S. Ouellette-Kobasa, personal communication, August 1987). Nevertheless, hardiness 'works' because it casts perceived control in a central role, yet recognizes that control does not work alone. Commitment (which, like reinforcement value, is a motivational construct) and challenge (a cognitive coping strategy) co-star along with control in the production of a superordinate construct that makes sense theoretically and can be validated empirically.

SUMMARY

This chapter draws upon fifteen years' worth of my research to illustrate the variety of ways with which aspects of control in health-care settings have been assessed. Three complex field studies in which we measured the desire for and perception of control over three different health-care settings were briefly presented. Our inability to document that we had, indeed, manipulated perceived control by giving enhanced choices to certain patients in those studies was pointed out, along with *ex post facto* explanations as to why those null findings might have come about. The Multidimensional Health Locus of Control Scale was discussed along with alternative methods of assessing perceived control over one's health status. The minimal role that MHLC scores have had in predicting health behavior was discussed, and a 'newly revised' modified social learning theory was presented in which assessments of self-efficacy beliefs (perceived control over one's behavior) play a central role. Finally, the important but non-singular role that perceived control plays in the construct of psychological hardiness was presented, and the notion of assessing health-related hardiness was discussed. Throughout the chapter, the advantages of 'domain-linked' (Bandura, 1986) over more generalized assessments of control have been stressed.

REFERENCES

Bandura, A. (1977). Self-efficacy: toward a unifying theory of behavior change. *Psychological Review*, **84**, 191–215.

Bandura, A. (1982). Self-efficacy in human agency. *American Psychologist*, **37**, 122–147.

Bandura, A. (1986). The explanatory and predictive scope of self-efficacy theory. *Journal of Social and Clinical Psychology*, **4**, 359–373.

Bradley, C., Brewin, C. R., Gamsu, D. R., and Moses, J. L. (1984a). Development of scales to measure perceived control of diabetes mellitus and diabetes-related health beliefs. *Diabetic Medicine*, **1**, 213–218.

Bradley, C., Gamsu, D. S., Moses, J. L., Knight, G., Boulton, A. J. M., Drury, J., and Ward, J. D. (1984b). Prediction of patients' treatment choice using diabetes-specific perceived control and health belief measures in a feasibility study of continuous subcutaneous insulin infusion. *Diabetologia*, **27**, 259A.

Bradley, C., Gamsu, D. S., Knight, G., Boulton, A. J. M., and Ward, J. D. (1986). Predicting risk of diabetic ketoacidosis in patients using continuous subcutaneous insulin infusion. *British Medical Journal*, **293**, 242–243.

Burish, T. G., Carey, M. P., Wallston, K. A., Stein, M. J., Jamison, R. N., and Lyles, J. N. (1984). Health locus of control and chronic disease: An external orientation may be advantageous. *Journal of Social and Clinical Psychology*, **2**, 326–332.

Condiotte, M.M., and Lichtenstein, E. (1982). Self-efficacy and relapse in smoking cessation programs. *Journal of Consulting and Clinical Psychology*, **49**, 648–658.

Hull, J. G., Van Trevren, R. R., and Virnelli, S. (1987). Hardiness and health: A critique and alternative approach. *Journal of Personality and Social Psychology*, **53**, 518–530.

Kaplan, R. M., Atkins, C. J., and Reinsch, S. (1984). Specific efficacy expectations mediate exercise compliance in patients with COPD. *Health Psychology*, **3**, 223–242.

Kobasa, S. (1979). Stressful life events, personality, and health: An inquiry into hardiness. *Journal of Personality and Social Psychology*, **37**, 1–11.

Kobasa, S. (1982). The hardy personality: Toward a social psychology of stress and health. In: J. Suls and G. Sanders (eds), *Social Psychology of Health and Illness* (pp. 3–32). Hillsdale, NJ: Erlbaum.

Kobasa, S. C., and Maddi, S. R. (1977). Existential personality theory. In: R. Corsini (ed.), *Current Personality Theories*. Itasca, IL: Peacock.

Krantz, D.S., Baum, A., and Wideman, M. W. (1980). Assessment of preferences for self-treatment and information in health care. *Journal of Personality and Social Psychology*, **39**, 977–990.

Kristiansen, C. M. (1986). A two value model of preventive health behavior. *Basic and Applied Social Psychology*, **7**, 173–183.

Langer, E. J. (1975). The illusion of control. *Journal of Personality and Social Psychology*, **32**, 311–328.

Lefcourt, H. M. (1976). *Locus of Control: Current Trends in Theory and Research*. Hillsdale, NJ: Erlbaum.

Maddi, S. R., Kobasa, S. C., and Hoover, M. (1979). An alienation test. *Journal of Humanistic Psychology*, **19**, 73–76.

Mills, R. T., and Krantz, D. S. (1979). Information, choice, and reactions to stress: A field experiment in a blood bank with laboratory analogue. *Journal of Personality and Social Psychology*, **37**, 608–620.

Peterson, C., Semmel, A., vonBaeyer, C., Abramson, L. Y., Metalsky, G. I., and Seligman, M. P. (1982). The attributional style questionnaire. *Cognitive Therapy and Research*, **6**, 287–300.

Phares, E. J. (1976). *Locus of Control in Personality*. Morristown, NJ: General Learning Press.

Pollock, S. E. (1986). Human responses to chronic illness: Physiologic and psychosocial adaptation. *Nursing Research*, **35**, 90–95.

Rock, D. L., Meyerowitz, B. E., Maisto, S. A., and Wallston, K. A. (1987). The derivation and validation of six multidimensional health locus of control scale clusters. *Research in Nursing and Health*, **10**, 185–195.

Rodin, J., and Langer, E. J. (1977). Long-term effects of a control-relevant intervention with the institutionalized aged. *Journal of Personality and Social Psychology*, **35**, 897–903.

Rokeach, M. (1973). *The Nature of Human Values*. New York: Free Press.

Rosenberg, M. (1965). *Society and the Adolescent Self-image*. Princeton, NJ: Princeton University Press.

Roskam, S. (1986). *Application of health locus of control typology approach toward predicting depression and medical adherence in rheumatoid arthritis*. Unpublished doctoral dissertation, Vanderbilt University, Nashville, TN.

Rotter, J. B. (1954). *Social Learning and Clinical Psychology*. Englewood Cliffs, NJ: Prentice-Hall.

Rotter, J. B. (1966). Generalized expectancies for internal vs. external control of reinforcement. *Psychological Monographs*, **80**, 1–28.

Rotter, J. B. (1979). Comments on Section IV: Individual differences and perceived control. In: L. C. Perlmuter and R. A. Monty (eds), *Choice and Perceived Control* (pp. 263–269). New York: Wiley.

Rotter, J. B. (1982). *The Development and Applications of Social Learning Theory: Selected Papers*. Brattleboro, VT: Praeger.

Schulz, R. (1976). The effects of control and predictability on the physical and psychological well-being of the institutionalized aged. *Journal of Personality and Social Psychology*, **33**, 563–573.

Smith, R. A., Wallston, B. S., Wallston, K. A., Forsberg, P. R., and King, J. E. (1984). Measuring desire for control of health care processes. *Journal of Personality and Social Psychology*, **47**, 415–426.

Smith, R. A. P., Woodward, N. J., Wallston, B. S., Wallston, K. A., Rye, P., and Zylstra, M. (1988). Health care implications of desire and expectancy for control in elderly adults. *Journal of Gerontology*, **43**, P1–P7.

Strecher, V. J., DeVellis, B. M., Becker, M. H., and Rosenstock, I. M. (1986). The role of self-efficacy in achieving health behavior change. *Health Education Quarterly*, **13**, 73–91.

Strickland, B.R. (1978). Internal–external expectancies and health-related behaviors. *Journal of Consulting and Clinical Psychology*, **46**, 1192–1211.

Taylor, S. E. (1979). Hospital patient behavior: Reactance, helplessness or control? *Journal of Social Issues*, **35**, 156–184.

Wallston, B. S., and Wallston, K. A. (1978). Locus of control and health: A review of the literature. *Health Education Monographs*, **6**, 107–117.

Wallston, B. S., and Wallston, K. A. (1981). Health locus of control. In: H. Lefcourt (ed.), *Research with the Locus of Control Construct* (Vol. 1). New York: Academic Press.

Wallston, B. S., Smith, R. A. P., Wallston, K. A., King, J. E., Rye, P. D., and Heim, C. (1987). Choice and predictability in the preparation for barium enemas: A person-by-situation approach. *Research in Nursing and Health*, **10**, 13–22.

Wallston, K. A., and Wallston, B. S. (1982). Who is responsible for your health? The construct of health locus control. In: G. Sanders and J. Suls (eds), *Social Psychology of Health and Illness* (pp. 65–95). Hillsdale, NJ: Erlbaum.

Wallston, K. A., Wallston, B. S., and DeVellis, R. F. (1978). Development of the multidimensional health locus of control (MHLC) scale. *Health Education Monographs*, **6**, 160–170.

Wallston, K. A., Wallston, B. S., Smith, M. S., and Dobbins, C. J. (1987). Perceived control and health. *Current Psychology Research and Reviews*, **6**, 5–25.

CHAPTER 6

Information, coping and control in patients undergoing surgery and stressful medical procedures

SUZANNE M. MILLER, CHRISTOPHER COMBS AND ELLEN STODDARD
Department of Psychology, Temple University, Philadelphia, USA

Despite decades of research and theorizing on the role of information, coping and control in patient response to aversive diagnostic and surgical procedures, little consensus exists as to the benefits of these interventions (Gil, 1984; Taylor and Clark, 1986; Schultheis *et al.*, 1987; Auerbach, in press). Further, a morass of studies has tended to yield a variety of conflicting findings. It has been difficult to find a conceptual framework or an empirically derived metric that can account for these inconsistencies. The present chapter attempts to delineate the conditions which do and do not lead to successful stress reduction. We first provide a definitional and theoretical framework for understanding and delineating the constructs of information, coping and control. Next, the literature in each of these areas is reviewed and its fit to the theories is examined. We conclude by presenting an integrative structure that helps to reconcile the inconsistencies in results and highlights areas for future research.

DEFINITIONAL AND THEORETICAL FRAMEWORK

While information, coping and control have often been construed so broadly as to render them indistinguishable, previous work suggests that it may be theoretically and empirically useful to keep them distinct (see Miller, 1979, 1980a,b, 1981; Miller and Birnbaum, 1989). Control is defined as the individual's

Stress, Personal Control and Health. Edited by A. Steptoe and A. Appels.
Published by John Wiley & Sons Ltd.

perception that he or she can execute (or has the potential to execute) some action that changes an aversive stimulus. In the medical context, this generally entails responses (e.g. pain management) that mitigate the severity or magnitude of the aversive event. In contrast, information (predictability) merely implies that the individual knows something about the event, whether or not he or she can do anything to change it. Such knowledge can include information about the disease, the staff, the specific medical procedures to be followed (procedural information) and the sensations to be experienced (sensory information). Finally, for the present purposes, coping is defined as the regulation of stressful emotions via attention deployment and the modulation of internal arousal. Relevant techniques include relaxation, distraction, reinterpretation, calming self-talk and so forth. This definition corresponds to Folkman and Lazarus' (1980) notion of emotion-focused coping, while information and control are viewed as orthogonal components of their notion of problem-focused coping.

Miller has specified two hypotheses to account for when information, coping and control are preferred and stress-reducing and when they are not. The first, the 'minimax' hypothesis, was devised primarily to address the issue of control (Miller, 1979, 1980a). It states that individuals are motivated by a desire to minimize the maximum danger to themselves. Therefore, they prefer and are less stressed by control, when having control allows them to put an upper limit on how bad the situation can become. Consider a patient who is faced with the prospect of an aversive diagnostic procedure but is instructed that if he or she breathes in a particular manner then discomfort will be minimized. This individual will perceive some control over the situation and be less stressed than a patient who believes that there is nothing he or she can do to reduce the level of discomfort.

Generally speaking, one's own responses are the most reliable and stable guarantees of a minimum upper limit of aversiveness. However, there are conditions under which another person's responses may be a better and more reliable guarantee of minimizing aversiveness than one's own. In these situations, having control will be dispreferred and stress-inducing. Hence, individuals will be more likely to relinquish control to the other, more competent, person. For example, when faced with a medical diagnosis with several treatment options, an unsophisticated lay person may well prefer to relinquish control over the decisional process to an identified expert.

The second view, the 'monitoring and blunting' hypothesis, seeks primarily to tie together the literatures on information, coping and stress (Miller, 1980b, 1981; Miller and Green, 1985; Miller and Birnbaum, 1988). This framework proposes an explicit interaction between control contingencies and informational and coping choices. Arousal remains high in aversive situations, the more the individual is 'monitoring' (information-seeking) and the less he or she is 'blunting' (cognitively avoiding and transforming) the negative aspects of the event. Arousal is reduced when he or she can psychologically blunt objective sources of danger. When an aversive event is controllable, high monitoring and low blunting are the main responses and information is preferred. Although this can heighten arousal, it enables the individual to execute controlling actions, which can be arousal-reducing as detailed by the minimax hypothesis. When an aversive event is uncontrollable, however, high monitoring and low blunting (which heighten arousal) have no offsetting instrumental value. Therefore, for many individuals, high blunting and low monitoring become the main response modes, since an individual without controlling actions can most effectively reduce stress by engaging in a variety of coping techniques. Here, information will be dispreferred and arousal-inducing, since it forces the individual back into the psychological presence of a danger he or she cannot avoid.

To illustrate, consider a patient whose physician warns him or her every time he or she is about to feel pain. The individual will be listening for the doctor's warnings and the warnings themselves will be invasive and intrusive, even if the individual is trying to block them out. In contrast, if the doctor were to provide no warning, threat-relevant information would be more diluted and less psychologically invasive and intrusive. This would make it easier for the individual to engage in a variety of coping techniques (e.g. relaxation) which help to minimize stress.

These coping techniques may have an additional advantage, in terms of minimax considerations. When an individual experiences a physically noxious aversive event against a background of bodily relaxation, it may reduce the impact of the event by attenuating perceptions of pain, reducing complications and facilitating recovery. For example, there is evidence that anxious patients run greater surgical risks because they need higher doses of anesthesia (Johnston, 1980; see also Carey and Burish, 1988). Thus, the provision of coping techniques to patients may provide them with an indirect means for minimizing the maximum aversiveness of the situation.

However, while some people will find it easy or desirable to use coping techniques (or difficult and inappropriate to seek information), others will find it difficult or inappropriate to use such techniques (or easy and desirable to seek information). For these latter individuals, information will be preferred and stress-reducing, because information provides them at least with environmental cues that reduce uncertainty and signal periods of safety (Weiss, 1970). That is, since they cannot place themselves in the 'psychological' presence of safety signals, they place themselves in the 'external' presence of such signals. In the case of a patient, if the physician always provides a warning before the individual is about to experience pain, then the high monitor/low blunter can at least be calm as long as the doctor is silent.

A second motivation among such individuals for seeking information in the face of uncontrollable threats may be related to the minimax hypothesis. That is, when another individual (e.g. the physician) is the most reliable and stable guarantee of minimal aversiveness, then some individuals may desire information as a means of seeking out and maintaining close contact with the identified expert.

THE EVIDENCE

This section presents evidence on the effects of information, coping and control on patient response to a variety of medical and surgical procedures. Inclusion criteria for studies were: (1) the use of adult populations; (2) the experimental manipulation of at least one of the three variables of interest; and (3) the use of an untreated or attention control group. Studies investigating adjustment to chronic or acute disease *per se* (without an explicit medical or surgical intervention) were omitted as were single case studies.

Information studies

General information

While the studies in this category often included sensory and procedural components in the information package, the actual content is typically not well described. Further, their results are less easy to interpret by virtue of their incorporation of additional sources of information. Therefore they are considered separately.

Two studies focused on patients undergoing cardiac catheterization. One of these compared a general information condition (detailing the disease, the procedure and related sensations), with both an attention and an untreated control (Kendall *et al.*, 1979). The information group showed better observed adjustment during the procedure, reported a decrease in anxiety after receiving the intervention (but not after catheterization), endorsed more positive self-statements and tended to be less likely to want to quit. There were no differences among groups in observer ratings of patient receptivity, irritation, denial and discomfort or in patient ratings of pain and anger. Finesilver (1978) found that a group receiving procedural, sensory and anatomical information as well as support and reassurance had lower observer ratings of distress during the procedure, received fewer medications and were more satisfied, compared with a control group (unspecified). No differences emerged in self-report measures of mood, before or after catheterization.

Six studies looked at patients undergoing minor and major elective surgery. Hysterectomy patients who received information (procedural, sensory and reassurance) were less annoyed about waking up at night in the hospital, had fewer days of pain in the three weeks after discharge and had marginally lower pre-surgery anxiety and worry than the no-information group (Ridgeway and Mathews, 1982). No effects obtained for self-reported mood, analgesics or symptoms (nausea, pain, vomiting, sleep disturbance) during the three days following the operation or in activity level, nausea, fatigue, depression and irritability after discharge. Vernon and Bigelow (1974) explored the impact of information (detailing the significant events and their rationalization) on hernia repair patients. Compared to a no-treatment control, informed patients were more satisfied and knowledgeable, more likely to anticipate pain and less likely to focus on the benefits of surgery or to deny thoughts of the operation. They also expressed less postoperative anger, greater confidence in doctors in general (but not their own doctor) before the surgery and greater confidence in their nurse after the surgery. The groups did not differ in pre- or post-self-report measures of affect or in observer measures of fear and hostility.

Among dental surgery patients, there were no differences in anxiety or observed adjustment between a group provided with disease, procedural and sensory information and a control group provided with details of the dental clinic and equipment (Auerbach *et al.*, 1976). However, 'internals' in the information condition showed better adjustment during surgery than internals in an attention control condition. The converse was true for 'external' subjects (Rotter, 1966). In a reanalysis of these data, those receiving information about tooth removal, procedures and postoperative instructions showed no benefits on anxiety and observer ratings of adjustment compared with an attention control group, although such information actually increased anxiety in females (Auerbach and Kendall, 1978).

While the above studies showed neutral to positive information effects, a study by Langer *et al.* (1975) found a more negative pattern of results. General surgery patients given information (reasons for preparatory practices, postoperative experiences, reassurance about hospital staff) received higher nurse ratings of anxiety and lower nurse ratings of ability to cope, compared to an attention control. The groups did not differ on mean number of pain relievers or sedatives requested, length of stay in the hospital or on physiological measures of blood pressure and pulse rate. Andrew (1970) looked at patients undergoing minor surgical and non-surgical procedures. She found that the impact of information was moderated by the patients' coping style (as assessed by Goldstein, 1959). 'Neutrals' (those showing no specific style) who received information had fewer days to discharge and used fewer medications. Conversely, information actually increased use of medications and had no effect on days to discharge for 'avoiders' (those showing denial or distancing). Information had no effect on sensitizers (those showing their feelings readily), presumably because those in the low-information condition spontaneously sought out and received high levels of information.

Finally, one study did not explicitly manipulate information, but focused cancer patients toward or away from chemotherapy by having them complete a questionnaire detailing the severity of their previous experience with the treatment or a questionnaire concerning parking facilities at the hospital, respectively (Gard *et al.*, 1988). Patients in the information condition rated the severity of their nausea as more severe than patients in the attention control. Interestingly, while a significantly larger number of the high monitors/low blunters (those who typically seek out threat-relevant information) than the low monitors/high blunters (those who typically distract from or avoid threat-relevant information) received antiemetic medication, they nonetheless experienced a higher incidence rate and longer episodes of nausea (Miller Behavioral Style Scale; Miller, 1987).

Sensory and preparatory information

Since general information contains a number of components, including reassurance and support, more recent studies have explicitly compared two particular subtypes of information relevant to the immediate medical context: sensory (which focuses on the sensations to be experienced) and procedural (which details the specific procedures to be followed). Five of these compared combined sensory and procedural information together with a no-treatment control.

Mills and Krantz (1979) found that when individuals donating blood received procedural (and sensory) information, it reduced nurse interventions and ratings of discomfort, increased ratings of pain, and had no effect on anxiety or the Stroop color–word test (a behavioral index of stress). Similarly, combined information reduced gagging and the amount of tranquilizer required during gastrointestinal endoscopy, but did not lower heart rate, overt signs of distress or time for tube passage (Johnson and Leventhal, 1974).

When patients undergoing cholecystectomy and abdominal hysterectomy were exposed to either sensory and procedural information or to the usual hospital care, they generally expressed a desire for the details provided (Wilson, 1981). However, the only main effect for information was a reduction in the length of hospital stay by an average of one day. For highly aggressive patients (assessed by a questionnaire designed for the study) information reduced self-reports of pain, negative moods, physical symptoms, use of medications and output of epinephrine, but had no effect on ambulation. Self-report measures of preoperative fear and denial had no impact on patient response.

A follow-up investigation of gastrointestinal endoscopy patients found that sensory and procedural information patients exhibited less distress during insertion, fewer insertion failures, and smaller heart rate increases during insertion, rated the procedure to be less uncomfortable than expected, perceived that they would be less uncomfortable in the future, and were marginally more accurate in their judgments of tube size (Wilson *et al.*, 1982). Avoiders (identified by a modified version of the original questionnaire) showed marginally less insertion and exploration distress when not exposed to information. No differences emerged for mood, valium, heart rate before and after the procedure, discomfort ratings or absolute judgments of tube size. In contrast, combined procedural and sensory information had no effects whatsoever on patients undergoing cholecystectomy and hysterectomy, including on measures of pain, state anxiety and analgesics (Scott and Clum, 1984). Contrary to predictions, sensitizers receiving information reported more pain than avoiders did (defined on the basis of Cohen and Lazarus, 1973).

Among the six studies comparing the impact of preparatory and sensory information with an attention control group, Anderson (1987) found that the combined group had lower pre- but not postoperative anxiety, lower pre-surgery specific fears and less negative affect after undergoing major cardiac surgery. Further, preparation was associated with less postoperative hypertension and with nurse ratings of better physical and psychological recovery by day 7, although no differences emerged on nurse-rated symptoms. There were also no differences between groups on various measures of recovery (analgesic use, days in hospital and a recovery index).

In a study of young women undergoing a routine pelvic examination, subjects who received sensory (and procedural) information showed less distress, as indicated by overt distress behaviors and pulse rates but not as measured by self-reported fear, than subjects who received general health education (Fuller *et al.*, 1978). In contrast, among patients undergoing their first cataract surgery, sensory information alone proved no better than general hospital and disease information in terms of mood, ambulation, days to discharge, first time ventured from home or cognitive orientation (Hill, 1982).

Auerbach *et al.* (1983) found that when dental extraction patients were presented with sensory and procedural information, they adjusted better (on dentist's ratings) than general information subjects. Further, subjects with a high preference for information (on the Krantz Health Opinion Survey; Krantz *et al.*, 1980) showed better adjustment when they received procedural and sensory v. general information; low-preference subjects adjusted slightly better with general information. Mode of presentation was unrelated to adjustment, although patients who received a personal delivery viewed the dentist more positively than those who received an impersonal delivery. A further study along these lines compared a cursory preoperative visit (presenting the barest outline of the forthcoming procedures) with a supportive visit (presenting fuller procedural details and establishing maximal rapport) prior to therapeutic abortion (Williams *et al.*, 1975). The cursory interviews increased preoperative induction dosages of thiopental sodium and eyelid reflexes in the patients with initially low anxiety, while both cursory and supportive information reduced induction dosages and eyelid reflexes of those patients with initially high anxiety.

When patients undergoing an aversive diagnostic procedure for cervical cancer were given procedural and sensory information, they showed marginally fewer overt signs of distress during the examination than those in a distracting attention-control condition (Miller and Mangan, 1983). However, combined information increased self-reports of depression and discomfort, both before and after the procedure. These data thus confirm previous studies, showing the strongest informational effects on measures of impact. Physiological indices, in contrast, were sensitive to person-by-situation influences as measured by the Miller Behavioral Style Scale (Miller, 1987). While high monitors /low blunters were generally more behaviorally and subjectively anxious than low monitors/ high blunters, low monitors/high blunters showed the lowest physiological arousal when they were not exposed to voluminous information than when it was provided. Conversely, high monitors/low blunters showed lower physiological arousal when information was made available than when it was withheld.

Six studies examined the differential effects of sensory v. procedural information. In an early study, both sensory and procedural messages reduced the amount of diazepam required during gastrointestinal endoscopy (Johnson *et al.*, 1973). In addition, patients in the sensory group showed less restlessness than those in the procedural group and fewer overt signs of tension than either of the other two groups. There were no differences in gagging or heart rate. A follow-up investigation of cholecystectomy patients revealed that sensory information (combined with procedural information) reduced the length of postoperative hospitalization and time after discharge before patients ventured from their homes compared to an untreated control, but not compared to procedural information. The groups were equivalent in terms of postoperative pain, ambulation and mood (Johnson *et al.*, 1978a, Experiment I). The positive effects were not replicated with a sample of herniorrhaphy patients (Experiment II; see also Johnson *et al.*, 1978b). In two studies of barium enema patients, those receiving sensory information reported that they had experienced less anxiety during the procedure than those receiving procedural information but not less than no-information controls (Hartfield and Cason, 1981; Hartfield *et al.*, 1982). A study of gynecological and gastrointestinal surgery patients failed to find any differences in postoperative pain, physical symptoms or distress between a procedural and a combined procedural and sensory condition (Ziemer, 1983).

Two additional investigations focused on the interacting effects of individual differences and information. Padilla *et al.* (1981) found equivalent self-reports of distress, discomfort, pain and anxiety between procedural and combined procedural/sensory groups undergoing nasogastric intubation. Procedural and sensory information led to a reduction in discomfort for patients who claimed to be high in control orientation but increased discomfort for patients low in control orientation ('Would you prefer to help with the procedure or to leave it up to the professionals?'). Finally, a study of patients undergoing cardiac catheterization found that high monitors/low blunters (Miller, 1987) who received combined sensory and procedural information reported less anxiety and had lower heart rates during the examination than those who received procedural information (Watkins *et al.*, 1986). Conversely, low monitors/high blunters receiving procedural information alone had lower anxiety and heart rates during the examination than those in the combined group. Further, while high monitors/low blunters in the procedural group were more likely to want more information than those in the combined group, low monitors/high blunters were generally satisfied with the level of information they received.

Conclusions

Overall, the effects of information on medical and hospital stress are not dramatic and are extremely uneven. In four studies, general information was found to have mixed effects, ranging from positive (especially on observer ratings of distress) to neutral (especially on self-report ratings of distress) (Kendall *et al.*, 1979; Ridgeway and Mathews, 1982; Vernon and Bigelow, 1974; Finesilver, 1978). General information had no effects at all in one study (Auerbach and Kendall, 1978) and neutral to negative effects in another (Langer *et al.*, 1975). Finally, two studies showed a role for individual differences, with internals and neutrals benefiting more from information than externals and avoiders (Andrew, 1970; Auerbach *et al.*, 1976).

When combined sensory and procedural information was compared with a no-treatment control, it produced some positive benefits, lowering observed indices of distress during impact but generally not affecting mood or physiological indices (Mills and Krantz, 1979; Johnson and Leventhal, 1974; Scott and Clum, 1984; Wilson 1981; Wilson *et al.*, 1982). These effects were stronger for aggressive and non-avoidant patients (Wilson, 1981; Wilson *et al.*, 1982). In comparison with an attention-control group, the effects of combined preparation ranged from neutral (Williams *et al.*, 1975; Hill, 1982) to somewhat positive (Auerbach *et al.*, 1983; Fuller *et al.*, 1978; Anderson, 1987). Results of a further study ranged from positive (on measures of overt behavior), to neutral (on physiological measures), to negative (on self-report measures) (Miller and Mangan, 1983). Two studies found that high-information-preference patients and monitors receiving sensory and procedural information showed better observed and/or physiological adjustment, in relation to low-information-preference patients and blunters (Auerbach *et al.*, 1983; Miller and Mangan, 1983; see also Williams *et al.*, 1975).

When the separate and interactive effects of procedural and sensory information are teased apart, sensory information alone was superior to procedural information alone in three studies (Johnson *et al.*, 1973; Hartfield and Cason, 1981; Hartfield *et al.*, 1982). Conversely, while procedural and sensory information combined was sometimes more effective than a no-pretreatment group, it was equivalent to procedural information (Johnson *et al.*, 1978a,b; Ziemer, 1983). A clearer pattern emerges when individual differences are considered: combined information was found to be superior to procedural information for high-control patients and monitors (Padilla *et al.*, 1981; Watkins *et al.*, 1986).

In summary, sensory information alone, and in combination with procedural information, appears to have the most benefits. However, it is difficult to account for the inconsistencies among studies in terms of situational variations, such as severity or type of medical condition or procedure under consideration (see also Suls and Wan, in press). In contrast, as predicted, dispositional factors appear to play an important moderating role, with certain individuals deriving more benefit from information—particularly sensory and procedural information —than others. Unfortunately, most of the instruments used to assess individual differences are unvalidated and/or conceptually flawed (e.g. Andrew, 1970; Padilla *et al.*, 1981; Wilson, 1981; Wilson *et al.* 1982). The two most promising measures are those of Krantz (Krantz *et al.*, 1980) and Miller (1987), which are both closely tied to behavior and have adequate psychometric properties.

Some researchers explain information-seeking as an attempt to achieve a perception of control over the situation (e.g. Thompson, 1981). However, information does not necessarily increase perceptions of control (e.g. Padilla *et al.*, 1981; cf. Anderson, 1987). Further, individuals often opt for information in explicitly uncontrollable contexts (cf. Miller, 1981). Recent research helps to shed some light on this issue. Miller *et al.* (1988) found that, while high monitors (and low blunters) typically preferred to have detailed information and reassurance about their medical condition, they did not appear to seek this information for its instrumental value. Indeed, compared to low monitors (and high blunters), they were more likely to desire to play a passive role in their medical care. These data are consistent with the predictions of the monitoring and blunting and the minimax hypotheses. First, information-seekers appear to prefer information in order to reduce uncertainty and thereby put themselves in the presence of safety signals. Second, seeking information enables patients to gain access to important sources of expertise (e.g. medical specialists) who, in turn, are in a critical position to minimize the maximum aversiveness of the situation for them. In support of this, Carver *et al.* (1989) found that high monitors not only tended to cope with stress by focusing on and ventilating their emotions, as would be expected, but they also became behaviorally disengaged (i.e. they gave up their goals and stopped trying to solve the problem) and instead sought out social support for instrumental reasons (i.e. they tried to get advice and find someone who could do something concrete about the problem).

From a practical standpoint, these data suggest a two-pronged approach to information delivery in medical contexts. For high monitors/low blunters, voluminous preparatory and sensory information should be made available, with an opportunity to express emotion and a focus on explicit reassurances about the external sources of competence available. Conversely, for low monitors/high blunters, more minimal procedural information should be made available, with an emphasis on the patient as an important self-resource in the situation.

One feature of virtually all of this literature is the limited amount of time devoted to information provision, in general averaging 10 minutes or less (14 studies). Only four studies spent between 20 and 45 minutes in information delivery and nine studies failed to specify information time. This means that patients typically may not have sufficient opportunity to cognitively rehearse and process the information they receive, even if they generally prefer and fare better with such information. This, in turn, can undermine the patient's sense of efficacy that he or she can use the information effectively (Bandura, 1985). While some evidence bears on this possibility (e.g. Shipley *et al.*, 1978, 1979), no study directly tests the possibility that the impact of information packages *per se* varies with the time allotted to the provision of this information.

Coping studies

Coping

Several investigations have examined the impact of a coping intervention on adaptation. Ten of these explored the effects of a relaxation intervention, typically progressive muscle relaxation. In an early study, Aiken and Henrichs (1971) found that, compared to a no-treatment control, relaxation significantly improved anesthesia time, cardiopulmonary bypass time and degree of hypothermia in open-heart surgery patients. It also reduced total units of blood required but did not affect duration of hypothermia or accomplishment of multivalve replacement. Similarly, cholecystectomy and hysterectomy patients taught to relax showed better recovery, less pain medication, greater output of epinephrine and quicker discharge than a no-treatment control (Wilson, 1981). No differences were observed in mood or ambulation. Low-fear subjects benefited more from the intervention than did high-fear subjects. In a follow-up study, relaxation training improved mood and reduced heart rate and observer ratings of distress during tube insertion in gastrointestinal endoscopy patients, but had no effect on valium usage or heart rate and distress during exploration (Wilson *et al.*, 1982). Relaxation was most effective with high-fear and avoidant subjects. Relative to an attention control, relaxation produced lower self-ratings of anxiety and marginally fewer requests to stop the examination in patients undergoing sigmoidoscopy, but did not alter heart rate or observer ratings (Kaplan *et al.*, 1982). A further study showed no benefits of relaxation on anxiety, pain or medication use in hysterectomy and cholecystectomy patients (Scott and Clum, 1984).

A number of these studies focused explicitly on cancer patients. For example, Domar *et al.* (1987) found that patients undergoing surgical removal of a skin cancer who were taught relaxation experienced their worst anxiety before entering the study. The attention-control group had their highest levels of anxiety during surgery and when facing the biopsy results. No clinically meaningful differences obtained on heart rate, respiratory rate or blood pressure. A series of investigations by Burish and his colleagues concentrated on patients undergoing chemotherapy (Burish and Lyles, 1981; Lyles *et al.*, 1982; Burish *et al.*, 1987; Carey and Burish, 1987). When trained in progressive muscle relaxation and guided imagery, patients showed reduced physiological arousal, reports of nausea and dysphoria, and nurse reports of nausea and anxiety in comparison with a no-treatment and an attention-control group. These benefits were typically stronger during the training period (under therapist guidance) than during follow-up.

In addition to relaxation alone, the use of deep muscle relaxation hypnosis has been shown to be effective in reducing nausea, gagging and retching in chemotherapy patients (e.g. Redd *et al.*, 1982). Further, systematic desensitization (involving relaxation and a graded hierarchy) has been found to reduce the occurrence, severity and duration of nausea (and vomiting) as compared to a counseling and a no-treatment control (Morrow and Morrell, 1982). Results of a subsequent study suggested that these results were not obtained when the relaxation component was taught by a tape-recording (Morrow, 1984). While both systematic desensitization and relaxation lowered post-treatment nausea and vomiting, only systematic desensitization led to decreases in anticipatory nausea and anxiety (Morrow, 1986).

The effectiveness of reinterpretation (selectively attending to the positive aspects of the procedure) has also been explored. Typically, reinterpretation interventions focus the patient on the more positive, beneficial components of the procedure and away from the more negative components of the situation (e.g. 'The medical staff is highly competent'; 'This won't last long'; 'It gives me a chance for a rest, which I needed', etc.). General surgery patients (e.g. hysterectomy, hernia repair, cholecystectomy) who received a reinterpretation intervention had improved nurse ratings of anxiety and ability to cope, requested fewer pain relievers relative to an attention control, and showed a trend toward fewer days to discharge (Langer *et al.*, 1975). There were no differences on physiological measures. Similarly, compared to an attention-control group, women undergoing hysterectomy had less sleep disturbance, had fewer oral and injected analgesics, and reported fewer days of pain when exposed to a reinterpretation intervention (Ridgeway and Mathews, 1982). There was a trend for reinterpretation to reduce number of symptoms and resumption of activities, although no differences emerged in mood.

When a combined coping intervention (including relaxation, reinterpretation and calming self-talk) was used with cardiac catheterization patients, it had positive effects on observed adjustment, anxiety and self-statements in relation to an untreated and an attention-control group, although it had no impact on self-ratings of pain and anger and observer ratings obtained after preparation (Kendall *et al.*, 1979). Similarly, Wells *et al.* (1986) found that general surgery patients (e.g. hysterectomy, cholecystotomy) exposed to a combined coping intervention (including self-monitoring, relaxation, distraction, self-statements) showed lower pre- and post-surgical anxiety, less post-surgical pain, better nurse ratings of adjustment and marginally lower use of analgesics and days to discharge than an untreated group.

Among studies teasing out the differential effects of diverse coping interventions, Kaplan *et al.* (1983) found that relaxation only, reinterpretation alone, and relaxation and reinterpretation combined were superior to an attention-only group on measures of observer distress, self-rated pain and benefits, and heart rate, in patients undergoing an electromyographic examination. No differences emerged among the three treatment groups. In contrast, with patients undergoing gall-bladder surgery, distraction reduced post-surgery anxiety and self-reports of pain compared with relaxation and a no-treatment group (Pickett and Clum, 1982).

A series of investigations explored the effectiveness of relaxation v. distraction in patients undergoing dental restoration. One study found that both relaxation and distraction improved patient and dentist ratings of discomfort (but not heart rate; Corah *et al.*, 1979a). However, while electrodermal activity was lower with relaxation, it actually increased with distraction. The results of one other study showed less observer distress for both distraction and relaxation, reduced anxiety for relaxation alone, and no differences for anesthesia or placement of amalgam (Corah *et al.*, 1979b). A final study showed that both relaxation and distraction decreased autonomic sensations but anxiety and helplessness were only reduced in relaxation patients. There were no differences in dentist ratings or electrodermal activity (Corah *et al.*, 1981). Comparing three different forms of distraction (audio comedy, video comedy, video game), Seyrek *et al.* (1984) found that each type reduced reports of physical sensations. While the video comedy and video game interventions decreased (or failed to increase) patient discomfort, they were also found to increase the frequency of non-specific electrodermal responses.

Coping v. information

Two studies presented endoscopy patients with a videotape depicting a patient undergoing the procedure, showing an average amount of distress and receiving calming talk by the nurse (combined information and coping) either zero, one or three times (Shipley *et al.*, 1978, 1979). With novice—but not experienced— patients, three viewings resulted in less tranquilizer required, lower self- and other-ratings of anxiety, and lower heart rate. Both novice and experienced sensitizers (based on Epstein and Fenz, 1967) showed decreased heart rate with more viewings, while repressors generally showed increased heart rate with exposure to the information/coping intervention. Further, experienced sensitizers—but not repressors—also had lower behavioral ratings of anxiety, with the three viewings. There was no effect on self-ratings of anxiety or discomfort or on amount of tranquilizer required. Finally, combined information and reinterpretation were found to be superior to information alone for general surgery patients, in terms of nurse ratings of anxiety and perceived ability to cope but not in terms of medication usage, discharge or physiological variables (Langer *et al.*, 1975).

Five studies compared the differential effectiveness of a pure information with a pure coping intervention. Among cholecystectomy and hysterectomy patients, sensitizers in the relaxation group reported less postoperative pain than sensitizers in an information and an information plus relaxation group (Scott and Clum, 1984). They also expressed lower anxiety than sensitizers in the combined group and received less analgesia than sensitizers in the information group. Similarly, avoiders in the relaxation group requested and received less combination medications than avoiders in the information group but showed equivalent postoperative pain and anxiety.

In a study of hysterectomy patients, those who received a reinterpretation-based coping intervention took fewer oral analgesics, were given fewer analgesic injections, had fewer post-discharge days of pain and tended to have fewer symptoms than those who received procedural, sensory and reassuring information. No differences emerged for self-reported mood or for post-discharge activity level (Ridgeway and Mathews, 1982). Similarly, Langer *et al.* (1975) found that, in comparison with general information, a reinterpretation coping device reduced observer ratings of preoperative fear and ability to cope, number of pain relievers requested and proportion of patients requesting sedatives, and tended to reduce hospital stay among patients undergoing major surgery. There were no differences in physiological measures. The coping intervention was also generally superior to a combined information and coping group.

With cardiac catheterization, results showed that patients receiving a combined coping intervention (emphasizing relaxation, reinterpretation and calming self-talk) were rated as better adjusted by the staff and showed more sustained reductions in self-ratings of anxiety than patients receiving general information, although no differences emerged on self-ratings of pain and anger or in observer ratings obtained after receiving the intervention (Kendall *et al.*, 1979). Among dental surgery patients, a coping intervention (consisting of relaxation, distraction, reinterpretation and calming self-talk) produced better observer ratings of adjustment than procedural and sensory information (Martelli *et al.*, 1987). Moreover, while high-information-preference patients showed better adjustment, less pain, greater satisfaction (and less anxiety) when they received the information v. coping intervention, low-information-preference patients showed a better overall response with the coping v. the information intervention.

Conclusions

The use of relaxation prior to aversive diagnostic and surgical procedures appears to be associated with a variety of benefits in comparison with both untreated and attention-control groups (Aiken and Henrichs, 1971; Burish and Lyles, 1981; Wilson, 1981; Kaplan *et al.*, 1982; Lyles *et al.*, 1982; Wilson *et al.*, 1982; Burish *et al.*, 1987; Carey and Burish, 1987; Domar *et al.*, 1987; cf. Scott and Clum, 1984). Variants on the relaxation technique, including deep muscle relaxation, hypnosis and systematic desensitization, also appear to be effective for patients (Morrow and Morell, 1982; Redd *et al.*, 1982; Morrow, 1984, 1986). While there is some suggestion that systematic desensitization may be more beneficial than relaxation alone (Morrow, 1986), this study differs from others along several dimensions, including the use of guided imagery and whether patients were specifically helped and instructed to use relaxation during chemotherapy.

In addition, positive outcomes are associated with the use of reinterpretation alone and reinterpretation in combination with relaxation and other coping techniques (Kendall *et al.*, 1979; Wells *et al.*, 1986). Investigations comparing the differential effectiveness of particular coping techniques are limited and the results are unclear. Findings range from no differences (Kaplan *et al.*, 1983), to a superiority of distraction over relaxation (Pickett and Clum, 1982), to a superiority of relaxation over distraction (Corah *et al.*, 1979a,b, 1981). It is difficult to make sense of these differences, since the studies vary in the amount of training and practice provided to subjects. When the effects of a coping intervention are compared to the effects of an information intervention, the former is generally found to produce more benefits for patients (Langer *et al.*, 1975; Kendall *et al.*, 1979; Ridgeway and Mathews, 1982; Martelli *et al.*, 1987). Combined coping and information are also somewhat more effective than information alone (Langer *et al.*, 1975).

Taken together, the results suggest that coping is successful in reducing anxiety (monitoring and blunting hypothesis) and in decreasing pain and speeding recovery (minimax hypothesis). Finally, consistent with the monitoring and blunting hypothesis, there appears to be a role for individual differences. While high-information-preference patients fare better with information, low-informa- tion-preference patients fare better with a coping intervention (Martelli *et al.*, 1987). Other studies have also found effects for high- v. low-fear subjects and sensitizers v. repressors (Shipley *et al.*, 1978, 1979; Wilson, 1981; Wilson *et al.*, 1982; Scott and Clum, 1984). However, the measures used are psychometrically inadequate or unexplored and the findings are somewhat inconsistent and difficult to interpret. A further methodological problem with virtually all of the studies is that while information patients typically receive a relatively brief, standardized protocol, the coping patients also receive personalized practice sessions and instructions to continue practicing (see Martelli *et al.*, 1987, for an exception). Thus, differences between information and coping interventions may, in part, be attributable to procedural differences such as the amount of personal attention and practice exposure the individual receives. To date, no evidence bears on this possibility.

It would seem useful to further explore and refine the efficacy of various coping interventions. In addition, there may be some important, but as yet unexamined, person by situation interactions. For example, some individuals—e.g. high monitors/low blunters—have been shown to engage in more scanning of internal cues than other individuals—e.g. low monitors/high blunters (Miller, 1989a, b; Miller *et al.*, 1988). Techniques such as progressive muscle relaxation, which require attention, discrimination and manipulation of bodily tension, may be more suitable for high monitors/low blunters, whereas low monitors/high blunters may fare better with relaxation procedures such as guided imagery that distract attention away from bodily cues of arousal. Similarly, low monitors/high blunters may benefit more from distraction than do high monitors/low blunters, since distraction allows them to effectively block out threat-relevant information. High monitors/low blunters, on the other hand, may benefit more from reinter- pretation, since it enables them to cognitively process information but restruc- tures it into a less threatening form.

Control studies

Control

Relative to a no-treatment group, one study found that a preoperative control-oriented intervention (the teaching of coughing and deep breathing) improved patients' ability to breathe and cough postoperatively but did not decrease days in hospital (King and Tarsitano, 1982). With a cholecystectomy and herniorrhaphy sample, no differences emerged between a pre-admission intervention (teaching such behaviors as breathing exercises and coughing) and a no-treatment control (Johnson *et al.*, 1978b; see also Johnson and Leventhal, 1974). Mills and Krantz (1979) found that blood donor patients, given a choice of arm, showed reduced nurse interventions and self-rated discomfort and pain relative to patients not offered a choice, but did not differ on performance under stress. In comparison with an attention group, control (self-help) had no impact on mood, days to discharge or time at home for cataract extraction patients (Hill, 1982).

Among patients undergoing dental restoration, provision of a control response (volume control) over distracting music reduced autonomic sensations but did not undercut feelings of helplessness and anxiety or change electrodermal responses, cavity preparation and amalgam placement (Corah *et al.*, 1981). Finally, when dental patients were provided with a button so that they could signal the dentist to stop (control), they actually showed more non-specific electrodermal responses (i.e. greater arousal) than a group not provided with a signalling device (Corah *et al.*, 1978). A follow-up study showed no effects of a signaling device on self- or observer-ratings of anxiety or on heart rate or electrodermal arousal (Corah *et al.*, 1979a).

Combined information, coping and control

Four studies explored the combined effects of an information/coping/control intervention on patient response, and compared it to a no-treatment control. In a classic study by Egbert *et al.* (1964), patients undergoing abdominal surgery received a combined message providing reassurance and describing postoperative pain, relaxation techniques and pain-controlling behaviors. The combined group showed less use of narcotics, fewer days in hospital and lower observer-, but not self-, rated pain.

An investigation of gynecological patients undergoing laparoscopy showed a number of benefits for patients receiving procedural, sensory and temporal information along with suggestions on how to cope with fear and speed recovery, including: less pre-surgical anxiety; less postoperative pain, thirst and nausea; greater vigor, and better recovery, time to drink and eat solids and return to activities (Wallace, 1984). Several variables showed no effects, including post-anxiety, four of the five affect scales, pre-surgical pain and pain at 2 hours after surgery, time to discharge, self-rated recovery, symptoms after surgery, blood pressure, heart rate, use of doctor-prescribed and over-the-counter medications and use of medical care. A combination intervention was also found to reduce the pain associated with IUD insertion (Newton and Reading, 1977). In contrast, when patients undergoing a routine pelvic examination were exposed to a combined information, coping and control message, it had no significant impact on overt distress, pulse rate or self-reported fear (Fuller *et al.*, 1978).

No differences emerged between surgery patients (gastrointestinal and gynecological) receiving a combined intervention (procedural and sensory information; coping by reappraisal, self-talk and distraction; and control via pain management and recovery exercises) and information alone on self-reported distress, pain, symptoms or reports of coping behaviors used (Ziemer, 1983). However, in a gastrointestinal endoscopy sample, a group given a combined intervention (procedural, sensory, relaxation, breathing and mouth behaviors) expressed less discomfort than a group given procedural and sensory information alone. Low-control subjects in the combined group experienced less discomfort, distress, pain and anxiety than those in the information-alone group (Padilla *et al.*, 1981).

When control and information were combined (without coping), Johnson and Leventhal (1974) found that it relieved gagging but increased time for tube passage in endoscopy patients, compared with an untreated group, and had no effect on tranquilizers, heart rate or signs of overt distress. Among cataract extraction patients, control (discomfort reduction and self-care) combined with sensory information reduced time at home but did not affect anxiety and depression, ambulation or days to discharge (Hill, 1982). While coronary artery bypass patients receiving either information alone or information plus control responses (oriented toward recovery and pain management) fared better than an attention-only group, no differences emerged between the two experimental groups (Anderson, 1987). In contrast, with blood donation subjects, while information (sensory and procedural) combined with control (choice of arm) reduced nurse interventions compared to a no-treatment control, it increased them in relation to either information or control alone (Mills and Krantz, 1979). Similar effects obtained for ratings of discomfort and pain.

Conclusions

Control—in the form of choice—showed significant benefits in the one study that explored this (Mills and Krantz, 1979). When control entails the management of pain and discomfort associated with the immediate and long-term impact of a medical procedure, it showed positive effects in one study (King and Tarsitano, 1982), but generally made no difference in three other studies (Johnson and Leventhal, 1974; Johnson *et al.*, 1978b; Hill, 1982). A further form of control, involving a device to stop an aversive procedure, generally did not seem beneficial (Corah *et al.*, 1978, 1979a) although having a device that controls a distractor fared somewhat better (Corah *et al.*, 1981).

In three of four studies, a combination of control, coping and information was generally found to have neutral to positive effects on patient outcomes (Egbert *et al.*, 1964; Newton and Reading, 1977; Wallace, 1984; cf. Fuller *et al.*, 1978), relative to an untreated comparison group. In relation to information alone, the combined intervention showed some advantage in one study (Padilla *et al.*, 1981) but not in a second study (Ziemer, 1983). Finally, combining information and control led to neutral to positive effects in two studies (Johnson and Leventhal, 1974; Hill, 1982), but to negative effects in another study (Mills and Krantz, 1979). This may be due to the type of control manipulated: simple choice combined with information seemed to have less impact than a combined information and pain management intervention.

Despite the widespread theoretical emphasis on control, and the demonstrated positive effects of having control in a variety of different domains, it is remarkable how few studies actually manipulate this variable in the medical context. This may reflect how difficult it is to find aspects of the procedure or environment over which patients can exert some meaningful control from a minimax perspective. In a laboratory setting, for example, subjects can be provided with a number of simple and complex responses to avoid, escape or reduce aversive events (Miller, 1979, 1980a). In a medical setting, where patients must, of necessity, undergo the aversive procedure, avoidance and escape are not generally viable options. Reduction of the aversive event is a more realistic goal. The only means to do this is via pain management, since the stimulus components of the procedure are medically determined and invariant. However, the teaching of breathing and other exercises to control pain may be generally ineffective without a certain level of training and practice, which is often impractical within the hospital setting.

In the absence of this, patients' self-efficacy expectations that they can successfully execute the required responses may be diminished (Bandura, 1985). This, in turn, may heighten anxiety and arousal, thereby offsetting any positive effects of the manipulation. Further, drawing patients' attention to the limited control that they are able to exert may, at the same time, make them exquisitely aware of all the variables that they cannot control (see also Folkman, 1984). This may be relevant to the other form of control available in medical settings, which is choice (e.g. over some particular aspect of the procedure). Adding information to choice appears to undercut its positive effects and this may be because informed patients realize how trivial their available control response is. The inclusion of coping instructions may help mitigate these effects. Finally, since individuals have been found to differ in their desires, expectations and attributions for control (Wallston *et al.*, 1987), the addition of relevant dispositional measures would be useful.

INTEGRATION OF THEORY AND EVIDENCE

Taken together, the data suggest a different pattern of results for information, coping and control interventions. While information (particularly procedural and sensory) and control (particularly pain management) can sometimes facilitate patient adjustment, they can also have the reverse effect. In contrast, the consequences of coping interventions, such as relaxation, are generally beneficial and superior to those of information. These discrepant findings can be integrated within the theoretical frameworks proposed here. Coping interventions, which enable individuals to selectively process aversive events in a less negative way, help them to reduce anxiety and manage their emotions in the face of threat (monitoring and blunting hypothesis). This, in turn, can attenuate the experience of pain and thereby may minimize the total aversiveness of the experience for the individual (minimax hypothesis). Information, on the one hand, generally focuses the individual on the negative aspects of the event and so interferes with anxiety reduction. However, for some individuals, this can be compensated for by the increased certainty that information allows (monitoring and blunting hypothesis) and/or by its utility in providing access to and contact with external sources of expertise (minimax hypothesis). Finally, while control should be stress-reducing when it enables the individual to provide an upper limit on how bad the situation can become (minimax hypothesis), direct forms of control are not generally available in a hospital setting, thereby undercutting the effectiveness of this manipulation.

Thus, in medical and surgical contexts, coping appears to be the most effective intervention for patients, by virtue of its implications for both arousal and adjustment. Information, on the other hand, may have particular value for a subset of patients, while control may have value when the response is a meaningful one. Future research should continue to untangle these effects, while simultaneously and systematically manipulating important situational variables (e.g. length of training) and dispositional tendencies (e.g. information, coping and control preferences). Finally, in terms of patient response, most of the current work assesses self- and other-rated distress and pain, various physical indices of impact and recovery and psychophysiological variables. It would also be informative to extend this network of measures to include assessments of immunological function (Levy, 1983).

ACKNOWLEDGEMENTS

We are indebted to Adina Birnbaum and Farah Quintos for their help. This chapter was partially supported by Temple University Research Incentive Fund to the first author.

REFERENCES

Aiken, L. H., and Heinrichs, T. F. (1971). Systematic relaxation as a nursing intervention technique with open heart surgery patients. *Nursing Research*, **20**, 212–217.

Anderson, E. A. (1987). Preoperative preparation for cardiac surgery facilitates recovery, reduces psychological distress, and reduces the incidence of acute postoperative hypertension. *Journal of Consulting and Clinical Psychology*, **55**, 513–520.

Andrew, J. M. (1970). Recovery from surgery, with and without preparatory instruction, for three coping styles. *Journal of Personality and Social Psychology*, **15**, 223–226.

Auerbach, S. M. (in press). Stress management and coping research in the health care setting: An overview and methodological commentary. *Journal of Consulting and Clinical Psychology*.

Auerbach, S. M., and Kendall, P. C. (1978). Sex differences in anxiety response and adjustment to dental surgery: Effects of general vs. specific preoperative information. *Journal of Clinical Psychology*, **34**, 309–313.

Auerbach, S. M., Kendall, P. C., Cuttler, H.F., and Levitt, N.R. (1976). Anxiety, locus of control, type of preparatory information, and adjustment to dental surgery. *Journal of Consulting and Clinical Psychology*, **44**, 809–818.

Auerbach, S. M., Martelli, M. F., and Mercuri, L. G. (1983). Anxiety, information, interpersonal impacts, and adjustment to a stressful health care situation. *Journal of Personality and Social Psychology*, **44**, 1284–1296.

Bandura, A. (1985). *Social Foundations of Thought and Action: A Social Cognitive Theory.* Englewood Cliffs, NJ: Prentice-Hall.

Burish, T. G., and Lyles, J. N. (1981). Effectiveness of relaxation training in reducing adverse reactions to cancer chemotherapy. *Journal of Behavioral Medicine*, **4**, 65–78.

Burish, T. G., Carey, M. P., Krozely, M. G., and Greco, F. A. (1987). Conditioned side effects induced by cancer chemotherapy: Prevention through behavioral treatment. *Journal of Consulting and Clinical Psychology*, **55**, 42–48.

Carey, M. P., and Burish, T. G. (1987). Providing relaxation training to cancer chemotherapy patients: A comparison of three delivery techniques. *Journal of Consulting and Clinical Psychology*, **55**, 732–737.

Carey, M. P., and Burish, T. G. (1988). Etiology and treatment of the psychological side effects associated with cancer chemotherapy: A critical review and discussion. *Psychological Bulletin*, **104** (3), 307–325.

Carver, C. S., Scheier, M. F., and Weintraub, J. K. (1989). Assessing coping strategies: A theoretically based approach. *Journal of Personality and Social Psychology*, **56** (2), 267–283.

Cohen, F., and Lazarus, R. S. (1973). Active coping processes, coping dispositions, and recovery from surgery. *Psychosomatic Medicine*, **35**, 375–389.

Corah, N. L., Bissell, G. D., and Illig, S. J. (1978). Effect of perceived control on stress reaction in adult dental patients. *Journal of Dental Research*, **57**, 74–76.

Corah, N. L., Gale, E. N., and Illig, S. J. (1979a). Psychological stress reduction during dental procedures. *Journal of Dental Research*, **58**, 1347–1351.

Corah, N. L., Gale, E. N., and Illig, S. J. (1979b). The use of relaxation and distraction to reduce psychological stress during dental procedures. *Journal of the American Dental Association*, **98**, 390–394.

Corah, N. L., Gale, E. N., Pace, L. F., and Seyrek, S. K. (1981). Relaxation and musical programming as means of reducing psychological stress during dental procedures. *Journal of the American Dental Association*, **103**, 232–234.

Domar, A. D., Noe, J. M., and Benson, H. (1987). The preoperative use of the relaxation response with ambulatory surgery patients. *Journal of Human Stress*, **13**, 101–107.

Egbert, L. D., Battit, G. E., Welch, E. C., and Bartlett, M. K. (1964). Reduction of postoperative pain by encouragement and instruction of patients. *New England Journal of Medicine*, **270**, 825–827.

Epstein, S., and Fenz, W. D. (1967). The detection of areas of emotional stress through variations in perceptual threshold and physiological arousal. *Journal of Experimental Research in Personality*, **2**, 191–199.

Finesilver, C. (1978). Preparation of adult patients for cardiac catheterization and coronary cineangiography. *International Journal of Nursing Studies*, **15**, 211–221.

Folkman, S. (1984). Personal control and stress and coping processes: A theoretical analysis. *Journal of Personality and Social Psychology*, **46**, 839–852.

Folkman, S., and Lazarus, R. S. (1980). An analysis of coping in a middle-age community sample. *Journal of Health and Social Behavior*, **21**, 219–239.

Fuller, S. S., Endress, M. P., and Johnson, J. E. (1978). The effects of cognitive and behavioral control on coping with an aversive health examination. *Journal of Human Stress*, **4**, 18–25.

Gard, D., Edwards, P. W., Harris, J., and McCormack, G. (1988). Sensitizing effects of pretreatment measures on cancer chemotherapy nausea and vomiting. *Journal of Consulting and Clinical Psychology*, **56**, 80–84.

Gil, K. M. (1984). Coping effectively with invasive medical procedures: A descriptive model. *Clinical Psychology Review*, **4**, 339–362.

Goldstein, M. J. (1959). The relationship between coping and avoiding behavior and response to fear-arousing propaganda. *Journal of Abnormal and Social Psychology*, **58**, 247–252.

Hartfield, M. J., and Cason, C. L. (1981). Effect of information on emotional responses during barium enema. *Nursing Research*, **30**, 151–155.

Hartfield, M. J., Cason, C. L., and Cason, G. J. (1982). Effects of information about a threatening procedure on patients' expectations and emotional distress. *Nursing Research*, **31**, 202–206.

Hill, B. J. (1982). Sensory information, behavioral instructions and coping with sensory alteration surgery. *Nursing Research*, **31**, 17–21.

Johnson, J. E., and Leventhal, H. (1974). Effects of accurate expectations and behavioral instructions on reactions during a noxious medical examination. *Journal of Personality and Social Psychology*, **29**, 710–718.

Johnson, J. E., Morrissey, J. F., and Leventhal, H. (1973). Psychological preparation for an endoscopic examination. *Gastrointestinal Endoscopy*, **19**, 180–182.

Johnson, J. E., Rice, V. H., Fuller, S. S., and Endress, M. P. (1978a). Sensory information, instruction in a coping strategy, and recovery from surgery. *Research in Nursing and Health*, **1**, 4–17.

Johnson, J. E., Fuller, S. S., Endress, M. P., and Rice, V. H. (1978b). Altering patients' responses to surgery: An extension and replication. *Research in Nursing and Health*, **1**, 111–121.

Johnston, M. (1980). Anxiety in surgical patients. *Psychological Medicine*, **10**, 145–152.

Kaplan, R. M., Atkins, C. J., and Lenhard, L. (1982). Coping with a stressful sigmoidoscopy: Evaluation of cognitive and relaxation preparations. *Journal of Behavioral Medicine*, **15**, 67–82.

Kaplan, R. M., Metzger, G., and Jablecki, C. (1983). Tolerance for a painful electromyographic examination. *Psychosomatic Medicine*, **45**, 155–162.

Kendall, P. C., Williams, L., Pechacek, T. F., Graham, L. E., Shisslak, C., and Herzoff, N. (1979). Cognitive–behavioral and patient education interventions in cardiac catheterization procedures: The Palo Alto Medical Psychology Project. *Journal of Consulting and Clinical Psychology*, **47**, 49–58.

King, I., and Tarsitano, B. (1982). The effect of structured and unstructured preoperative teaching: A replication. *Nursing Research*, **31**, 324–329.

Krantz, D. S., Baum, A., and Wideman, M. (1980). Assessment of preferences for self-treatment and information in health care. *Journal of Personality and Social Psychology*, **39**, 977–990.

Langer, E. J., Janis, I., and Wolfer, J. (1975). Reduction of psychological stress in surgical patients. *Journal of Experimental Social Psychology*, **11**, 155–165.

Levy, S. M. (1983). Behavioral medicine and cancer: An emerging field of inquiry. *Behavioral Medicine Update*, **5**, 7–11.

Lyles, J. N., Burish, T. G., Krozely, M. G., and Oldham, R. K. (1982). Efficacy of relaxation training and guided imagery in reducing the aversiveness of cancer chemotherapy. *Journal of Consulting and Clinical Psychology*, **50**, 509–524.

Martelli, M. F., Auerbach, S. M., Alexander, J., and Mercuri, L. G. (1987). Stress management in the health care setting: Matching interventions with patient coping styles. *Journal of Consulting and Clinical Psychology*, **55**, 201–207.

Miller, S. M. (1979). Controllability and human stress: Method, evidence and theory. *Behavior Research and Theory*, **17**, 287–304.

Miller, S. M. (1980a). Why having control reduces stress: If I can stop the roller coaster I don't want to get off. In: M. Seligman and J. Garber (eds), *Human Helplessness: Theory and Applications*. New York: Academic Press.

Miller, S. M. (1980b). When is a little knowledge a dangerous thing? Coping with stressful life-events by monitoring vs. blunting. In: S. Levine and H. Ursin (eds), *Coping and Health*, Proceedings of a NATO conference. New York: Plenum Press.

Miller, S. M. (1981). Predictability and human stress: Towards a clarification of evidence and theory. In: L. Berkowitz (ed.), *Advances in Experimental Social Psychology* (Vol. 14). New York: Academic Press.

Miller, S. M. (1987). Monitoring and blunting: Validation of a questionnaire to assess different styles for coping with stress. *Journal of Personality and Social Psychology*, **52**, 345–353.

Miller, S. M. (1989a). To see or not to see: Cognitive informational styles in the coping process. In: M. Rosenbaum (ed.), *Learned Resourcefulness: On Coping Skills, Self-Regulation, and Adaptive Behavior*. New York: Springer.

Miller, S. M. (1989b). Individual differences in the coping process: what to know and when to know it. In: B. Carpenter (ed.) *Personal Coping: Theory, Research and Application*. New York: Praeger.

Miller, S. M., and Birnbaum, A. (1988). Putting the life back into life events: Toward a cognitive social learning analysis of the coping process. In: S. Fisher and J. Reason (eds), *Life Stress, Cognition, and Health*. Chichester: Wiley.

Miller, S. M., and Birnbaum, A. (1989). When to whistle while you work: A cognitive social learning approach to coping and health. In: J. J. Hurrell, S. L. Sauter and C. Cooper (eds), *Job Control and Worker Health*. Chichester: Wiley.

Miller, S. M., and Green, M. (1985). Coping with threat and frustration: Origins, nature and development. In: M. Lewis and C. Saarni (eds), *Socialization of Emotions* (Vol. 5). New York: Plenum Press.

Miller, S. M., and Mangan, C. E. (1983). The interacting effects of information and coping style in adapting to gynecologic stress: Should the doctor tell all? *Journal of Personality and Social Psychology*, **45**, 223–236.

Miller, S. M., Brody, D. S., and Summerton, J. (1988). Styles of coping with threat: Implications for health. *Journal of Personality and Social Psychology*, **54**, 345–353.

Mills, T., and Krantz, D. S. (1979). Information, choice, and reaction to stress: A field experiment in a blood bank with laboratory analogue. *Journal of Personality and Social Psychology*, **37**, 608–620.

Morrow, G. R. (1984). Appropriateness of taped versus live relaxation in the systematic desensitization of anticipatory nausea and vomiting in cancer patients. *Journal of Consulting and Clinical Psychology*, **52**, 1098–1099.

Morrow, G. R. (1986). Effect of cognitive hierarchy in the systematic desensitization treatment of anticipatory nausea in cancer patients: A component comparison with relaxation only, counseling, and no treatment. *Cognitive Therapy and Research*, **10**, 421–446.

Morrow, G. R., and Morrell, C. (1982). Behavioral treatment for the anticipatory nausea and vomiting induced by cancer chemotherapy. *The New England Journal of Medicine*, **307**, 1476–1480.

Newton, J. R., and Reading, A. E. (1977). The effects of psychological preparation on pain at intrauterine device insertion. *Contraception*, **16**, 523–532.

Padilla, G. V., Grant, M. M., Rains, B. L., Hansen, B. C., Bergstione, N., Wong, H. L., Hanson, R., and Kubo, W. (1981). Distress reduction and the effects of preparatory teaching films and patient control. *Research in Nursing and Health*, **4**, 375–387.

Pickett, C., and Clum, G. A. (1982). Comparative treatment strategies and their interaction with locus of control in the reduction of postsurgical pain and anxiety. *Journal of Consulting and Clinical Psychology*, **50**, 439–441.

Redd, W. H., Andresen, G. V., and Minigawa, R. Y. (1982). Hypnotic control of anticipatory emesis in patients receiving cancer chemotherapy. *Journal of Consulting and Clinical Psychology*, **50**, 14–19.

Ridgeway, V., and Mathews, A. (1982). Psychological preparation for surgery: A comparison of methods. *British Journal of Clinical Psychology*, **21**, 271–280.

Rotter, J. B. (1966). Generalized expectancies for internal versus external control of reinforcement. *Psychological Monographs*, **80**, (whole No. 609).

Schultheis, K., Peterson, L. and Selby, V. (1987). Preparation for stressful medical procedures and person × treatment interactions. *Clinical Psychology Review*, **7**, 329–352.

Scott, L. E., and Clum, G. A. (1984). Examining the interaction effects of coping style and brief interventions in the treatment of postsurgical pain. *Pain*, **20**, 279–291.

Seyrek, S. K., Corah, N. L., and Pace, L. F. (1984). Comparison of three distraction techniques in reducing stress in dental patients. *Journal of the American Dental Association*, **108**, 327–329.

Shipley, R. H., Butt, J. H., Horwitz, B., and Farbry, J. E. (1978). Preparation for a stressful medical procedure: Effect of amount of stimulus preexposure and coping style. *Journal of Consulting and Clinical Psychology*, **46**, 499–507.

Shipley, R. H., Butt, J. H., and Horwitz, E. A. (1979). Preparation to reexperience a stressful medical examination: Effect of repetitious videotape exposure and coping style. *Journal of Consulting and Clinical Psychology*, **47**, 485–492.

Suls, J., and Wan, C. K. (in press). The effects of sensory and procedural information on adaptation to stressful medical procedures and pain: A meta-analysis. *Journal of Consulting and Clinical Psychology*.

Taylor, S. E., and Clark, L. F. (1986). Does information improve adjustment to noxious medical procedures? In: M. J. Saks and L. Saxe (eds), *Advances in Applied Social Psychology* (Vol. 3). Hillsdale, NJ: Erlbaum.

Thompson, S. C. (1981). Will it hurt less if I can control it? A complex answer to a simple question. *Psychological Bulletin*, **90**, 89–101.

Vernon, D. T. A., and Bigelow, D. A. (1974). Effect of information about a potentially stressful situation on response to stress impact. *Journal of Personality and Social Psychology*, **29**, 50–59.

Wallace, L. M. (1984). Psychological preparation as a method of reducing the stress of surgery. *Journal of Human Stress*, **10**, 62–79.

Wallston, K. A., Wallston, B. S., Smith, S., and Dobbins, C. J. (1987). Perceived control and health. *Current Psychological Research and Reviews*, **6**, 5–25.

Watkins, L. O., Weaver, L., and Odegaard, V. (1986). Preparation for cardiac catheterization: Tailoring the content of instruction to coping style. *Heart and Lung*, **15**, 382–389.

Weiss, J. M. (1970). Somatic effects of predictable and unpredictable shock. *Psychosomatic Medicine*, **32**, 397–409.

Wells, J. K., Howard, G. S., Nowlin, W. F., and Vargas, M. J. (1986). Presurgical anxiety and postsurgical pain and adjustment: Effects of a stress inoculation procedure. *Journal of Consulting and Clinical Psychology*, **54**, 831–835.

Williams, J. G. L., Jones, J. R., Workhoven, M. N., and Williams, B. (1975). The psychological control of preoperative anxiety. *Psychophysiology*, **12**, 50–54.

Wilson, J. F. (1981). Behavioral preparation for surgery: Benefit or harm? *Journal of Behavioral Medicine*, **4**, 79–102.

Wilson, J. F., Moore, R. W., Randolph, S., and Hanson, B. J. (1982). Behavioral preparation of patients for gastrointestinal endoscopy: Information, relaxation, and coping style. *Journal of Human Stress*, **8**, 13–23.

Ziemer, M. M. (1983). Effects of information on postsurgical coping. *Nursing Research*, **32**, 282–287.

CHAPTER 7

Perceived control and the experience of pain

ARNOUD ARNTZ AND ANTON J. M. SCHMIDT
Department of Medical Psychology, University of Limburg, Maastricht, The Netherlands

INTRODUCTION

Pain can have uncontrollable aspects. Not only medical treatment, but also traditional ways of dealing with pain (taking rest, avoidance of activities) can fail to produce pain relief. Sometimes, pain results from medical treatment or from natural processes, such as childbirth, which are largely beyond the influence of the subject. Although it may seem self-evident that the experience of having no control over pain is a source of suffering in itself, the question can be posed whether having no control intensifies the experienced pain itself, and conversely, whether experiencing control over pain can diminish the pain experience. Besides the possible direct relationship between control and pain, the long-term consequence of failing to acquire control over prolonged pain is of interest, since many patients have to deal with chronic pain. Some chronic pain patients seem to suffer in a manner that is disproportionate to medical findings and display very helpless behaviour, whereas others lead fairly undisturbed lives. As will be seen, these differences may be explained by the lack of control and the associated learned helplessness experienced by the former group. Before discussing the relationship between controllability and pain, two general issues are treated. First, what is meant by 'perceiving control'? Second, what is pain and why can psychological factors influence it?

Stress, Personal Control and Health. Edited by A. Steptoe and A. Appels.
Published by John Wiley & Sons Ltd.
© ECSC–EEC–EAEC, Brussels–Luxembourg, 1989

The perception of control

Very generally, control can be defined as some behaviour (overt or covert) that reliably changes something else. Thus, when a subject is exerting control over pain, he or she behaves in a certain way that alters the pain experienced. In this chapter, control is largely taken to imply ways of decreasing, limiting or preventing aversive experiences such as pain. Thus, its use is confined to the cases where control has positive consequences. Interestingly, various studies have shown that actual control does not have any effect in the absence of the perception of a reliable relationship between the controlling response and its outcome. Control can be perceived even when it is not actually present, but may still have the same effect as real control. Thus, the belief that pain can be controlled may have positive consequences, even when the controlling response is not used. What is important, then, is the perception of control.

The experience of pain

Pain can be defined as 'an unpleasant sensory and emotional experience, associated with actual or potential tissue damage or described in terms of such damage' (IASP, 1986). This broad definition does justice to the many aspects of pain. Nociception, the sensory detection, transduction and neural transmission of noxious events, forms the basis for pain sensation. It is doubtful whether, even in the most controlled laboratory conditions, a linear relationship is demonstrable between peripheral, nociceptive activity and the pain experienced, because the nociception can be modified strongly at low levels within the nervous system (Wall and Melzack, 1985). This means that the signal that finally leads to the awareness of pain can be amplified or reduced by higher processes. Nociception and the experience of pain may even be totally unrelated: pain can be reported without nociception, as in phantom pain (Sherman *et al.*, 1987); or there can be noxious stimulation without pain sensations (Wall, 1979). Assuming that pain is a subjective sensory and emotional experience, it is clear that pain can be modified to a high degree by influencing factors such as the external environment or the focus of concentration (Sternbach, 1978). Thus, psychological factors play a very important role in the experience of pain. Analogous to (other) emotions, pain has various aspects that are not necessarily strongly interrelated, since subjective–emotional, cognitive, behavioural and physiological reactions can be distinguished.

Conclusion

A relationship between controllability and pain can be postulated on theoretical grounds. Having established this, two main questions can be raised. First, does perceiving control actually diminish pain? Second, if this is the case, why does perceived control have this influence? In addressing the first issue, a distinction should be made between various kinds of pain. The first category that will be discussed pertains to *laboratory pain*. It must be separated from naturally occurring pain, because its validity with respect to clinical pain may be questionable. However, studies of laboratory pain do allow the researcher to control pain stimulation in a systematic fashion. As will be seen, elegant experiments have been done on the influence of control over laboratory pain. In addition, *pain coping strategies* have been extensively studied in the laboratory, and the influence of perceived control on the efficacy of these will also be discussed.

The second category is *acute clinical pain*, which must be distinguished from *chronic clinical pain*. The lower boundary for chronicity is usually taken to be 6 months. It is generally accepted that the distinction between acute and chronic pain is not only of diagnostic value but also has far-reaching therapeutic consequences. It will be argued that, on balance, despite the differences between various kinds of pain, the first question can be answered in the affirmative. Finally, the last section of the chapter outlines various explanations that can be offered to explain this effect.

DOES PERCEIVED CONTROL REDUCE THE EXPERIENCE OF PAIN?

Does perceived control reduce the negative effects of laboratory pain?

As early as 1949 (Haggard, 1949), positive effects of having control over a painful stimulus upon reactions to pain in the laboratory were reported. Previous reviews on the effects of control over aversive stimuli in general have come to different conclusions. Averill (1973) and Thompson (1981) concluded that controllability does not reliably decrease the impact of aversive events. However, both reviews used broad definitions of control, which may have obscured positive effects of control defined in more restricted ways. Miller (1979) applied a more restricted definition of control and concluded that controllable aversive events may have less negative effects. In contrast with these reviews, this section is restricted to control over *noxious, painful* stimuli. Animal research, where the subjective experience of pain cannot be assessed, is not discussed. In this section, the question will be addressed whether behavioural control over the pain stimulus itself reduces the effects of laboratory pain. Controllability of aversive events is here defined as the availability of an overt response that actually modifies the event, or the perception of or belief in the availability of this response. Different modifying responses have been the object of research, e.g. escape from the event, changing its probability of occurrence or self-administration of the event (cf. Miller, 1979).

Experimental studies on controllability and pain: types of control and designs

As Miller (1979) has argued, several different types of behavioural control can be distinguished. The first is *self-administration* (SA), where subjects administer the painful stimulus to themselves, in contrast to administration by the experimenter. The second type of control is *instrumental control* (I), where the subject can (partially) avoid, escape or reduce the stimulus by some response (actual control); or believes that he or she can do so, but objectively cannot because the experimenter controls the stimulus (perceived control). In this class of experiments, the subject can, for instance, terminate the shock. In the actual control design, the group that has no control is a yoked one (every subject in the no-control group is yoked to a subject in the experimental condition so that the total amount of aversive stimulation is equal). The perceived control design is similar, except that the experimenter determines the amount of aversive stimulation, so each pair of subjects experiences the same stimulation. The third type distinguished by Miller is '*actual control equated for predictability*' (CP). Predictability can be defined as the availability of a sign that reliably signals the start, end, increase or decrease of the noxious stimulus. Predictability has been found to influence reactions to painful stimuli, and in many experiments the experimental manipulation of control is confounded with effects of predictability. For instance, when the subject can reliably stop a painful stimulus, the subject can also reliably predict *when* it stops. The subject that has no control cannot predict the end of stimulation. Therefore, designs have been developed where predictability is controlled for (for instance by providing an external cue that signals when the stimulus stops in both conditions—the only difference between conditions is that subjects in the control condition believe that they caused the termination of the stimulus, whereas subjects in the no-control group do not have this belief). The fourth type, *potential control* (P), refers to conditions where subjects believe or know that there is a controlling response available but they do not use it. Examples are studies where subjects are told that they can withdraw their hand out of the ice-water, but are (sometimes emphatically) asked not do so. There is also another design, not mentioned by Miller. In the *loss of control* design, subjects are first given control and later on deprived of it. This group is contrasted to a group that never had had control (e.g. Staub *et al.*, 1971, Exp. I).

Indices of effects of controllability

Different indices of effects of controllability have been investigated. In the present context, the following will be discussed: subjective and physiological distress during anticipation; subjective and physiological impact of the painful stimulus; tolerance/endurance of the painful stimulus; and post-exposure performance. Following Miller (1979), skin conductance responses (SCR) during anticipation and impact, as well as heart rate (HR) during impact, are summarized here as most important physiological indices. Although not strictly an *effect* of controllability, preference (subjectively expressed or actual choice) for control will also be discussed, since it highlights an important aspect of control.

Table 1 summarizes the findings of 34 studies with respect to these indices. The studies are clustered according to the type of control.

Self-administration

Eight studies investigated the effects of self-administration contrasted with administration by the experimenter (Table 1). Although preferred, self-administration does not appear to have a powerful positive effect on anticipation and on pain. However, it does not have negative effects.

Instrumental control

Instrumental control was defined as the subject's perception that he or she avoids, reduces or stops the painful stimulation by an overt response. Results of 17 studies (Table 1) indicate that instrumental control reduces anticipatory distress, increases tolerance/endurance of pain and fosters post-exposure performance. The impact of painful stimuli can be less distressing when the subject has control. However, very difficult responses or high uncertainty about the outcome of the response may lead to less positive and even negative effects of controllability, especially on physiological impact reactions (cf. Miller, 1979). For instance, the negative effect of control on SCR in the Gatchel studies has been attributed by Miller (1979) to the fact that subjects had to learn what the escape response was. In the present context, subjective impact is an important issue. Only one study (Weisenberg *et al.*, 1985, condition 1) reports a negative effect of control on experienced pain. The study has, however, several methodological shortcomings (no pre-test to assess subjective pain level; a small number of trials where control could be employed; a weak manipulation of control; and an unclear definition of the controlling response). The most conservative conclusion, then, is that controllability is certainly not worse than no control with respect to subjective pain and is superior with respect to tolerance.

Control equated for predictability

Theoretically, this design is very important, since it differentiates the effects of instrumental control over the termination of the noxious stimulation from effects of predictability. There are, indeed, indications that control can have positive effects above predictability on experienced pain, and on physiological reactions during anticipation and impact (Table 1).

Does the difficulty of the controlling response influence the effects of control on subjective pain? This question was addressed in a recent study by Arntz and De Jong (1989). Subjects had to perform IQ test-like tasks in two series, each task followed by painful electric shock. In the perceived-control condition, subjects were told that they could decrease the duration of the shock in the second series

TABLE 1. Summary of laboratory studies on the effect of control over painful stimuli

Study	Type of control	Stimulus	Preference Subjective	Preference Choice	Anticipation Subjective	Anticipation SCR	Impact Subjective	Impact SCR	HR	Tolerance/ endurance	Post-exposure performance	Other findings
Ball and Vogler (1971)	SA	S		+								
Haggard (1949)	SA	S				+[a]		+				
Pervin (1963)	SA	S	+		ns							
Staub et al. (1971, Exp. I)	SA	S					ns					
Weisenberg et al. (1985, condition 3)	SA	S					ns	ns	−	ns		
Zimbardo et al. (1966)	SA	S					+	+				
Weisenberg et al. (1985, condition 4)	SA + I	S					+	ns	+			
Bjorkstrandt (1973)	SA + CP	S				ns[a]		+				
Averill et al. (1977)	I	S		+	+							With control, Ss report more distraction and displayed lower SCL
Averill and Rosenn (1972)	I	S			ns		ns					
Bowers (1968)	I	S			+		+	ns				
Champion (1950)	I	S						+				
Corah and Boffa (1970)	I	N					+	+		+		
De Good (1975)	I	S					+					Decreased blood pressure with control
Elliott (1969)	I	S	ns[c]		ns				−			
Gatchel et al. (1977)	I	N			+			−			+	
Gatchel and Proctor (1976)	I	N				+		−	ns		+	
Hokanson et al. (1971)	I	S										Decreased blood pressure with control
Houston (1972)	I	S			+							
Lepanto et al. (1965)	I	H								+		
Pennebaker et al. (1977, Exp. I)	I	N					ns	ns				Fewer physical symptoms

Study	Type of control	Stimulus						Positive effect on performance during exposure
Sherrod et al. (1977)	I	N			ns			+
Staub et al. (1971, Exp. II)	I	S			+	+	+	
Szpiler and Epstein (1976)	I	S	+	+	−			
Weisenberg et al. (1985, condition 1)	I	S			ns	ns	−	
Arntz and De Jong (1989)	CP	S			+	+		
Geer et al. (1970)	CP	S		+	ns	ns	ns	
Glass et al. (1973)	CP	S		ns	+	ns		+
Corah and Boffa (1970)[b]	P	N			+	+	+	+
Glass et al. (1969)	P	N			+	ns	+	+
Glass et al. (1971)	P	N			ns	ns		
Pennebaker et al. (1977, Exp. II)	P	N			ns		Fewer physical symptoms	
Kilminster and Jones (1986)	P + C	CPT				ns		Higher frontalis EMG
Mills and Krantz (1979, Exp. II)	P + C	CPT			ns			+

Blank denotes not measured.
+ denotes a positive effect of controllability.
− denotes a negative effect of controllability.
ns denotes a non-significant effect of controllability.
Type of control:
SA = self-administration.
I = instrumental control.
CP = control equated for predictability.
P = potential control.
C = choice of hand (to emerge in cold water).
Stimulus:
S = shock (electric shock).
N = noise (loud noise).
H = heat.
CPT = cold pressor test (ice-water).
[a] SCR to warning signal (others are spontaneous SCRs).
[b] Here the no escape–choice v. no escape–no choice conditions are considered (choice that was not effectuated is considered as potential control).
[c] N too small

from 6 seconds to 3 seconds by giving the right answer. Actually, they always received shocks of 3 seconds. Subjects in the no-control condition also performed this task, but they were simply told that shock duration would be reduced irrespective of their performance. Thus, subjects in the no-control condition had equal or even higher predictability of the stopping of the stimulus than subjects in the perceived-control condition (who believed that shock duration would only decrease if they choose the right answer).

Figure 1 illustrates the results on subjective pain (corrected for pre-test level). Subjects in the perceived-control condition rated the shocks significantly less painful than subjects who did not believe that they could control shock duration. This study illustrates that even difficult controlling responses can lead to reduced pain experience.

Potential control

With potential control, subjects clearly tolerate more pain and perform better after pain exposure (Table 1). It is, however, notable that subjective pain is not consistently influenced by potential control. Physiological data sometimes indicate no effects of potential control. There are, however, methodological problems with the potential control design. The effect of controllability depends, of course, on the actual and perceived differences between potential control and no-control control conditions. Subjects are with varying degrees of emphasis asked, or even instructed, to refrain from using the controlling response. Thus, the experienced controllability can be limited by strong experimenter demands. Sometimes subjects who use the response are replaced by new subjects (e.g. Corah and Boffa, 1970). In the cold pressor test studies, subjects always have the option to

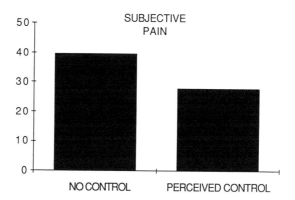

FIGURE 1. Subjective pain with and without perceived control over the termination of painful electric shock ($p < 0.05$). (Arntz and De Jong, 1989.)

withdraw their hands from the ice-water, giving them considerable potential control. Thus, clearer results may be found when the difference in controllability between conditions is maximized.

Loss of control

One study investigated the effect of loss of control (Staub *et al.*, 1971). Subjects who could control increases in shock intensity were later on deprived of control. Compared with the group who had never had control, they rated pain higher and showed lower shock tolerance. This study indicates that loss of control may be even worse than never having had control.

Conclusions

The question whether perceived control reduces the negative effects of laboratory pain can be answered with a qualified yes: perceived control *can*, but not always does, reduce the negative effects of laboratory pain. Its effects depend on a number of factors, including the effect measure, the type of control and its salience.

Concerning the different measures, the dissociation between physiological, subjective and behavioural indices is remarkable. On the behavioural level, unequivocal positive effects are found on pain tolerance/endurance and on post-exposure performance. Physiological anticipation effects indicate that, with control, anticipatory distress is equal to or less than that present without control. Physiological impact data show equivocal results, with the negative effects of control possibly depending on uncertainty about the success of the controlling response in some studies. Nevertheless, there is a tendency towards a positive effect of having control on physiological impact reactions. At the subjective level, the effects of control on anticipation and impact appear to be equal to or less than those experienced without control: if control does not do any good, it does not do any harm either. In the present context tolerance/endurance and subjective pain are most important: people are more disturbed by their experience of pain than by physiological reactions. Therefore, our conclusions with respect to the effects of control on laboratory pain must be more positive than those of Averill (1973) and Thompson (1981).

The effects of control appear to vary with different types of control. Control over the initiation of a painful stimulus has only a limited positive effect on the impact of the stimulus. In contrast, control over the end of stimulation or over increase of noxious stimulation has more powerful positive effects. The effects on tolerance are most clear: when the subject can terminate the stimulus or control its maximum intensity, tolerance and endurance are higher. This finding is of great clinical importance in itself, for in clinical pain, tolerance and endurance of experienced pain influence to what extent patients can function normally or see themselves as ill, disabled, in need of medication or restricted. Theoretically, this observation indicates *why* control can have positive effects on the experience of pain. We will return to this issue later.

The positive effects of perceived control clearly depend on the degree of certainty the subject has that the behavioural response will have an effect. Thus, Averill (1973) and Miller (1979) conclude that only when there is high certainty that the controlling response will be efficacious do positive effects of perceived control emerge.

In conclusion, the inference that 'if control does not do any good, it does not do any harm either' could be more positive if experimental studies were more rigorous methodologically. First, the intensity of the pain stimulus should be individually adjusted, since subjects differ enormously in experienced pain intensity. Without controlling the individual level, inter-subject variance can obscure the effects of control versus no-control. Second, predictability should be controlled. Third, only behavioural responses that have a salient relationship with their presumed effects should be used. Fourth, the differences between control and no-control manipulations should be maximized (this is certainly not the case in cold pressor test studies). Last, and most important: the positive effects of having control depend on the subject's perception that he or she can limit or terminate the noxious stimulation. Therefore, experimental manipulations should concentrate on optimizing these differences.

Pain coping strategies and perceived control in the laboratory

If the source of pain cannot be controlled, the experience of pain seems to be inevitable. However, it has been shown that various pain coping strategies can be employed to promote pain endurance and to reduce suffering. In the following, the role of perceived control in the application of such strategies will be discussed. In this context, perceived control is defined as the perception that coping methods can be applied during pain, and will have positive effects on the subjective pain experience, on pain tolerance or on pain endurance.

Pain coping strategies

A variety of pain coping strategies have been investigated in the laboratory: relaxation, distraction, positive self-statements, imagery strategies, hypnosis, stress inoculation training, cognitive transformation of the situation, etc. Research comparing several strategies indicates that vivid distracting mental activity (via internal or external stimuli) is a superior strategy (Kanfer and Goldfoot, 1966; Grimm and Kanfer, 1976; Worthington, 1978; Beers and Karoly, 1979; for reviews: Tan, 1982; Turk *et al.*, 1983). Investigation of spontaneous coping strategies also indicates that vivid distraction is most powerful (Rosenbaum, 1980). Tolerance is found to be the most sensitive parameter, while pain threshold and subjective discomfort seem to be less influenced by these strategies.

Perceived control and pain coping strategies

Several forms of control that the subject can exercise over the application of coping strategies have been investigated. In general, from this research it can be concluded that perceiving control over the practice of the strategy is a powerful factor, and is probably a necessary condition for demonstrating its effectiveness.

To begin with, various kinds of *choice* are found to have positive effects. Choice of coping strategy enhances pain tolerance compared with prescribed strategies (Avia and Kanfer, 1980). Choice of elements of the coping method is also important. The effects of vivid imagination of distracting scenes on pain tolerance and on subjective pain were higher when subjects could choose the content of what should be imagined, compared to prescribed content (Worthington, 1978). It is interesting to note that subjects who chose the imagery content had more vivid imagery, and that vividness correlated with increased tolerance ($r = 0.41$) and decreased subjective pain ($r = -0.30$). Personal influence over the timing of external distraction has also been found to be important: subjects who could advance distracting slides at their own rate tolerated cold pressor pain longer than yoked volunteers (Kanfer and Seidner, 1973).

These findings might be attributed to the more powerful distracting properties of self-chosen and self-paced stimuli, rather than perceived control over the strategy. However, several studies have found that perceived control itself is important. In a second experiment, Kanfer and Seidner (1973) showed that contingent positive reinforcement of a coping response enhanced cold pressor tolerance more than mere distraction or non-contingent positive reinforcement. Thus controllability of reinforcement (controllability defined in terms of learning theory as contingency between response and reinforcement) of a pain coping response enhances pain tolerance. It can be concluded that control over reinforcement of coping fosters the belief in the ability to self-control the coping strategy.

Comparable findings are reported in studies employing bogus feedback about pain coping techniques. Positive bogus feedback about relaxation performance as a coping response for cold pressor pain has been shown to increase pain tolerance (Neufeld and Thomas, 1977). Since physiological arousal and subjective discomfort were not different between conditions, the authors concluded that the increased tolerance was not caused by more effective relaxation, but was actually caused by the subjects' belief in their ability to apply the technique. Positive bogus biofeedback about hand-warming ability has also been shown to increase cold pressor pain tolerance, as compared with negative bogus biofeedback (Litt, 1988, Exp. II). Interestingly, subjects preferred termination of the cold pressor test to be contingent on hand-warming performance only when they were led to believe in high ability. It is unlikely that success v. failure feedback *per se* causes different pain tolerances; bogus feedback about ability to endure cold pressor pain did not reliably affect subsequent tolerance in a study by Litt (1988, Exp. I). In addition to perceiving control over the use of a coping technique, subjects have to believe in its pain-decreasing properties; when told the rationale of technique, volunteers benefited more from a pain coping technique than when they were asked just to apply it as a task (without a rationale) during the experiment (Girodo and Wood, 1979).

Attribution and pain coping

As we have seen, perceiving pain coping strategies as effective and under voluntary control is essential. This can be restated in attributional terms: the person has to perceive a stable, internal source that can positively influence the pain experience. Attributional research has further substantiated this view. Davison and Valins (1969) gave subjects a 'drug' and had them believe that it decreased the pain of electric shock by manipulating the shock level. Half of the subjects were told that they had been given a placebo; these people subsequently tolerated higher shock levels than those who believed that the drug had caused the pain relief. It can be concluded that experimental subjects attributed pain relief to their own pain coping abilities (a stable, internal source) and that this attribution promoted pain tolerance.

External but controllable attributions can also promote pain tolerance. Nisbett and Schachter (1966) led subjects to attribute the physiological symptoms of painful shock to a (harmless) drug. These people then tolerated higher shock levels than controls. It seems that participants perceived the drug-induced symptoms as being less harmful and more controllable. An experiment by Friedman *et al.* (1985) supports this interpretation: giving people the opportunity to ascribe uncomfortable sensations to a non-damaging process increased pain tolerance.

Thus two attributions have positive effects on pain tolerance: (1) a stable, internal attribution of pain tolerance or pain relief to high levels of ability in coping with pain; and (2) external attribution of sensations to a non-harmful and controllable cause. Interestingly, the first attribution may also suggest to the individual that the cause of the pain is not actually harmful, since something can be done about the pain experience by means of coping strategies ('if the cause is truly harmful, then nothing can be done about it').

Conclusions

There are several successful coping strategies that can be employed to decrease suffering and to increase pain tolerance and endurance. It is most likely that powerful distraction from pain awareness is the essential factor in these strategies.

In order to be effective, subjects have to believe that the strategy helps and that they actually have the ability to use it at will during the painful experience. Without these beliefs, the positive effects disappear. Thus, perceiving control over application as well as perceiving controllable effects of coping strategies are essential. Perceiving control over pain through the use of coping techniques can be promoted by:

(1) choice of technique;
(2) influence on the timing of elements of the technique;
(3) contingent reinforcement of the use of the technique, either through pain relief or other reinforcers;
(4) attribution of pain coping to stable, internal sources;
    in addition, attribution of pain sensations to non-harmful, controllable sources also promotes pain tolerance.

Acute clinical pain

Various authors have stressed the importance of perceived control with respect to acute pain and its treatment (Turk *et al.*, 1983; Chapman and Turner, 1986; Weisenberg, 1987). In the following, we will review empirical studies on the relationship between perceived control and acute clinical pain. It is important to make a distinction between various aspects of the acute pain situation: the subjective experience of pain, the subjective emotional experience (worry, anxiety), physiological arousal, and behaviours like pain endurance and medication use. There are two main areas in which research has been conducted: dental pain and pain during childbirth.

Dental pain

A number of correlational studies have examined the ways in which patients deal with stress and pain during dental treatment. From this research, which has mainly focused on dental anxiety—and not on dental pain—it can be concluded that there is clear evidence of a relationship between anxiety or the stress experienced during dental treatment and the disproportional expectation of pain and other negative, catastrophizing thoughts about the treatment. The more that patients experience a loss of control over their negative thoughts, as well as over other symptoms, the more anxiety they experience during treatment. There also seems to be a relationship between the degree to which the treatment is experienced as an event outside personal control and aversiveness. Strong support for this conclusion comes from research by Chaves and Brown (1987), who found that 44% of patients employed cognitive strategies to minimize pain and stress, while 37% catastrophized, e.g. exaggerated the negative aspects of the experience. Catastrophizing was related to experiencing more stress during treatment but not to higher levels of reported pain. In line with these findings is a study by Prins (1985), who interviewed 40 children referred for dental treatment to a specialized clinic because of their high anxiety. Only half of the children were actually anxious, and for most of them dental anxiety was based on fear of pain. Prins concluded that 'for most children a visit to the dentist is one undifferentiated aversive event about which not much can be done. Their behaviour is mainly controlled by external contingencies and to a lesser extent by their own plans or rules' (p. 650). There was a clear relationship between the child's sense of self-control over his or her fear sensations and the degree of anxiety. Highly anxious children were preoccupied with external, aversive stimuli, with the threat of pain and with escape fantasies. Unfortunately, the study did not report relationships with experienced pain. Similar findings were reported by Kent (1987).

Besides these correlational studies, there are several experimental studies that have investigated the effect of perceived control manipulations on pain as well as on anxiety. In this setting, perceived control is usually manipulated by giving a group of patients a standardized way to signal to the dentist when they want the current activity (like drilling) to stop. This group is compared with patients treated in the usual way.

In general, it seems that giving patients a way to control the pain-causing activity decreases the experienced discomfort and subjective pain. The objective (behavioural) pain and fear measurements, however, are less clearly linked to the presence of perceived control. This also applies to psychophysiological reactions, and to subjective fear.

Illustrative for these findings is Corah's work. In 1973 he reported an unpublished study by Kruger. Paedodontic patients were given a two-stage signalling device to inform the dentist when they were experiencing discomfort. Thus, patients with this device may have experienced *some* control over the dentist's activities by informing him about the level of discomfort. Behaviour ratings indicated that patients with the signalling device were more cooperative and were not as restless as the control patients. Subjective experiences were not reported in this experiment.

In a later study, Corah (1973) heightened controllability in a group of young (6–11 years) dental patients. Here, the device had two buttons; the first to inform the dentist with a green light that the procedure was bothering the child, but not at such a level that he or she wanted the dentist to stop. The second button turned on a red light and a buzzer, upon which the dentist stopped until the child felt more comfortable. The contrast group received the usual treatment. In the experimental group, only half of the patients actually used the control device. The experimental group showed fewer spontaneous SCR fluctuations during high-stress procedures (injections of analgesia, high-speed drilling) but slightly more during low-stress procedures. Behavioural ratings of patients' anxiety and cooperativeness were not significant between groups, nor were head and body movements. Unfortunately, no subjective measures of anxiety and pain were taken. Perhaps because of the disappointing findings Corah *et al.* (1978) tried to replicate this study in a group of adult dental patients, with even more contradictory results: the perceived-control group now displayed *more* spontaneous SCR fluctuations during high-stress procedures. Again, dentists' ratings of anxiety yielded no significant results.

Finally, Corah *et al.* (1979) compared three experimental groups (relaxation by means of instruction via headphones, perceived control by means of the signalling device, and active distraction by means of playing a video game) with normal treatment. Subjective anxiety was significantly lower in the relaxation and distraction groups, but the perceived control condition did not differ significantly from normal treatment. Patients expressed a clear preference for active distraction, but not for other conditions. Physiological responses did not show any superiority of perceived control. Unfortunately, again no ratings of pain intensity–pain discomfort were taken. These were, however, included in the studies of Thrash *et al.* (1982) and Wardle (1983). Thrash *et al.* used the signalling device discussed above. Dental patients were asked to indicate their level of discomfort continuously by pressing one of three buttons, connected to green, yellow and red lights. In one condition (actual feedback, the proper perceived control condition) the dentist stopped when the red light was on, and patients knew that the dentist would stop in the event of a red light. In a second condition (belief in feedback), subjects were shown the device, and were led to believe that the dentist could see the lights. They were not, however, told that the dentist would react to their feedback; the lights were actually disconnected, so the dentist could not react. In a third condition (no feedback), subjects were asked to monitor their level of discomfort by the device, but there were no lights so they had no feedback opportunities. Results show that the actual feedback group experienced less discomfort and less pain during injection and also used the red button significantly less frequently than the no-feedback group. The group who believed (at first) in feedback fell between the proper perceived-control group and the no-feedback group. Thus, strong evidence was found for the positive effect of perceived control on experienced pain and discomfort.

Finally, in accordance with Corah *et al.* (1979), Wardle contrasted three experimental conditions. Dental patients were given either distraction (pictures on the ceiling), detailed information about procedures and the sensations they could expect, perceived control (the patients were asked to raise an arm if they wanted a pause) or none of these. Procedural/sensations information and perceived control were equally effective on subjective pain. However, only information reduced subjective anxiety significantly. Dentist's ratings of pain and anxiety gave no significant results. The different effects of control and information on anxiety are intriguing. It must be stressed that the control that patients could exercise was not very powerful in this Wardle study (compared to the red lights in the dentist's line of vision or the sound of a buzzer) and patients may have been anxious whether the dentist would see the signal and would react fast enough.

Childbirth and perceived control

Childbirth is a very important experience for many women and men. In contrast with medical treatments, the pain stimulus is not external, and a method to acquire direct control over the presence of the stimulus is not available. Nevertheless, many women and men take classes to prepare themselves for the event. Various methods are described for childbirth preparation and many of these attempt to assist women to have relatively painless childbirths (see Mulcahy and Janz, 1973). Most methods give information about the processes of childbirth and give training in timing, relaxation, breathing and pain-control techniques. Thus, various theoretical ideas on pain control can be found in these methods: breaking the (supposed) fear–tension–pain cycle by relaxation techniques; pairing a breathing response with uterine contractions to replace the experience of pain; knowledge about processes and sensations that might reduce uncertainty; concentration on other aspects than pain (distraction); control of the behaviour in labour, etc. Mulcahy and Janz (1973) state that the integrated 'Erna Wright method emphasizes that the individual remains in complete control of the situation by knowledge of what is to occur, utilizing concentration with controlled breathing and active relaxation combined with cognitive and motor activity' (p. 423). Numerous studies have shown that learning and applying these techniques results in the use of less medication during childbirth compared with unprepared childbirth (see Manning and Wright, 1983, for a short review).

In correlational studies, it has been found that the confidence of the woman in the childbirth training (rather than formal characteristics of the training) is related to experienced pain and use of medication (Cogan *et al.*, 1976) and that internals (locus of control) benefit more from these methods than externals (Willmuth *et al.*, 1978). Interestingly, Felton and Segelman (1978) found that the Lamaze childbirth training changed the women's beliefs about personal control.

Brewin and Bradley (1982) investigated the relationship between perceptions of personal and staff control over labour discomfort and over labour duration, and experienced labour pain/discomfort. Women who had followed childbirth preparation classes perceived higher levels of personal as well as staff control. In the group who attended classes, perceived personal control over labour duration was associated with less pain/discomfort during childbirth. This relationship was not found in the group of non-attenders, in which perceived control by the staff over labour discomfort was related to reduced labour pain/discomfort. This study indicates that perceptions of internal control as well as of control by others can have pain-reducing effects. Manning and Wright (1983) investigated the relationship of expectancy for ability to control pain without medication during the early stages of labour with actual medication use and medication-free labour time. All women had followed childbirth classes. The belief in the capacity to control the pain correlated with medication use ($r = -0.47$) and the percentage of time in labour without medication ($r = 0.42$). The general belief that the training would make it possible to have medication-free childbirth was an almost equally strong predictor.

Thus, childbirth training methods seem to result in higher levels of internal control with regard to pain and the process and duration of labour. The level of perceived control varies, however, and the strength of the belief seems to be related to medication use, medication-free labour time, and to reports of pain and discomfort. In addition to these effects of personal control, perceived control by professional staff over childbirth discomfort seems to be related to a reduction in experienced pain.

Conclusions

Perceived control seems to be an important issue with respect to acute pain. The notion of control is, however, used in very different ways: controllability of various pain symptoms, controllability of the pain stimulus, or controllability of the internal process that causes the pain. Symptoms may be distinguished in cognitive (catastrophizing, attention), physiological (breathing, heart rate, sweating, muscle tension, etc.), emotional (anxiety, worry, distress) and behaviour (endurance, medication use, crying, yelling, moving, etc.). Training in methods for limiting these symptoms leads to higher levels of perceived control over symptoms, and this probably increases pain tolerance, reduces medication use, and may also blunt the pain experienced. Giving the subject control over the pain stimulus seems to have clear positive effects on pain and discomfort. However, the effect of this type of control on anxiety and physiological responses is less clear. Probably, the effect depends on various aspects of the control response and how they are perceived: the difficulty of the response, belief in the power of the response and belief in the rapidity of beneficial effects from the response. For instance, dental patients who are told that the dentist will stop drilling when they raise their arm may be anxious about whether the dentist will see the arm and will stop promptly.

Research on dental pain indicates that the effects of perceived control over the dentist's behaviour and the effects of procedure/sensation information are comparable. The methods have similarities in that: (1) they decrease the uncertainty about possible future worsening of pain or damage; and (2) they increase confidence that the experience can be endured without fatal damage (since controllability increases self-confidence, while information increases confidence in the professional helper). In sum, perceived control in the acute-pain situation decreases the intensity of pain, aversiveness and discomfort by decreasing uncertainty.

Chronic pain

The potential for developing learned helplessness (Abramson *et al.*, 1978) is strong among chronic-pain patients. This results from their repeated experience of failing to attain control over pain either by personal action or by medical treatment. In this section, research into the perception of control in chronic pain is first described. Then several aspects of learned helplessness shown by chronic-pain patients, namely generalized perceptions of uncontrollability, lowered self-esteem and depression, decreased ability and motivation to learn, are outlined. Finally, the relationship between perceived control and the treatment of chronic pain will be discussed.

Chronic pain and perceived control over pain

The present authors asked 22 chronic low back pain patients to rate two types of perceived control: (1) the ability to decrease pain when it is present; and (2) the ability to prevent back pain. Patients perceived relatively low levels of control over both aspects. The ability to *prevent* back pain appears to be the most important dimension of controllability: it correlates negatively with back pain intensity ($r = -0.54$, $p < 0.01$) and with negative evaluation of having chronic pain ($r = -0.50$, $p < 0.01$). Lack of perceived control over pain appears to be an important characteristic of those chronic-pain patients who experience pain disproportionate to organic causes (Reesor and Craig, 1987). These ('non-organic') patients felt more ineffective and overwhelmed in their attempts to cope with pain than did organic-pain patients. Interestingly, during an experimental pain induction the former group reported few cognitions reflecting perceived control and manifested more catastrophizing. Thus, these patients showed a generalized tendency to react helplessly to pain.

The perception of uncontrollability of pain can aggravate beliefs that one is disabled and incapable of work and other activities. Arthritic-pain patients who believe that they can exercise little influence over how much their illness affects them lead less-active lives and experience more pain than others (Shoor and Holman as cited by Bandura, 1986). Disability beliefs are associated with more severe suffering in chronic-pain patients (Dolce, 1987; Feuerstein *et al.*, 1987; Reesor and Craig, 1987). Sampling the daily experiences of patients with chronic low back pain, Arntz *et al.* (1989a) found that these patients perceive themselves as helpless, disabled and weak. Avoidance of activities that are (mostly falsely) believed to increase pain is an important characteristic of chronic-pain patients (Philips, 1987). Avoidance has been found to be strongly correlated with beliefs in the lack of ability to self-control pain ($r = -0.62$; Philips, 1987).

It is clear that chronic pain is associated with perceptions that pain is largely uncontrollable. The extent of suffering, disability beliefs and passive avoidance are all associated with lack of perceived control. The avoidance behaviour of chronic-pain patients is more reminiscent of the passivity of depressives than the avoidance behaviour of phobics. This similarity between chronic pain and depression is in line with learned helplessness theory.

The learned helplessness of chronic-pain patients is characterized by several factors, which will be discussed one by one.

Generalized perception of uncontrollability

Chronic-pain patients appear to be characterized by a generalized tendency to perceive their activities and their lives as uncontrollable by themselves as well as by others. In their view chance is an important causal agent.

Empirical evidence for generalized perceptions of uncontrollability comes from Srivastava (1983), McGreary and Turner (1984) and Skevington (1979, 1983a): chronic-pain patients seem to have external loci of control and high beliefs in chance. There may be an alteration from personal helplessness (attribution of uncontrollability to oneself) in early phases of treatment to universal helplessness (nobody has control) as chronicity progresses (Skevington, 1983b). The generalized lack of control is apparent in a recent study of the daily experiences of chronic low back pain patients. Compared with normals, these patients report less control over ordinary events and activities during the day (Arntz *et al.*, 1989a). In addition, chronic-pain patients experience high levels of environmental stress, like low work satisfaction, no influence over work characteristics, divorce, death of partner, accidents, etc. (Feuerstein *et al.*, 1987), that are partly objectively uncontrollable, and partly can be perceived as uncontrollable. Prospective research is needed to establish whether environmental stress that is perceived as uncontrollable is a risk factor in the transition from acute to chronic pain. In sum, there is a relationship between chronic pain and generalized perceptions of no control, but it is not clear whether this is a causal factor or a consequence of chronic pain.

Self-esteem and depression

It is frequently reported that chronic-pain patients have lowered self-esteem (Schmidt & Arntz, 1987) although this is not always marked (Skevington, 1979; Arntz *et al.*, 1989c). The moderately lowered self-esteem is in agreement with the external-chance attributions that chronic-pain patients make: they do not blame themselves for their pain.

Depressive symptoms appear to be more profound. Depression, as well as anxiety, is related to perceiving that pain coping strategies are ineffective in patients with chronic low back pain (Rosenstiel and Keefe, 1983). Hopelessness and depression may well be both a consequence and a cause of the continuation of perceived uncontrollability.

Decreased ability and motivation to learn

Learned helplessness theory predicts that chronic-pain patients will show decreased ability and motivation to learn to control their pain and to learn to increase physical functioning. Research on physical performance does indeed indicate that chronic low back pain patients do not show learning and are less influenced by external information about their performance (Schmidt, 1985). These patients have difficulties in learning to alter activities in circumstances that cause low levels of back pain, and may therefore over-exert until pain becomes very intense (Nalibof *et al.*, 1981). A related characteristic of chronic-pain patients is the combination of *increased* pain threshold and *decreased* pain tolerance (Schmidt and Arntz, 1987). It is as yet unclear whether this characteristic has always been there or is caused by chronic pain. There are clinical indications that chronic-pain patients had increased pain thresholds before chronicity, and had a tendency to over-exert without feeling physical warning signals. Probably, these patients have formerly experienced high levels of control over physical functioning. In any case, increased pain threshold and decreased pain tolerance may be important factors in maintaining the perceived uncontrollability of pain: at lower levels of noxious stimulation nothing is felt, so that patients cannot learn pain prevention responses; and very quickly the pain is experienced as intolerable and overwhelming, making the patient a helpless victim.

Perceived control and the treatment of chronic pain

It appears from the above that the behaviour of chronic-pain patients can partially be explained using the learned helplessness concept. This implies that controllability will also play an important role in treatment. In fact, it has been reported that chronic-pain patients with severe learned helplessness deficits show less improvement with psychological or medical treatment (Thomas and Lyttle, 1980; Chapman and Brena, 1982). When improvement takes place, it appears to be especially large in perceived control over pain and in related areas (Phillips, 1987; Flor *et al.*, 1983). Before further elaboration, the special situation of the chronic-pain patient who appeals for treatment should be emphasized.

First, there are clinical indications that chronic-pain patients perceive that they formerly had high levels of control over physical functioning. Experiencing severe acute pain and the associated physical limitations may have resulted in a major loss of control for these subjects. From laboratory research, it is known that loss of control is more stressful than never having had control at all (Overmier *et al.*, 1980; Staub *et al.*, 1971).

Second, chronic-pain patients are known to strive for total pain relief, viewing pain as primarily a medical problem that should be medically treated. As long as chronic-pain patients try to acquire this kind of control, they are doomed to experience repeated failures, continuing their helplessness. The kind of control that can be acquired first requires an acceptance by the patient of having pain. One cannot learn pain coping or prevention strategies without accepting that one has pain. There are indications that subjects who do not accept unchangeable aversive facts suffer more, and adapt less (Silver *et al.*, 1982; Rothbaum *et al.*,

1982). Thus, it appears to be necessary to refrain from trying to acquire total control of what cannot be controlled, in order to perceive the availability of control over what can be controlled.

The relationship between chronic pain, low perceived control and the other factors discussed above can be integrated in a hypothetical model (Figure 2). The core of the model is the vicious circle between low perceived control and the experience of pain and depression.

Of the many different chronic pain treatments, such as operant reinforcement of non-pain behaviour, relaxation training, cognitive-behavioural therapy, EMG biofeedback, exposure to pain-increasing stimuli, etc., one is especially suited to illustrate the role of perceived control in treatment: this is EMG biofeedback training for tension headache and chronic low back pain.

Although the rationale seems clear (muscle tension leads to pain), no stable relationships between EMG decreases and decreased subjective pain have been found (see Turner and Chapman, 1982, for a review). However, EMG biofeedback has been found to be superior to placebo treatment or no treatment. Thus there seem to be other factors that result in pain relief. Nouwen and Solinger (1979) found that those chronic low back pain patients who experienced successful EMG decreases coupled with reductions in experienced pain showed stable improvement at follow-up. Those patients who were less successful did not show improvement. However, at follow-up there was no relationship between EMG and improvement in back pain. This paradox led Nouwen and Solingen to

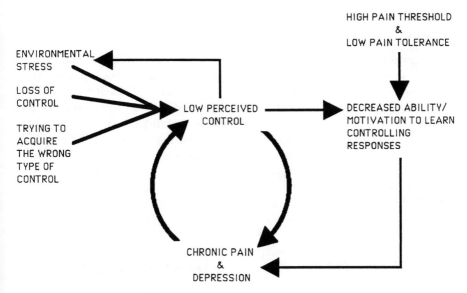

FIGURE 2. A hypothetical model of the relationship between chronic pain and low perceived control.

hypothesize that the successful patients perceived control over tension and pain, and that this control mediated final success. Holroyd *et al.* (1984) tested this hypothesis in a fascinating experiment. In a two by two design, headache patients received either audio feedback (lower tones suggesting tension decrease) contingent on *decreased* EMG or on *increased* EMG. The second factor was the degree of success (high v. low), and this was experimentally manipulated by means of bogus graphic display of EMG activity during and across sessions. High success feedback, regardless of direction of actual EMG, produced significantly greater improvement in headache complaints and medication use. Again, improvement was not related to EMG. Interestingly, high-success feedback also caused changes in locus of control and in self-efficacy. Bush *et al.* (1985) report similar findings, in that paraspinal EMG feedback and bogus feedback produced equal improvement in chronic low back pain patients. Another study (Biederman *et al.*, 1987) manipulated the size of the feedback scale on the apparatus (but in all conditions feedback correlated with actual EMG decrease) and did not find significant effects. However, in this study, the number of patients was very small and the success manipulation relatively weak.

In summary: patients' helplessness and perceived uncontrollability are central themes in psychological treatment of chronic pain. They are areas in which much progress in treatment can be achieved. It is very probable that improvement during and after treatment is mediated by perceived control over pain and other problems. The important factor appears not to be the actual technique that is applied, but whether the patient perceives it as helpful and applicable.

Conclusions

It appears that chronic-pain patients show characteristics of learned helplessness as a result of experiencing chronic uncontrollable pain and stress. They perceive low control over pain and life and are avoidant in their behaviour. Thus, the relationship between low perceived control, learned helplessness and psychological suffering is apparent. It may be hypothesized that these patients suffer especially from failing to acquire total control (and complete pain relief). Instead of accepting pain and trying to acquire some control by means of coping strategies, they become helpless and think that nobody can do anything. On the other hand, psychological treatments can be effective in reducing pain and psychological suffering. Letting the patient perceive control over pain seems to be an essential mediator of treatment success.

WHY DOES PERCEIVED CONTROL REDUCE PAIN?

Previous reviews of the effects of perceived control on the experience of aversive events (not restricted to pain) have come to different conclusions. Averill (1973) concluded that controllability does not reliably decrease the impact of aversive events. He states that effects of controllability depend upon the *meaning* of the controlling response for the subject, but theoretical predictions about the determinants of meaning and implications of different meanings remain vague. Miller (1979) concluded that controllable events may hurt less. She discussed ten theories that purported to explain the positive effects of control and concluded that seven are based on circular reasoning (e.g. explaining why control reduced physiological anticipatory arousal by stating that controllable stress is less arousing, without explaining why this is). However, the three remaining theories cannot explain all findings, most importantly the effect of controllability above predictability. Miller proposed a new theory (the 'minimax' hypothesis), which explains positive effects of control as follows (see also Chapter 6). In controllable conditions, the subject can rely on a stable, reliable source (his or her own response) that can modify the aversive event. Therefore, future danger can reliably be kept below an acceptable maximum level. When you have no control, there is no guarantee that future danger will be restricted. The hypothesis explains why subjects prefer control and show less anticipatory arousal. However, according to Miller the minimax hypothesis cannot explain the decreased *impact* of aversive events.

Finally, Thompson(1981) concluded in her review that controllability does *not* influence aversiveness. Thompson states that the *meaning* of the aversive event is the important issue, but remains (like Averill) rather vague about implications of this assertion.

In this chapter the focus was on pain, and other types of aversive events were excluded. Laboratory as well as clinical studies were discussed. There appears to be ample evidence that controllability *can* reduce the experience of pain and *can* promote tolerance and endurance.

The question will now be addressed of why perceived control may have these effects.

With the exception of one theory, no theories that are circular according to Miller will be discussed. In addition, no theories will be discussed that cannot explain the superior effects of controllability above predictability. Five explanations can be put forward.

Anxiety increases the experience of pain and controllability reduces anxiety

Although a rather popular explanation, there are two problems with it. First, is it true that anxiety (or the associated physiological arousal) increases pain? Second, does control always reduce anxiety in cases where it reduces pain?

Does anxiety increase pain?

The frequently observed correlation between acute pain and anxiety (Chapman and Turner, 1986) should not be confused with a causal effect of anxiety on pain. Chapman and Turner (1986) state that anxiety has physiological effects that increase the pain response: increased sympathetic activity and the release of epinephrine at the sympathetic terminals may sensitize or directly activate nociceptors; increased muscle tension, especially near the site of the wound, may cause additional pain. A psychological explanation might be that intense anxiety causes loss of control over thinking (Kent, 1987), which deprives the person of one of the most powerful coping strategies—distraction. Bolles and Fanselow (1980), however, have proposed a controversial theory, which implies that fear and pain are mutually exclusive states. Fear is assumed to decrease the experienced pain and to activate the organism (flight–fight response), whereas pain is assumed to deactivate the organism, promoting healing. Their theory is based on findings in animal studies and the applicability to human pain is not clear yet.

In humans, research findings give conflicting results. Kleinknecht and Bernstein (1978), Dougher (1979), Weisenberg *et al.* (1985), Ahles *et al.* (1987) and Malow *et al.* (1987) report positive correlations between state anxiety and subjective (externally caused or internal spontaneous) pain. Klepac *et al.* (1982) found that dental patients who avoided treatment showed reduced pain tolerance, but that pain threshold and subjective pain were not different from those of dental fearless patients. Two studies have investigated the effect of experimentally induced anxiety on pain. In the first (Malow, 1981), anxiety induction was related to a greater tendency to report pain. In the second (Dougher *et al.*, 1987), only anxiety that had as its focus the pain stimulus had a pain-increasing effect.

In contrast to these positive findings, many studies found no significant relationships (Arntz *et al.*, 1989a; Arntz *et al.*, 1989b; Bowers, 1968; Chaves and Brown, 1987; Klepac *et al.*, 1980), or even negative relationships, as in a study of Kent (1984), who found that highly anxious dental patients experienced *less* pain during treatment than low-anxious patients.

Also in contradiction to the hypothesis, reducing anxiety and physiological arousal does not necessarily have strong pain-relieving effects, as the research on relaxation shows. The effects of relaxation and biofeedback seem not to be mediated by decreased physiological arousal (see above). Positive effects are probably caused by distraction from pain by actively involving the subject in various exercises.

Thus, on the one hand it is generally accepted that, in human beings, acute pain can be accompanied by subjective anxiety and physiological arousal. On the other hand, it is not clear whether anxiety and physiological arousal increase the experience of pain. It might be hypothesized, however, that when the focus of anxiety is on pain, the pain experience is more intense and tolerance is lower. The critical factor therefore seems to be attention, and not anxiety. A frightened wounded soldier who runs for his life will probably experience no pain when he tries to escape the battleground.

Does control always reduce anxiety in cases where it reduces pain?

Laboratory studies indicate that this is not always the case (see Table 1). As has been discussed above, research on coping strategies shows that when subjective pain and pain tolerance are positively affected, anxiety and physiological arousal are not always reduced. Similarly, anxiety during dental treatment does not seem to be reliably influenced by giving the subject control over the dentist's behaviour, whereas pain is affected. In short, perceiving control over pain or its cause can lead to pain relief and enhanced pain tolerance without any associated decrease in physiological arousal or subjective anxiety.

Since both parts of this anxiety-reduction hypothesis appear to be questionable, it seems unlikely that positive effects of perceived control are mediated by decreased anxiety or decreased physiological arousal.

Perceiving control promotes endogenous opioid release

This explanation presumes that control promotes the release of natural analgesic opioids that reduce the experience of pain. Several arguments can be made against this explanation.

First, perceiving *no* control over stress appears to be related to endogenous opioid release, in contrast to perceiving control, as basic animal research has shown (Maier *et al.*, 1983; Watkins and Mayer, 1982; see Chapter 13). It has been argued that the same processes that lead to learned helplessness deficits trigger endogenous opioid release (Maier *et al.*, 1983). Moreover, chronic-pain patients who suffer disproportionally to somatic causes display heightened opioid levels as do depressed patients (Terenius, 1985; Almay *et al.*, 1978), probably as a result of experiencing chronic uncontrollable pain. Thus, endogenous opioid release seems to be related to uncontrollable pain, and not to perceived control over pain.

Second, since the organism develops tolerance for endogenous opioids (Terman *et al.*, 1984), the pain-decreasing effects of control would be only temporary if they were based on endogenous opioids. Treatment studies of chronic pain patients have, however, shown that increased control can have long-lasting positive effects.

Third, it seems unlikely that the chronic-pain patients who suffer emotionally and behaviourally most from pain, and already have very high levels of endogenous opioids, can profit from still higher levels. Perceiving control can, however, help those patients. Most likely perceiving control is related to a *decrease* in opioid levels caused by a diminution of perceived uncontrollability.

Thus, it is unlikely that the effects of control are mediated by increased endogenous opioid release. However, other endogenous analgesic mechanisms may play a role, although research has not yet demonstrated such effects.

Controllability changes the meaning of pain or the meaning of the cause of the pain

The experience of pain depends strongly on cognitive-emotional factors. On the basis of the meaning of the pain or its inferred cause, pain can be felt in very different degrees (Beecher, 1956). We hypothesize that the inferred harmfulness of the pain or its cause is a central issue. It can be argued that control over pain or its cause changes the meaning of the pain and hence the way it is experienced. Pain that cannot be controlled may be appraised as caused by a harmful process. Pain that can be controlled may be appraised as non-harmful and hence will have a different significance for the subject. Thus, the subject may reason that if the pain (or cause) is truly harmful, nothing can be done about it. And conversely, if something can be done to decrease it (leading to perceived control), that it means that the pain (and its cause) is not truly harmful. Some evidence for this explanation has been discussed. However, its role in the effects of controllability deserves fuller investigation. It may apply especially to clinical pain or possibly harmful laboratory pain, but it cannot explain all laboratory findings on the effects of behavioural control over an external pain stimulus, such as control over the duration of the stimulation.

Perceived control is a positive experience *per se* which can compensate negative experiences

Several authors have proposed that acquiring and exercising control is a positive experience *per se*, and that having no control or losing control is a negative experience. Averill (1973) argues that controllability has acquired these qualities in evolution (because of its survival value). Psychoanalytical authors have stressed its value for the development of the child (Fisher, 1986). Control has also been seen as a primary pleasure (Fisher, 1986) or an unconditioned reinforcer (Miller, 1979). What is not implied in this explanation is the reinforcement the subject experiences when he or she actually stops or decreases pain. What is meant is that knowing that the pain can be controlled or perceiving control without actually exercising it has a positive effect by itself. Miller argues that this explanation is a circular one. However, there seems to be no reason why it cannot be tested empirically.

Perceiving control allows people to distract themselves from pain

The core of this explanation is the simple fact that pain cannot be felt when it is not in awareness. Perceiving control over pain gives the subject certainty that the pain (or its cause) will not exceed unbearable or unacceptable limits. Hence, subjects do not have to attend continuously to internal signals of impending danger and can distract themselves. Attention to pain increases the pain experience; distraction decreases it. This explanation is actually an extension of Miller's minimax hypothesis. It is a parsimonious explanation and can be empirically tested. Like Miller's minimax hypothesis, it can account for the fact that under certain circumstances subjects choose to give others control (e.g. to the professional doctor), when these others are perceived as more reliable sources of control.

It can also explain why subjects are willing to tolerate or endure more pain when having control (because they have higher certainty that they can end the pain than when having no control), as well as why the experience of pain can be less intense and less emotional under these circumstances. It may account for the observation that the effects of perceived control over the dentist's behaviour and the effects of procedural and sensation information are comparable: the interventions are similar: (1) in that they decrease the uncertainty of the subject about future worsening of pain or damage (control by giving the subject an opportunity to stop the cause of the pain, information by establishing the limits of treatment and its sensory effects); and (2) in that they increase confidence that the experience can be endured without fatal damage (control increases self-confidence, information increases confidence in the professional helper). Thus both procedures probably decrease uncertainty and increase confidence, and these allow the subjects to distract themselves.

The last three explanations may in fact all play a role in the effects of controllability. It certainly seems worth while investigating them. For too long have the positive effects of perceived control over pain been taken for granted.

REFERENCES

Abramson, L. Y., Seligman, M. E. P., and Teasdale, J. D. (1978). Learned helplessness in humans: Critique and reformulation. *Journal of Abnormal Psychology*, **78**, 49–74.

Ahles, T. A., Cassens, H. L., and Stalling, R. B. (1987). Private body consciousness, anxiety and the perception of pain. *Journal of Behavior Therapy and Experimental Psychiatry*, **18**, 215–222.

Almay, G. L., Johansson, F., and Knorring, von L. (1978). Endorphins in chronic pain. I. Differences in CSF endorphin levels between organic and psychogenic pain syndromes. *Pain*, **5**, 153–162.

Arntz, A., and De Jong, P. J. (1989). CLBP and perceived control: An experimental study (in preparation).

Arntz, A., DeVries, M., and Schmidt, A. J. M. (1989a). Daily experiences of chronic low back pain patients (in preparation).

Arntz, A., Heijmans, M., and Van Eck, M. (1989b). Predictions of dental pain: the fear of any expected evil is worse than the evil itself. *Behaviour Research and Therapy* (in press).

Arntz, A., Merckelbach, H., Peters, M., and Schmidt, A. J. M. (1989c). Chronic low back pain, response specificity and habituation to painful stimuli (submitted for publication).

Averill, J. R. (1973). Personal control over aversive stimuli and its relationship to stress. *Psychological Bulletin*, **80**, 286–303.

Averill, J. R., and Rosenn, M. (1972). Vigilant and nonvigilant coping strategies and psychophysiological stress reactions during the anticipation of an electric shock. *Journal of Personality and Social Psychology*, **23**, 128–141.

Averill, J. R., O'Brien, L., and DeWitt, G. W. (1977). The influence of response effectiveness on the preference for warning and on psychophysiological stress reactions. *Journal of Personality*, **45**, 395–418.

Avia, M. D., and Kanfer, F. H. (1980). Coping with aversive stimulation: The effects of training in a self-management context. *Cognitive Therapy and Research*, **4**, 73–81.

Ball, S., and Vogler, R.E., (1971). Uncertain pain and the pain of uncertainty. *Perceptual and Motor Skills*, **33**, 1195–1203.

Bandura, A. (1986). Self-efficacy mechanism in physiological activation and health-promoting behavior. In: J. Madden IV, S. Matthysse and J. Barchas (eds), *Adaptation, Learning and Affect*. New York: Raven Press.

Beecher, H. K. (1956). Relationship of significance of wound to pain experienced. *Journal of American Medical Association*, **161**, 1609–1613.

Beers, T. M., and Karoly, P. (1979). Cognitive strategies, expectancy, and coping style in the control of pain. *Journal of Consulting and Clinical Psychology*, **47**, 179–180.

Biederman, H. J., McGhie, A., Monga, T. N., and Sharks, G. L. (1987). Perceived and actual control in EMG treatment of back pain. *Behaviour Research and Therapy*, **25**, 137–147.

Björkstrand, P. (1973). Electrodermal responses as affected by subject—versus experimenter—controlled noxious stimulation. *Journal of Experimental Psychology*, **97**, 365–369.

Bolles, R. C., and Fanselow, M. S. (1980). A perceptual–defensive–recuperative model of fear and pain. *Behavioral and Brain Sciences*, **3**, 291–323.

Bowers, K. S. (1968). Pain, anxiety, and perceived control. *Journal of Consulting and Clinical Psychology*, **32**, 596–602.

Brewin, C., and Bradley, C. (1982). Perceived control and the experience of childbirth. *British Journal of Clinical Psychology*, **21**, 263–269.

Bush, C., Ditto, B., and Feuerstein, M. (1985). A controlled evaluation of paraspinal EMG biofeedback in the treatment of chronic low back pain. *Health Psychology*, **4**, 307–321.

Champion, R. A. (1950). Studies of experimentally induced disturbance. *Australian Journal of Psychology*, **32**, 596–602.

Chapman, C. R., and Brena, S. F. (1982). Learned helplessness and responses to nerve blocks in chronic low back pain patients. *Pain*, **14**, 355–364.

Chapman, C. R., and Turner, J. A. (1986). Psychological control of acute pain. *Journal of Pain and Symptom Management*, **1**, 9–20.

Chaves, J. F., and Brown, J. M. (1987). Spontaneous cognitive strategies for the control of clinical pain and stress. *Journal of Behavioral Medicine*, **10**, 263–276.

Cogan, R., Hennebron, W., and Klopfer, F. (1976). Predictors of pain during prepared childbirth. *Journal of Psychosomatic Research*, **20**, 523–533.

Corah, N. L. (1973). Effects of perceived control on stress reductions in pedodontic patients. *Journal of Dental Research*, **52**, 1261–1264.

Corah, N. L., and Boffa, J. (1970). Perceived control, self-observation, and response to aversive stimulation. *Journal of Personality and Social Psychology*, **16**, 1–4.

Corah, N. L., Bissell, D., and Illig, S. J. (1978). Effect of perceived control on stress reduction in adult dental patients. *Journal of Dental Research*, **57**, 74–76.

Corah, N. L., Gale, E. N., and Illig, S. J. (1979). Psychological stress reduction during dental procedures. *Journal of Dental Research*, **58**, 1347–1351.

Davison, G. C., and Valins, S. (1969). Maintenance of self-attributed and drug-attributed behavior change. *Journal of Personality and Social Psychology*, **11**, 25–33.

DeGood, D. E. (1975). Cognitive control factors in vascular stress response. *Psychophysiology*, **12**, 399–401.

Dolce, J. J. (1987). Self-efficacy and disability beliefs in behavioral treatment of pain. *Behaviour Research and Therapy*, **25**, 289–299.

Dougher, M. J. (1979). Sensory decision theory analysis of the effects of anxiety and experimental instructions on pain. *Journal of Abnormal Psychology*, **88**, 137–144.

Dougher, M. J., Goldstein, D., and Leight, K. A. (1987). Induced anxiety and pain. *Journal of Anxiety Disorders*, **1**, 259–264.

Elliott, R. (1969). Tonic heart rate: Experiments on the effects of collative variables lead to a hypothesis about its motivational significance. *Journal of Personality and Social Psychology*, **12**, 211–228.

Felton, G., and Segelman, F. (1978). Lamaze childbirth training and changes in belief about personal control. *Birth and the Family Journal*, **5**, 141–150.

Feuerstein, M., Papciak, A. S., and Hoon, P. E. (1987). Biobehavioral mechanisms of chronic low back pain. *Clinical Psychology Review*, **7**, 243–273.

Fisher, S. (1986). *Stress and Strategy*. London: Lawrence Erlbaum.

Flor, H., Haag, G., Turk, D.C., and Koehler, H. (1983). Efficacy of EMG biofeedback pseudotherapy, and conventional medical treatment for chronic rheumatic back pain. *Pain*, **17**, 21–31.

Friedman, H., Thompson, R. G., and Rosen, E. F. (1985). Perceived threat as a major factor in tolerance for experimentally induced cold-water pain. *Journal of Abnormal Psychology*, **94**, 624–629.

Gatchel, R. J., and Proctor, J. D. (1976). Physiological correlates of learned helplessness in man. *Journal of Abnormal Psychology*, **85**, 27–34.

Gatchel, R. J., McKinney, M. E., and Koebernick, L.F. (1977). Learned helplessness, depression and physiologic responding. *Psychophysiology*, **14**, 25–31.

Geer, J. H., Davison, G. C., and Gatchel, R. J. (1970). Reduction of stress in humans through nonveridical perceived control of aversive stimulation. *Journal of Personality and Social Psychology*, **16**, 731–738.

Girodo, M., and Wood, D. (1979). Talking yourself out of pain: The importance of believing that you can. *Cognitive Therapy and Research*, **3**, 23–33.

Glass, D. C., Singer, J. E., and Friedman, L. N. (1969). Psychic cost of adaptation to an environmental stressor. *Journal of Personality and Social Psychology*, **12**, 200–210.

Glass, D. C., Reim, B., and Singer, J. E. (1971). Behavioral consequences of adaptation to controllable and uncontrollable noise. *Journal of Experimental and Social Psychology*, **7**, 244–257.

Glass, D. C., Singer, J. E., Leonard, H. S., Krantz, D., Cohen, S., and Cummings, H. (1973). Perceived control of aversive stimulation and the reduction of stress responses. *Journal of Personality*, **41**, 577–595.

Grimm, L., and Kanfer, F.H. (1976). Tolerance of aversive stimulation. *Behavior Therapy*, **7**, 593–601.

Haggard, E. A. (1949). Experimental studies in affective processes. I. Some effects of cognitive structure and active participation on certain autonomic reactions during and following experimentally induced stress. *Journal of Experimental Psychology*, **33**, 257–284.

Hokanson, J. E., DeGood, D. E., Forrest, M. S., and Brittain, T. M. (1971). Availability of avoidance behaviors in modulating vascular-stress responses. *Journal of Personality and Social Psychology*, **19**, 60–86.

Holroyd, K. A., Penzien, D. B., Hursey, K. G., Tobin, D. L., Rogers, L., Holm, J. E., Mancille, P. J., Hall, J. R., and Chila, A. G. (1984). Change mechanisms in EMG biofeedback training: Cognitive changes underlying improvements in tension head-ache. *Journal of Consulting and Clinical Psychology*, **52**, 1039–1053.

Houston, B. K. (1972). Control over stress, locus of control, and response to stress. *Journal of Personality and Social Psychology*, **21**, 249–255.

International Association for the Study of Pain, Subcommittee on Taxonomy. Classification of chronic pain; descriptions of chronic pain syndromes and definitions of pain terms. (1986). *Pain* (Suppl. 3).

Kanfer, F. H., and Goldfoot, D. A. (1966). Self-control and tolerance of noxious stimulation. *Psychological Reports*, **18**, 79–85.

Kanfer, F. H., and Seidner, M. L. (1973). Self-control: Factors enhancing tolerance of noxious stimulation. *Journal of Personality and Social Psychology*, **25**, 381–389.

Kent, G. (1984). Anxiety, pain and type of dental procedure. *Behaviour Research and Therapy*, **22**, 456–469.

Kent, G. (1987). Self-efficacious control over reported physiological, cognitive and behavioural symptoms of dental anxiety. *Behaviour Research and Therapy*, **25**, 341–347.

Kilminster, S. G., and Jones, D. M. (1986). Perceived control and the cold pressor test. *Stress Medicine*, **2**, 73–77.

Kleinknecht, R. A., and Bernstein, D. A. (1978). The assessment of dental fear. *Behavior Therapy*, **9**, 626–634.

Klepac, R. K., McDonald, M., Hange, G., and Dowling, J. (1980). Reactions to pain among subjects high and low in dental fear. *Journal of Behavioral Medicine*, **3**, 373–384.

Klepac, R. K., Dowling, J., and Hange, G. (1982). Characteristics of clients seeking therapy for the reduction of dental avoidance: Reactions to pain. *Journal of Behavior Therapy and Experimental Psychiatry*, **13**, 293–300.

Lepanto, R., Moroney, W., and Zenhausern, R. (1965). The contribution of anxiety to the laboratory investigation of pain. *Psychonomic Science*, **3**, 475–476.

Litt, M. D. (1988). Self-efficacy and perceived control: Cognitive mediators of pain tolerance. *Journal of Personality and Social Psychology*, **54**, 149–160.

Maier, S. F., Sherman, J. E., Lewis, J. W., Terman, G. W., and Liebeskind, J. C. (1983). The opioid/nonopioid nature of stress-induced analgesia and learned helplessness. *Journal of Experimental Psychology, Animal Behavior Processes*, **9**, 80–90.

Malow, R. M. (1981). The effects of induced anxiety on pain perception: A signal detection analysis. *Pain*, **11**, 397–405.

Malow, R. M., West, J. A., and Sutker, P. B. (1987). A sensory decision theory analysis of anxiety and pain responses in chronic drug abusers. *Journal of Abnormal Psychology*, **96**, 184–189.

Manning, M. M., and Wright, T. L. (1983). Self-efficacy expectancies, outcome expectancies, and the persistence of pain control in childbirth. *Journal of Personality and Social Psychology*, **45**, 421–431.

McGreary, C., and Turner, J. (1984). Locus of control, repression-sensitization, and psychological disorder in chronic pain patients. *Journal of Clinical Psychology*, **40**, 897–901.

Miller, S. M. (1979). Controllability and human stress: Method, evidence and theory. *Behaviour Research and Therapy*, **17**, 287–304.

Mills, R. T., and Krantz, D. S. (1979). Information, choice and reactions to stress: A field experiment in a blood bank with laboratory analogue. *Journal of Personality and Social Psychology*, **4**, 608–620.

Mulcahy, R. A., and Janz, N. (1973). Effectiveness of raising pain perception threshold in males and females using a psychoprophylactic childbirth technique during induced pain. *Nursing Research*, **22**, 423–427.

Nalibof, B. D., Cohen, M. J., Schandler, S. L., and Heinrich, R. L. (1981). Signal detection and threshold measures for chronic back pain patients, chronic illness patients, and cohort controls to radiant heat stimuli. *Journal of Abnormal Psychology*, **90**, 271–274.

Neufeld, R. W. J., and Thomas, P. (1977). Effects of perceived efficacy of a prophylactic controlling mechanism on self-control under pain stimulation. *Canadian Journal of Behavioural Science*, **9**, 224–232.

Nisbett, R. E., and Schachter, S. (1966). Cognitive manipulation of pain. *Journal of Experimental Social Psychology*, **2**, 227–236.

Nouwen, A., and Solinger, J. W. (1979). The effectiveness of EMG biofeedback training in low back pain. *Biofeedback and Self-Regulation*, **4**, 103–111.

Overmier, J. B., Patterson, J., and Wielhiewicz, R. M. (1980). Environmental contingencies as sources of stress in animals. In: S. Levine and H. Ursin (eds), *Coping and Health* (pp. 1–38). New York: Plenum Press.

Pennebaker, J. W., Burnam, M. A., Schaeffer, M. A., and Harper, D. C. (1977). Lack of control as a determinant of perceived physical symptoms. *Journal of Personality and Social Psychology*, **35**, 167–174.

Pervin, L. A. (1963). The need to predict and control under conditions of threat. *Journal of Personality*, **31**, 570–587.

Philips, C. (1987). Avoidance behavior and its role in sustaining chronic pain. *Behaviour Research and Therapy*, **25**, 273–279.

Prins, P. J. M. (1985). Self-speech and self-regulation of high and low-anxious children in the dental situation: An interview study. *Behaviour Research and Therapy*, **23**, 641–650.

Reesor, K. A., and Craig, K. P. (1987). Medically incongruent chronic back pain: Physical limitations, suffering, and ineffective coping. *Pain*, **32**, 35–45.

Rosenbaum, M. (1980). Individual differences in self-control behaviors and tolerance of painful stimulation. *Journal of Abnormal Psychology*, **89**, 581–590.

Rosenstiel, A. K., and Keefe, F. J. (1983). The use of coping strategies in chronic low back pain patients: Relationship to patient characteristics and current adjustment. *Pain*, **17**, 33–44.

Rothbaum, F., Weisz, J. R., and Snyder, S. S. (1982). Changing the world and changing the self: A two-process model on perceived control. *Journal of Personality and Social Psychology*, **42**, 5–37.

Schmidt, A. J. M. (1985). Performance level of chronic low back pain patients in different treadmill test conditions. *Journal of Psychosomatic Research*, **29**, 639–645.

Schmidt, A. J. M., and Arntz, A. (1987). Psychological research and chronic low back pain: A stand-still or breakthrough? *Social Sciences and Medicine*, **25**, 1095–1104.

Sherman, R. A., Sherman, C. J., and Bruno, G. M. (1987). Psychological factors influencing chronic phantom limb pain: An analysis of the literature. *Pain*, **28**, 285–295.

Sherrod, D. R., Hage, J. N., Halpern, P. L., and Moore, B. S. (1977). Effects of personal causation and perceived control on responses to an aversive environment: The more control, the better. *Journal of Experimental Social Psychology*, **13**, 14–27.

Silver, R. L., Wortman, C. B., and Klos, D. S. (1982). Cognitions, affect and behavior following uncontrollable outcomes: A response to current human helplessness research. *Journal of Personality*, **50**, 480–514.

Skevington, S. M. (1979). Pain and locus of control: A social approach. In: D. J. Oborne, M. M. Gruneberg and J. R. Eisen (eds), *Research in Psychology and Medicine* (Vol. 1, pp. 61–69). London: Academic Press.

Skevington, S. (1983a). Social cognitions, personality and chronic pain. *Journal of Psychosomatic Research*, **27**, 421–428.

Skevington, S. (1983b). The changing beliefs, attributions and expectations of early synovitis patients: A longitudinal study of the effects of chronic pain and hospitalization. *Pain* (Suppl. 2), S180.

Staub, E., Tursky, B., and Schwartz, G. E. (1971). Self-control and predictability: Their effects on reactions to aversive stimulation. *Journal of Personality and Social Psychology*, **18**, 157–162.

Sternbach, R. A. (ed.) (1978). *The Psychology of Pain*. New York: Raven Press.

Srivastava, A.K. (1983). Locus of control in migraine patients. *Pain* (Suppl. 2), S181.

Szpiler, J. A., and Epstein, S. (1976). Availability of an avoidance response as related to autonomic arousal. *Journal of Abnormal Psychology*, **85**, 73–82.

Tan, S. Y. (1982). Cognitive and cognitive-behavioral methods for pain-control: A selective review. *Pain*, **12**, 1–21.

Terenius, K. (1985). Families of opioid peptides and classes of opioid receptors. In: H. C. Fields *et al.* (eds), *Advances in Pain Research and Therapy* (Vol. 9). New York: Raven Press.

Terman, G. W., Lewis, J. W., and Liebeskind, J. C. (1984). Endogenous pain inhibitory substrates and mechanisms. In: C. Benedetti *et al.* (eds), *Advances in Pain Research and Therapy* (Vol. 7). New York: Raven Press.

Thomas, M. R., and Lyttle, D. (1980). Patient explanations about success of treatment and reported relief from low back pain. *Journal of Psychosomatic Research*, **24**, 297–301.

Thompson, S. C. (1981). Will it hurt less if I can control it? A complex answer to a simple question. *Psychological Bulletin*, **90**, 89–101.

Thrash, W. J., Marr, J. N., and Boone, S. E. (1982). Continuous self-monitoring of discomfort in the dental chair and feedback to the dentist. *Journal of Behavioral Assessment*, **4**, 273–284.

Turk, D. C., Meichenbaum, D., and Genest, M. (1983). *Pain and Behavioral Medicine*. New York: Guilford Press.

Turner, J. A., and Chapman, C. R. (1982). Psychological interventions for chronic pain: A critical review. II. Operant conditioning, hypnosis and cognitive therapy. *Pain*, **12**, 23–46.

Wall, P. D. (1979). On the relation of injury to pain. *Pain*, **6**, 253–264.

Wall, P. D., and Melzack R. (eds) (1985). *Textbook of Pain*. Edinburgh: Churchill Livingstone.

Wardle, J. (1983). Psychological management of anxiety and pain during dental treatment. *Journal of Psychosomatic Research*, **27**, 399–402.

Watkins, L. R., and Mayer, D. J. (1982). Organization of endogenous opiate and nonopiate pain control systems. *Science*, **216**, 1185–1192.

Weisenberg, M. (1987). Psychological intervention for the control of pain. *Behaviour Research and Therapy*, **25**, 301–312.

Weisenberg, M., Wolf, Y., Mittwoch, F., Mikulincur, M., and Aviram, O. (1985). Subject versus experimenter control in the reaction to pain. *Pain*, **23**, 187–200.

Willmuth, L., Weaver, L., and Borenstein, J. (1978). Satisfaction with prepared childbirth and locus of control. *Journal of Obstetrical and Gynaecological Nursing*, **7**, 33–37.

Worthington, E. L. (1978). The effects of imagery content, choice of imagery content, and self-verbalization on the self-control of pain. *Cognitive Therapy and Research*, **2**, 225–240.

Zimbardo, P. G., Cohen, A. R., Weisenberg, M., Dworkin, L., and Firestone, I. (1966). Control of pain motivation by cognitive dissonance. *Science*, **151**, 217–219.

CHAPTER 8

The relationship between anxiety, lack of control and loss of control

SUSAN MINEKA AND KELLY A. KELLY
Department of Psychology, Northwestern University, Evanston, USA

INTRODUCTION

The importance of experiencing a sense of control over various aspects of one's environment to the organism's general physical and emotional health is well documented by the wide range of topics covered in this volume. The present chapter focuses on the effects of experience with control, lack of control, and loss of control on the origins and maintenance of fear and anxiety. Experience with control and lack of control have been implicated as important factors in several different emotional and motivational states, most notably fear, anxiety and depression. Indeed, it has been argued that control and lack of control are important in mediating these emotions not only within the range of normal day-to-day fluctuations of these mood states, but also in the expression of more pathological forms of these emotions such as occur in clinical disorders ranging from simple phobias, to generalized anxiety states, panic disorder and certain forms of unipolar depression. Thus, for example, Lang sees control as one of the three fundamental dimensions of human emotion (1979, 1984, 1985), whereas other theorists focus on the role of lack or loss of control in the origins and maintenance of clinical anxiety and depressive disorders (e.g. Abramson *et al.*, 1978; Barlow, 1988; Garber *et al.*, 1980; Mineka, 1985a,b; Seligman, 1975).

From a historical standpoint, it is perhaps interesting to note that the role of uncontrollability (experience with lack of control) in the origins of depression has generally received more attention in the past fifteen years than has its role in the origins of fear and anxiety disorders. This is in spite of the fact that some theorists

Stress, Personal Control and Health. Edited by A. Steptoe and A. Appels.
Published by John Wiley & Sons Ltd.
©ECSC–EEC–EAEC, Brussels–Luxembourg, 1989

had argued for the importance of lack or loss of control in fear and anxiety well before it was strongly implicated in depression (e.g. Mandler, 1966, 1972; Masserman, 1971; Mowrer and Viek, 1948). The reason for this historical accident is probably not that uncontrollability is really more important in depression than in fear and anxiety. Rather, the first truly systematic and programmatic research on the effects of control and lack of control, which stemmed out of the learned helplessness paradigm (Overmier and Seligman, 1967; Seligman and Maier, 1967), led several years later to the development of an influential experimental model of human depression (e.g. Seligman, 1975). The powerful statements of this helplessness theory of depression, and the large amount of empirical research directed toward testing it, may have masked the importance of lack of control in the origins of fear and anxiety. In a recent review discussing research and theory on the role of uncontrollability in anxiety and depression, Barlow (1988) stated 'but what has happened to anxiety?' (p. 268). It seems, to use Barlow's terms, that research implicating lack of control in depression has 'overshadowed' work implicating lack of control in fear and anxiety.

An additional factor contributing to this historical accident is that, although the overlap or comorbidity between anxiety and depression has long been noted, it has only recently received a significant amount of attention in either empirical or theoretical work (cf. Maser and Cloninger, 1989). Several theoretical articles have now attempted to discuss the origins and maintenance of anxiety and depressive disorders in a unified framework in which perceptions of lack of control play a shared role in anxiety and depression (and mixed anxiety/ depressive states) (e.g. Alloy *et al.*, 1989; Garber *et al.*, 1980). Certain forms of depression are also thought to be caused and characterized by hopelessness (certainty of negative outcome), in addition to helplessness (perceived lack of control) (see Abramson *et al.*, 1989, for a discussion of the hopelessness theory of depression). Thus, in these current theories perceived lack of control may underlie what anxiety and depression share in common; hopelessness may be, at least in part, what distinguishes them from one another.

The present chapter will review animal and human research implicating lack or loss of control in the origins and maintenance of fear and anxiety, both as a normal mood state and in clinical anxiety disorders. Our general framework will be to first discuss research demonstrating how a *prior* history of control or lack of control over important life events can affect how much fear or anxiety is created by a given stressful situation. Second, we will discuss the importance of control and lack of control *during* exposure to aversive or stressful experiences in determining the immediate, short-term and long-term, affective, behavioral and physiological consequences of those stressors. Finally, we will discuss how, *after* fear or anxiety has been acquired, actual or perceived control over the sources of fear or anxiety can be helpful in reducing the fear or anxiety. Indeed, in this latter context we will discuss current research and theory suggesting the importance of instilling a sense of perceived control during cognitive-behavioral therapies for anxiety disorders.

IMPORTANCE OF A PRIOR HISTORY OF CONTROL IN MEDIATING FEAR/ANXIETY RESPONSES TO STRESSORS

Positive effects of experience with control

The origins of generalized expectancies for control have long been thought to derive from experience during early development with response-contingent stimulation, and such expectancies have been thought to have profound effects on social, emotional and cognitive functioning (e.g. Lewis and Goldberg, 1969; Mineka *et al.*, 1986; Seligman, 1975; Watson, 1979; White 1959). Developmental psychologists have especially noted the importance of control over social stimulation in promoting secure attachments and the balance of fearful versus exploratory responses to novel and arousing situations (e.g. Ainsworth *et al.*, 1978; Sroufe *et al.*, 1974). In general, it has been thought that the responsiveness of care-givers to their infants' signals forms the basis for such expectations for control, and correlational studies have indeed corroborated that infants with more responsive care-givers do show more secure attachments, and less fearful reactions to novel or frightening situations. Unfortunately, such correlational studies confound care-giver responsiveness with other care-giver characteristics, such as warmth and lovingness, which would also be thought to promote positive developmental outcomes (e.g. Ainsworth *et al.*, 1978; Clarke-Stewart, 1973; see Mineka *et al.*, 1986, for a review).

Mineka *et al.* (1986) reasoned that a useful way to test this hypothesis more directly was through the use of a primate model in which long-term experimental manipulations of control could be made, unconfounded with other care-giver characteristics which might also promote more secure attachment relationships and lower levels of fear and anxiety in novel and threatening situations. In their experiments Mineka *et al.* used five groups of infant peer-reared rhesus monkeys (four per group) that had been separated from their mothers at birth. Between 6 weeks and 11 months of age, each group lived in a standard group cage for infant monkeys. In their cages the two master groups had a number of different operant manipulanda (chains, keys, levers) which, at specified times cued by discriminative stimuli, could be operated to deliver a variety of reinforcers, such as Similac, water, sugar pellets and other food treats. The two yoked groups lived in identical environments except that their manipulanda were inoperative; whenever a monkey from the master group successfully operated its manipulandum a comparable reinforcer was delivered to a member of the yoked group non-contingently. Thus master and yoked groups were equated on number of reinforcers received, and differed only in whether they had control over receipt of these reinforcers. In the second replication, an additional no-stimulation control group was added. This group did not have access to the operant manipulanda, or to the variety of reinforcers received by the other four groups. This group was included to determine whether any differences that were obtained between the master and yoked groups were due to positive effects of having experience with control and mastery, or to negative consequences of having experience with uncontrollable positive reinforcers. Between $6\frac{1}{2}$ and 11 months of age, all five groups were tested in several different situations to assess their reactions to a variety of fear-provoking, novel and stressful events.

Starting at $6\frac{1}{2}$ months of age, three biweekly fear tests were conducted. During these tests a toy monster that had flailing arms and legs, and that made a loud noise, was turned on and off in front of the infant monkeys' home cage for a 30-minute period. In each replication, master monkeys showed significantly less fear of the toy monster than yoked or no-stimulation monkeys on two of the three tests. Fear was indexed by retreat to the back of the cage away from the monster, and by amount of time spent clinging to one another. Thus, master monkeys spent less time clinging to one another, and spent more time in the front of the cage near the toy monster.

Following the three fear tests in the home cage, three tests were conducted to assess fear/exploratory behavior in a novel environment—a large primate playroom with 12 different objects to explore. Each group was first placed in a transport cage with its door open in the middle of the playroom to determine whether spontaneous emergence into the playroom would occur. If the monkeys had not spontaneously emerged in 10 minutes, they were taken out of the cage and left in the playroom for 30 minutes, during which time their behavior was carefully observed and scored. Results from the spontaneous emergence test were quite striking. On the first test none of the monkeys emerged spontaneously, but by the second and third tests master monkeys were all emerging spontaneously (on the average, in less than 4 minutes), whereas only one yoked monkey (and zero no-stimulation control monkeys) ever emerged spontaneously within the 10-minute period allotted by the experiment (see Figure 1). Striking behavioral differences also were noted once the monkeys were in the playroom. Again, these differences were not especially striking on the first test, but certainly were by the second and third tests—a point at which the playroom was no longer a totally novel environment because the monkeys had all spent 30–60 minutes there during the previous test(s). During these latter two tests, master monkeys spent more time locomoting, less time clinging to one another, touched more different objects, and touched objects more times than did the yoked and no-stimulation control monkeys (see Figures 2 and 3). Thus, master monkeys were not only more eager to enter the novel playroom situation, but also showed far more exploratory behavior once in it.

Finally, all monkeys were subjected to several 3-day separations from peers (during which they were housed individually) between $8\frac{1}{2}$ and 10 months of age. Further, one of the master and one of the yoked groups from replication 2 were

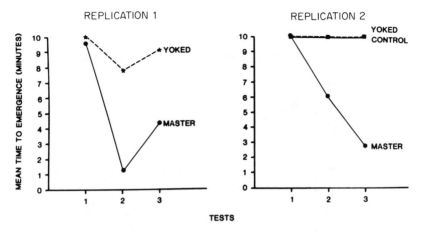

FIGURE 1. Mean number of minutes to emerge from the transport cage during the three group playroom tests of both replications 1 and 2 (10 is maximum possible). From Mineka *et al.* (1986). By permission of the Society for Research in Child Development.

GROUP PLAY ROOM TESTS

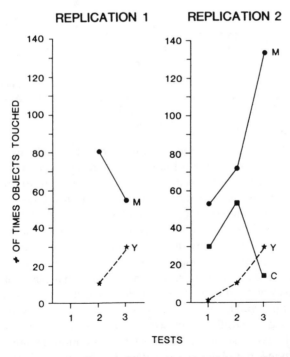

FIGURE 2. Mean number of times objects were touched during two of the group playroom tests of replication 1 and the three group playroom tests of replication 2. From Mineka *et al.* (1986). By permission of the Society for Research in Child Development. M = master; Y = yoked; C = non-stimulated control.

GROUP PLAY ROOM TESTS
REPLICATION 2

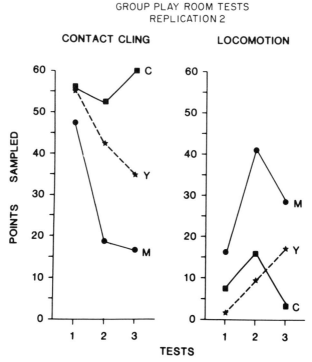

FIGURE 3. Mean number of points sampled for contact cling and locomotion during the three group playroom tests of replication 2 (60 is maximum possible). Abbreviations as in Figure 2. From Mineka *et al.* (1986). By permission of the Society of Research in Child Development.

also subjected to several 'intruder' separations during which one member of the master group at a time was placed in the yoked group, and vice versa. Intruder tests were conducted in order to determine whether the groups differed in their abilities to cope with the difficult task of integrating themselves into a new peer group, while also undergoing the stress of separation from their own peers. Results of the individual separation tests did not reveal any striking differences between groups in the ability to cope and adapt to these highly stressful separations during which the monkeys were alone in their home cages. However, in replication 2 the monkeys were also given individual playroom tests during individual separations to determine whether the differences seen during group playroom testing would be maintained when the animals were in a state of distress following separation and were being tested by themselves. Results indicated that master subjects continued to show more exploratory behavior during these individual playroom tests than did the other groups. Furthermore, the results of the 'intruder' separation tests also suggested that master subjects coped better with being the intruder in the yoked group than vice versa. In particular, masters as intruders explored the environment more, and ate and drank more than did yoked subjects as intruders. Furthermore, the host groups' behaviors also differed, with the yoked group showing more fearful/submissive behaviors on the first day when a master intruder was present, than did the master group toward the yoked intruders. As Mineka *et al.* conclude, 'these results suggest that when the separation environment is enriched to provide more varied response options and demands [than a solitary home cage], a history of prior control may well permit the primate infant to cope more effectively with separation from attachment figures' (p. 1255). These results should, however, be seen as tentative and in need of replication because these tests were only conducted in the second replication of the experiment.

In summary, the results of Mineka *et al.*'s studies with infant monkeys strongly implicate the importance of a prior history of control over appetitive events in one's environment in mitigating the impact of a variety of fear- and stress-provoking situations. These results are quite consistent with those obtained from correlational studies on human infants discussed above. It is also important to note that the effects observed were *mastery* effects rather than helplessness effects as have more often been observed in the literature on the impact of uncontrollable aversive events. That is, master subjects showed a superior ability to adapt to, or cope with, novel and stressful situations relative to both yoked and no-stimulation control subjects, which generally did not differ. By contrast, in the majority of experiments using a yoked design with aversive stimulation, yoked subjects show deficits relative to both master and no-stimulation control subjects. It is also important to note that these effects were obtained even when the experience with control and mastery was over inanimate aspects of the environment (e.g. food and treats), rather than over sources of social stimulation as have more often been implicated in the child development literature. Thus, at least to some extent the effects of control may be able to operate independently of the attachment relationship. As Mineka *et al.* concluded, 'Given this, increasing the controllability of the inanimate environment may prove to be a viable means of facilitating the development of human infants who, because of the need for long-term hospitalization or institutional care, or because their care-givers are emotionally unable to provide sufficient response-contingent stimulation, would otherwise experience few opportunities to learn to master the environment' (p. 1255).

These results are also certainly strongly suggestive, although by no means conclusive, that an early history of control may play a significant role in reducing susceptibility to fear and anxiety disorders in adulthood. Limitations of this experiment in this regard derive from the fact that it only dealt with the effects of experimental manipulations of control in the first year of life, and from the fact that only control over positive, inanimate aspects of the environment was studied. Ideally, primate studies should be done using even more long-term manipulations of control, over both appetitive and aversive events, of both a non-social and a social nature (e.g. control over reunions following separations). Such studies could help to delineate the role of different types of control and mastery experiences in reducing susceptibility to a range of stressful experiences in adulthood known to be implicated in the origins of fear and anxiety disorders (see Barlow, 1988; Marks, 1987, for recent reviews).

Loss of control and increased anxiety/stress

In the above section we have reviewed evidence that extensive experience with control, perhaps through instilling a sense of mastery, often has beneficial effects in reducing the impact of fear and anxiety-provoking situations. However, there are some situations in which the loss of control over environmental stressors, after having once had it, may be more stressful than never having had control (see Mineka, 1982; Mineka and Hendersen, 1985, for reviews). Stroebel (1969), for example, showed that when a lever that had previously controlled several noxious stimuli was removed, rhesus monkeys showed signs of intense disturbance and stress, even though no further noxious stimuli were presented. Although Stroebel did not have a comparison group that never had control over the noxious stimuli, his results nonetheless suggest that loss of control can sometimes create intense distress.

   This suggestion was corroborated in a more well-controlled experiment by Hanson *et al.* (1976). Using a strictly yoked design in rhesus monkeys, Hanson *et al.* found that when a lever that had previously controlled loud noise was removed, the monkeys showed greater elevations in cortisol levels than did monkeys that never had control over the noise. To the extent that cortisol levels are a reliable measure of stress, these results suggest that loss of control may be more stressful in some circumstances than never having had it. Unfortunately, the boundary conditions determining whether a prior history of control will have beneficial versus deleterious consequences are not well understood, in part because very little work has been directed at studying loss of control directly (see also Mineka and Kihlstrom, 1978; Mineka and Hendersen, 1985, for discussion of these issues). One possibility is that increased anxiety/stress may be a likely consequence of direct removal of the availability of an instrumental response that had previously been effective in controlling aversive stimulation as long as the organism remains in the situation where the aversive stimulation had been delivered; in such cases the organism may continue to expect occurrence of the aversive stimulation even if it is no longer delivered (as in Stroebel's experiment). By contrast, beneficial consequences of a prior history of control may be more likely to be observed when the organism is studied in different situations or contexts that do not involve direct removal of the availability of an instrumental response that was previously effective in controlling aversive stimulation.

IMPORTANCE OF CONTROL DURING AVERSIVE OR
STRESSFUL SITUATIONS IN REDUCING
FEAR AND ANXIETY

Animal studies

As discussed in the Introduction, there is not only evidence that a prior history of
control and mastery can reduce the impact of fear and anxiety-provoking
situations, but also evidence that the ability to control the occurrence of aversive
environmental stimulation can reduce both the immediate and the short-term
impact of that stimulation. Early hints of such effects can be derived from a
review of the early literature on experimental neurosis in animals (see Broadhurst, 1961, 1973; Mineka and Kihlstrom, 1978). Although a multitude of
sometimes rather idiosyncratic experimental procedures were used by a wide
range of investigators to induce 'neurotic' behavior in many different species
(dogs, sheep, pigs, rats, cats, monkeys), the majority of the procedures used
involved either variants on classical conditioning or punishment of consummatory behavior (see Mineka and Kihlstrom, 1978, for a review). Furthermore,
although a wide range of 'neurotic' behaviors were described as following from
these myriad procedures, the majority of the affective and somatic symptoms
could be described as falling into one of two classes: either excessive agitation,
activity and autonomic arousal (increased breathing rate, piloerection, strug-
gling, howling, etc.), or decreased activity, passivity and withdrawal, sometimes
accompanied by social isolation. Some animals appeared to experience both
kinds of symptoms at different times. As argued by Mineka and Kihlstrom
(1978), these symptoms appear to be prototypes for what in humans might be
described as chronic fear or anxiety, and passivity or depression, respectively.

What is important from the standpoint of the present review is the suggestion
of Mineka and Kihlstrom (1978) that the common theme running through the
diverse experimental procedures used to induce experimental neurosis was that in
each case 'environmental events of vital importance to the organism became
unpredictable, uncontrollable, or both' (p. 257). Indeed, as noted by Mineka
and Kihlstrom, paradigms used in the study of classical conditioning necessarily
involve strong elements of uncontrollability. Classical conditioning as traditionally studied since Pavlov (1927) involves experimenter-controlled delivery of
conditioned and unconditioned stimuli, and so when aversive unconditioned
stimuli are used the subject is being exposed to uncontrollable (although
predictable) aversive events. Why classical fear conditioning does not always
produce 'experimental neurosis' probably derives from threshold effects (e.g.
number of CS–US pairings, and/or US intensity) and from ways in which
uncontrollability interacts with unpredictability (e.g. as uncontrollable events
become increasingly unpredictable, the likelihood of 'experimental neurosis' may

increase; this was especially notable in the experiments of Liddell (cf. Mineka and Kihlstrom, 1978)).*

The importance of control in fear conditioning was first studied experimentally by Mowrer and Viek (1948), who found that rats exposed to inescapable or uncontrollable shocks acquired more fear than did rats exposed to the same amount of escapable or controllable shocks. This 'fear from a sense of helplessness' has since been replicated by a number of different investigators using a number of different paradigms and indices for assessing fear (e.g. Brennan and Riccio, 1975; Desiderato and Newman, 1971; Mineka *et al.*, 1984; Osborne *et al.*, 1975). For example, Mineka *et al.* (1984) found approximately two-fold differences in the amount of fear that was conditioned to a neutral tone in rats as a function of whether the tone was paired with escapable or inescapable shock. Master rats received 50 fear conditioning trials in which a tone was paired with electric shock that could be escaped (terminated) after a minimum 1-second duration. Yoked rats also received 50 fear conditioning trials but with inescapable shocks of the same duration and intensity as that of the masters (i.e. each rat in the yoked group had a partner in the master group whose escape latency determined the amount of shock the yoked rat received on that trial). The amount of fear conditioned to the CS was assessed in a different context over the next three days, using freezing during and following CS presentations as an index of fear. During testing, yoked rats showed approximately twice as many freezing responses in the presence of the CS, and immediately following its termination, as did the master rats; these differences persisted across three days of testing.

In addition to replicating prior demonstrations of the importance of control over US termination in determining the amount of fear conditioned to a CS, Mineka *et al.* also attempted to address the question of what mechanisms mediated these effects of control. Generally such results have been interpreted in terms of the increased aversiveness or stressfulness of uncontrollable shocks (e.g. Maier *et al.*, 1969; Seligman *et al.*, 1971). However, an alternative idea was proposed by Averill (1973), who argued that the beneficial effects of having control over the offset of aversive events stem primarily from the added predictability inherent in having a controlling response. That is, organisms with control also know when the aversive event will end, and have a salient marker of the ensuing interval in which the aversive event will not occur. In order to explore this hypothesis as to the mechanism through which control mediates its effects on fear conditioning, Mineka *et al.* used additional groups of yoked rats that had no control over shock termination, but which were provided with an exteroceptive feedback signal when the master rats made their escape response. In several different kinds of experiments, using both signalled and unsignalled escape learning paradigms, strong support was found for the idea that control *per*

---

* Because the present review focuses on the role of uncontrollability in fear/anxiety, the interrelated concept of unpredictability will not be extensively discussed. See Mineka and Kihlstrom (1978), Mineka and Hendersen (1985), Seligman (1975) for reviews.

se is not necessary to produce the lower level of fear characteristic of subjects with control. This conclusion derived from results of yoked groups which received an exteroceptive feedback signal (lights off)whenever the master subjects made their escape response. These yoked-feedback groups showed comparable, low levels of fear conditioned to the CS as the master groups. Thus, simply 'mimicking' the response of the master subjects by presenting an exteroceptive feedback signal to the yoked subjects without control whenever the master subject made an escape response was sufficient to produce the lower level of fear in the yoked-feedback subjects (see Figure 4). Mineka *et al.* hypothesized that escape responses and feedback stimuli may both operate to reduce fear through the acquisition of fear-inhibitory properties because they are both salient predictors of relatively long shock-free intervals intertrial (see also Warren *et al.*, in press).

One issue highlighted by these results is the importance of examining the dynamics of fear conditioning in more complex contexts than has been done in the past. The great majority of conclusions about the dynamics of Pavlovian conditioning have been derived from the traditional paradigm in which the subject has no control over the US and no feedback about the offset of the US.

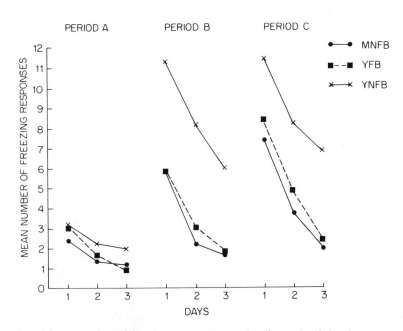

FIGURE 4. Mean number of freezing responses per day for each of the three groups of experiment 3, summed across the test trials of each day, separately for periods A, B and C. (MNFB = master–no feedback group; YFB = yoked–feedback group; YNFB = yoked–no feedback group; period A = 20 s before tone onset; period B = 20 s during tone; period C = 20 s after tone offset.) From Mineka *et al.* (1984). By permission of the American Psychological Association.

However, many of the everyday events where Pavlovian conditioning occurs are situations in which subjects have some control over the US and/or some feedback that the US has terminated and will not occur again for awhile. The results of Mineka *et al.* highlight the fact that such factors can play an important role in how much fear conditioning occurs to the neutral stimuli paired with such USs, with less fear being conditioned when the organism has added control or predictability. Because conditioned excitors of fear are generally well maintained over time (Hendersen, 1978; Mineka and Tomarken, 1989), these results also suggest that control over the US during conditioning may have long-term as well as short-term consequences.

Human research: laboratory studies

Laboratory studies with humans, like laboratory studies with animals, have found control to have profound effects on fear and anxiety. On the average, human subjects prefer control, find control to reduce anticipatory anxiety, and find control to reduce the impact of aversive events. One prominent hypothesis put forth to explain all these effects of control on fear and anxiety in humans is Miller's minimax hypothesis (1979, 1980). Miller has proposed that individuals consider personal control over aversive events to be an internal, stable attribute that allows them to minimize the maximum danger, at any given time and in the future. Miller hypothesizes that:

> If a subject attributes the cause of relief to a stable, internal factor—such as his own response—he has a reliable predictor that in the future danger will only occur up to some relatively low, maximum amount. In contrast, if the attribution is to some unstable, external factor—such as the experimenter's whims—future danger is not guaranteed to be restricted to a relatively low maximum. (Miller, 1979; p. 295)

The minimax hypothesis predicts that to the extent that an individual believes that he or she possesses the most reliable reponse(s) to minimize the maximum danger, then control will be preferred, and perceiving oneself to be in control over an aversive event will result in less arousal, less anticipatory anxiety, and less anxiety at impact. When an individual believes that another person possesses a more reliable control response than any of his or her own, then the individual would be expected to prefer not to have control. In the latter case the perception of control would result in more arousal and anxiety. Miller's hypothesis appears to be able to account for the majority, but perhaps not all, of the relevant laboratory research on the relationship between anxiety and control in humans. We will discuss the highlights of this area of research. A more comprehensive treatment of this literature can be found in Miller (1979).

With human subjects, the assessment of anxiety is less straightforward than it is in animal research. Lang (1968, 1971) has advocated the use of multiple response measures in the study of emotions. According to Lang, emotional responses occur in three loosely coupled systems: the physiological, the cognitive and the behavioral. Exposure to uncontrollable aversive events has been found to have impact on all three of the response systems, leading to increases in autonomic arousal, self-reported anxiety and disruption of ongoing behavior. Our review of the relationship between control and anxiety in experimental laboratory studies with non-clinical subjects will be organized according to Lang's three-response system approach.

The physiological response system

The assessment of anxiety within the physiological response system has traditionally consisted of measures of autonomic arousal, such as skin conductance. Several investigators have observed that, compared with those who possess control, individuals exposed to uncontrollable aversive stimuli show skin conductance responses of greater magnitude. For instance, Geer and Maisel (1972) presented slides depicting dead bodies to two groups of subjects. One group was informed that they could turn the slides off if the slides became too aversive. The other group was not allowed to shorten viewing time but was told how long each slide would be displayed. Subjects in the latter group were yoked to subjects in the former group so as to equate the viewing times. Subjects who viewed the slides for a predictable, but uncontrollable, length of time exhibited more arousal/anxiety as measured by spontaneous galvanic skin responses when compared with individuals who were in control of the slides. There is also evidence that self-administered shock is preferred to (Ball and Vogler, 1971; Pervin, 1963), and produces less arousal than, shock administered by another (Björkstrand, 1973; Haggard, 1943; but also see Staub *et al.*, 1971).

There is some evidence suggesting that the arousal-reducing effect of control will not be found when the correct control response is unknown and difficult to determine. For example, Gatchel and Proctor (1976) exposed groups of subjects to a series of aversive tones. One of the groups was informed that there was some response they could make to escape the noise. The correct control response consisted of pressing a switch four times, and took several trials to learn. Another group was not led to believe control was possible; they were instructed to passively listen. Under these conditions the escapable noise subjects showed higher skin conductance responses than the passive subjects. It seems, however, that the escapable noise subjects began to exhibit less arousal as they mastered the escape response; the frequency of spontaneous fluctuations in skin conductance decreased during the later trials.

Geer *et al.* (1970) sought to determine whether one's perception of control, versus the actual contingencies as arranged by the experimenter, was responsible for the stress-reducing effects of control over an aversive stimulus. In their perceived-control paradigm, all subjects initially participated in a reaction time task in which they were instructed to respond at the onset of a 6-second shock, although reaction time had no effect on shock duration. After a number of such trials, half of the subjects were told that the duration of shock would be reduced to 3 seconds if their reaction times reached a criterion. The other subjects were merely informed that shocks would be shorter. In actuality, all subjects received 3-second-long shocks during the second part of the experiment, non-contingent on reaction time. Geer *et al.* (1970) found that subjects in the perceived-control condition showed fewer spontaneous skin conductance responses during the intertrial intervals, and smaller electrodermal responses to shock onset, than did subjects who did not perceive themselves to be in control of shock duration.

Unfortunately, perception of control was confounded with actual reduction in shock duration in Geer *et al.*'s perception of control paradigm. That is, all subjects actually received reduced shock duration. In order to assess the effects of perception of control *per se*, Glass *et al.* (1973) included four groups of subjects in a variant on the Geer *et al.* (1970) paradigm. In addition to the two conditions included by Geer *et al.* (1970), Glass *et al.* (1973) included two groups who experienced no reduction in shock duration, one of which received the perception of control instructions while the other was informed that shocks would be shorter. Thus, the main effects of perception of control and reduction of shock (and the effect of their interaction) on arousal could be separately assessed. The skin conductance results failed to replicate those of Geer *et al.* (1970); subjects were equally aroused in all groups. Consequently, no conclusions regarding the effect of mere perception of control on the physiological response system can be drawn from this study. Differences in behavioral after-effects were observed, however, and will be discussed below.

Some investigators have studied the effects of potential control on anxiety. In a typical potential control paradigm, one group of subjects receives instructions describing some condition under which they will be able to exert control over an aversive stimulus, such as shock, but is asked by the experimenter not to do so unless they feel it is absolutely necessary. The potential control paradigm differs from the perceived control paradigm in two ways. In potential control studies, the subject is actually able to exert control while perceived control subjects' responses do not actually affect the aversive stimuli. In addition, perceived control subjects are not usually discouraged from attempting to exert control, as is the case in the potential control paradigm. The results of studies of potential control have been mixed. Glass and his colleagues found that the knowledge that one has an escape response available, even if it is never exercised, was sufficient to reduce anticipatory arousal (Glass *et al.*, 1971) and arousal following uncontrollable noise among college students (Reim *et al.*, 1971) and older urban residents (Glass *et al.*, 1971). Corah and Boffa (1970) also found potential control to lower physiological responses to shock but Glass *et al.* (1969) failed to find this effect.

The cognitive response system

The cognitive components of anxiety include thoughts, feelings, and images of threat, fear, helplessness or danger, which are usually assessed by self-report. Self-reports of anxiety and related emotions have been found to increase following exposure to uncontrollable negative events. Interestingly, many of the studies described below employed learned helplessness paradigms, designed to relate helplessness to depression. As noted below and in the Introduction, self-reported affect following exposure to uncontrollable negative events in these paradigms reveals that anxiety is at least as prominent, if not more prominent, than depression.

For example, an early study by Bowers (1968) found that subjects who expected to be able to avoid shock were less anxious before shock delivery than were subjects who believed the shocks to be uncontrollable. In a later study, Miller and Seligman (1975) administered the Multiple Affect Adjective Checklist (Zuckerman and Lubin, 1965) to subjects before and after exposure to escapable or inescapable noise. Subjects who could not control the noise (i.e. those for whom the noise was inescapable) rated themselves as more anxious, depressed and hostile after exposure than did subjects who could terminate the noise. Using a similar experimental paradigm, Gatchel et al.(1975) also observed increases in self-reported anxiety, depression and hostility among subjects exposed to uncontrollable noise. Furthermore, Gatchel et al. found the group differences had disappeared after subjects were provided with a mastery experience (solving anagrams). More recently, Brier et al. (1987) found that exposure to inescapable noise, but not exposure to escapable noise, led to increased reports of both depression and anxiety, but the increase in depression was of a relatively small magnitude compared to the increase in anxiety.

The behavioral response system

In addition to increased autonomic arousal and self-reported negative affect, a third consequence of exposure to uncontrollable aversive stimuli, behavioral disturbance, has been observed by several investigators (e.g. Glass et al., 1973; Reim et al., 1971). For example, in a perceived control study by Glass et al. (1971), subjects were given a seven-page paper to proofread after having been exposed to noise that was perceived to controllable versus uncontrollable. On average, subjects in the perceived control condition exhibited superior proofreading performance (i.e. overlooked fewer errors to be found in the passage) as compared to subjects in the no-perceived control condition.

Similarly, impaired Stroop color-naming performance was found by Glass et al. (1973) to follow exposure to uncontrollable, but not controllable, shock. The behavioral disturbances in the Stroop task were originally attributed to the effects of uncontrollable shock producing increased psychological stress, but some recent research on the role of attentional biases in anxiety suggests a possible alternative explanation in which the effects are mediated by the anxiety following uncontrollable shock.

Mathews and MacLeod (1985) administered a modified version of the Stroop color-naming task to anxious out-patients and non-patient controls. The subjects were required to name the color of ink in which physical or social threat-relevant words and non-threat-related words were printed. The anxious subjects were slower in general at the color naming but they were particularly slow with the threat-related words. In addition, current level of anxiety was found to be the best predictor of extent of interference. Mathews and MacLeod suggest that the emotional arousal produced by the threat words in the anxious patients may disrupt their attentional sets, diverting attention from the nominal task of color naming to the content of the threat words. A similar interpretation would seem applicable to the Glass *et al.* (1973) results described above. That is, the uncontrollably shocked subjects were probably more anxious than the controllably shocked subjects (see discussion above). This anxiety may then have produced the impaired performance on the Stroop task. It would be interesting to assess whether the Glass *et al.* (1973) manipulation would have an especially strong effect for threat-related Stroop words, as would be suggested by the results of the Mathews and MacLeod study.

Human research: clinical phenomena and clinical studies

The results of the animal and human laboratory studies discussed above strongly suggest that more fear and anxiety is experienced when stressors are uncontrollable. Many theories have also implicated uncontrollable stressors as important in the etiology of full-blown anxiety disorders (e.g. Alloy *et al.*, in press; Barlow, 1988; Foa *et al.* 1989; Mineka, 1985a,b). For example, as briefly discussed in the introduction, Alloy *et al.* have presented a helplessness/hopelessness perspective on the etiologies of a range of anxiety disorders, mixed anxiety and depression, and pure depression. In their theory, perceptions of certain or uncertain helplessness (i.e. low to high estimates of how likely it is that one will not be able to control important outcomes) are implicated in the origins of anxiety disorders. Anxiety accompanies uncertain and certain helplessness as long as one still maintains some hope that negative outcomes may not occur, even though one cannot actually control these outcomes. They also hypothesize, however, that the more certain one is of one's helplessness, the more likely it is that depressive symptomatology will be mixed with the anxiety symptoms. Alloy *et al.*'s hypothesis is in keeping with the findings of differential comorbidity among the different anxiety disorders and depression (cf. Barlow, 1985; DiNardo and Barlow, in press). In this theory, anxiety symptoms are thought to sometimes wane and be replaced by pure depression when certainty that one is powerless to control outcomes is accompanied by certainty that negative outcomes will indeed occur (i.e. when one becomes hopeless).

There are also some suggestions in the literature that when uncontrollable and unpredictable aversive events are actually involved in the etiology of anxiety disorders the degree of uncontrollability and/or unpredictability may, in part, determine which anxiety disorder emerges. For example, post-traumatic stress disorder (PTSD) and simple phobias are similar in that they often develop following traumatic events. Foa *et al.* (1989) have recently hypothesized that PTSD, a much more severe and pervasive disorder, is more likely than simple phobia to result when the traumas are more highly unpredictable and/or uncontrollable (e.g. rape, war, torture, natural disaster). Başoğlu and Mineka (in preparation) have also argued that the emergence of PTSD in torture victims may stem in large part from the uncontrollable, unpredictable nature of the stressors involved in torture.

Control has been implicated as important in clinical anxiety disordered patients in two ways. First, individuals with anxiety disorders often report feeling helpless to cope in the face of the sources of their fears, such as phobic stimuli or panic attacks (e.g. Bandura, 1977; Beck and Emery, 1985; Barlow, 1988). Another type of helplessness found among anxious patients is a fear of future helplessness, as in the worry of persons with generalized anxiety disorder and obsessive-compulsive disorder, or the anticipatory anxiety in panic disorder with or without agoraphobia (Barlow, 1988; Mavissakalian and Barlow, 1981; Klein, 1964). These two aspects of helplessness probably should not be thought of as completely independent. It seems likely that fear of future helplessness may be based, in part, on past experiences of the former type of helplessness.

Some investigators have found evidence of a correlation between anxiety and feelings of control in clinically anxious samples. Williams and his colleagues have investigated the role of perceptions of self-efficacy in approach behavior among phobics. Bandura (1982) has defined self-percepts of efficacy as 'judgments of how well one can execute courses of action required to deal with prospective situations' (p. 122). For instance, Williams and Watson (1985) obtained ratings of perceived self-efficacy from acrophobics at progressively greater heights before and after treatment. Both before and after treatment, perceptions of self-efficacy strongly predicted approach behavior. In a somewhat different vein, Rachman *et al.* (1986) found in a study with agoraphobic patients that almost 50% of their subjects reported a decline in feelings of control during weeks in which they had experienced at least one panic attack. Only 25% of the sample reported an increase in feelings of control during weeks in which they had panicked. In panic-free weeks, only 22% of the agoraphobics reported feeling less in control, while 42% indicated that they felt more efficacious. Telch *et al.* (in press) studied the appraisals of perceived self-efficacy in coping with panic in patients with pure panic disorder versus patients with panic disorder with moderate to severe agoraphobic avoidance. They found that the agoraphobics reported more dysfunctional appraisals of their ability to cope with panics than did the pure panic disorder subjects, i.e. agoraphobics have less confidence in their personal resources to manage panic. Telch and his colleagues hypothesized that the lower perceptions of efficacy in coping with panic among the agoraphobics may have had some etiological significance in the development of their avoidance. That is, agoraphobic avoidance may be more likely to develop in patients with panic attacks if they perceive themselves as being unable to cope with the panic attacks that they may experience in public places.

Loss of control, rather than simply a lack of control, seems to be a particularly important factor in the etiology and maintenance of panic disorder (Barlow, 1988). For example, a sense of, or fear of, loss of control has been found to be among the most common and most severe of symptoms reported to be present during panic attacks (Sanderson *et al.*, 1987, cited by Sanderson *et al.*, 1989). To the extent that patients with panic attacks are accurate in their perceptions of loss of control, laboratory situations designed to increase these perceptions would be expected to cause an increase in the anxiety symptoms that are experienced. Such has been found to be the case in laboratory panic-induction studies.

A large number of pharmacological and behavioral procedures have been found capable of inducing increased anxiety, and sometimes full-blown panic attacks, among patients with panic disorder (see Barlow, 1988, and Margraf *et al.*, 1986, for thorough reviews of the panic-induction literature). The list of panic-provocation agents includes adrenaline, isoproterenol, yohimbine and lactate infusions, caffeine consumption, hyperventilation, carbon dioxide inhalation and even relaxation (Barlow, 1988). No single biological mechanism is able to account for the effects of these diverse panic-provoking procedures. But as Barlow (1988) has noted, two common factors do appear to be present in all of the different procedures. First, subjects who experienced acute increases in anxiety during these challenges are those who are most anxious at baseline. The second commonality is more relevant to our discussion. As Barlow (1988) concludes, in all types of panic-producing procedures, there is 'the elicitation of a specific somatic response that is associated with a sense of loss of control' (p. 155). That is, the physical sensations produced by the various provocation procedures are perceived by panic-prone individuals as representing *loss* of control over one's own body. The fear associated with the belief that one is losing control leads to an increase in these somatic symptoms, which in turn strengthens the perception of losing control, perpetuating a positive feedback loop.

A few preliminary studies have found support for the hypothesis that fear of losing control is implicated in the increased anxiety caused by the provocation procedures described above. For example, Heide and Borkovec (1983), studying relaxation-induced anxiety in patients with generalized anxiety disorder, found the fear of losing control to be strongly associated with increased *tension* during the relaxation exercises. Adler *et al.* (1987) studied the responses of patients with panic disorder to each of the following: a relaxation tape that included suggestions of giving up control of one's muscles; a tape with muscle tension instructions; and a tape of a passage of prose. More panic disorder subjects reported experiencing moderately severe panic symptoms during the relaxation tape than during either of the other two tapes. A third study investigating the role of control in panic-provocation procedures will be described in more detail because it is the only one to have actually manipulated perceptions of control.

Using a clever variation on the perceived control paradigm, Sanderson *et al.* (1989) examined the effect of an illusion of control on laboratory-induced anxiety among 20 patients presenting for treatment who had diagnoses of panic disorder with agoraphobia. After a 5-minute baseline period, during which the subjects received compressed air, there was a 15-minute induction trial, which consisted of breathing 5.5% carbon-dioxide-enriched air, a known panic-provoking agent. Before beginning the experimental procedures, all subjects were told that whenever a signal light was lit they could use a dial on their chair to reduce the concentration of carbon dioxide they received. Subjects were strongly encouraged, however, to resist adjusting the carbon dioxide mixture when the opportunity was present. In actuality, the dial was inoperative and adjusting it had no effect on the amount of carbon dioxide delivered. Half of the patients were assigned at random to the illusion-of-control group; for this group the signal light remained lit during the entire carbon dioxide trial. The remaining ten patients comprised the no-illusion-of-control group; for these subjects, the signal light remained unlit during the entire carbon dioxide trial. Hence, a perception of control was induced in the illusion-of-control group but not in the no-illusion group.

Sanderson *et al.* (1989) collected subjective anxiety ratings from all subjects every $2\frac{1}{2}$ minutes during the experiment. At the completion of the 20-minute experiment, or whenever it was terminated by the subject, patients indicated whether any panic symptoms were experienced during the procedure and, if so, their intensity. Subjects reported on the presence of several catastrophic and non-catastrophic thoughts accompanying the symptoms experienced. In addition, the investigators wished to determine which patients had actually experienced a panic attack. Rather than relying on patients' self-reports of panic, the above information was used to determine whether a panic attack had occurred (using criteria comparable to those of DSM-III). Subjects were also asked to rate the similarity of symptoms occurring in the laboratory to those during a typical panic attack. A manipulation check was performed to determine if indeed the groups differed in perceptions of control.

The experimental manipulation of perceptions of control was found to be effective. The illusion-of-control group reported having significantly greater control over the symptoms produced by carbon dioxide inhalation than did the no-illusion-of-control group. The results indicate that perception of control also had an effect on symptomatology experienced during carbon dioxide inhalation. As compared to the illusion-of-control group, the no-illusion subjects reported a greater number of panic symptoms, rated the symptoms experienced as more severe, endorsed more catastrophic thoughts, and reported more subjective distress. In fact, while the subjective anxiety ratings among the no-illusion group increased by nearly two points on a nine-point scale, anxiety ratings among the illusion group decreased by almost a full point (see Figure 5).

In addition, 8 out of the 10 no-illusion subjects, but only 2 out of the 10 illusion subjects, met criteria for a panic attack. The no-illusion subjects perceived their

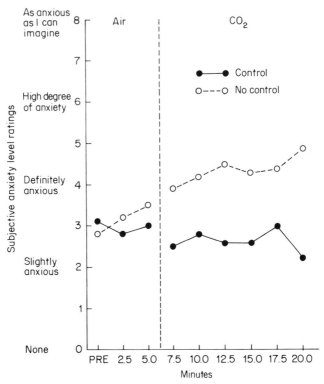

FIGURE 5. Mean subjective anxiety ratings of the control group and the no-control group taken every 2.5 minutes during the inhalation of air for 5 minutes followed by 15 minutes of CO_2-enriched air. From Sanderson *et al.* (1989). By permission of the American Medical Association.

symptoms to be 'quite' similar to their typical panic attacks but illusion subjects perceived only a slight similarity. Finally, the groups differed in their willingness to tolerate the induction procedure. Two of the ten no-illusion patients terminated the session before the end of the 15-minute inhalation period, but none of the illusion patients did so.

The results of the Sanderson *et al.* study provide the most direct evidence to date that perceptions of control can attenuate the effects of exposure to anxiety-provoking stimuli among clinically anxious individuals. In summary, they found evidence that, at least among patients with panic disorder, perceptions of control mediate the experience of anxiety in each of the three emotional response systems previously described. With respect to the physiological system, patients with an illusion of control experienced fewer and less severe somatic symptoms of panic and fewer met criteria for a panic attack. In the cognitive/affective realm, the illusion patients experienced fewer catastrophic thoughts, less subjective distress during inhalation, and perceived their laboratory-induced symptoms as less similar to naturally occurring panics than did the no-illusion patients. Finally, the illusion group was less likely than the no-illusion group to exhibit escape behavior during carbon dioxide inhalation, as evidenced by their greater willingness to complete the procedure. Because of the wide-ranging implications of this study, replication with a larger number of patients seems to be an important next step in this area of research. Furthermore, given the high incidence of at least infrequent panic attacks among all types of anxiety-disordered patients (Barlow, 1988), it would be interesting to replicate this study using patients with other anxiety disorder diagnoses.

IMPORTANCE OF CONTROL FOLLOWING THE ACQUISITION OF FEAR/ANXIETY IN ITS REDUCTION

Thus far, we have discussed research implicating a role for prior experience with control and mastery in reducing the impact of a variety of fear- and anxiety-provoking situations. In addition, we have discussed animal and human research implicating the importance of control during the experience of aversive stimulation in reducing the immediate and short-term impact of that aversive stimulation, using physiological, behavioral and cognitive/subjective levels of analysis. Long-term benefits from having control over aversive stimulation may also accrue in that substantially less fear is conditioned to neutral stimuli present at the time of the stimulation (e.g. Mineka *et al.*, 1984). In this section, we review evidence that once fear or anxiety has been acquired (either as occurs in a laboratory setting, or as occurs in a full-blown anxiety disorder), experience with control over the source of the fear/anxiety can be helpful in reducing the fear/anxiety.

Animal studies

In the Mineka *et al.* (1984) experiments discussed above, we saw that less fear was conditioned to a neutral stimulus paired with escapable as opposed to inescapable shocks. Here we discuss the importance of what happens *following* conditioning for the level of fear that is maintained over time. These experiments employed an avoidance-learning paradigm—that is, one where the organism can learn not only to escape an aversive stimulus but also to avoid it completely by responding shortly after a signal for the impending aversive stimulus comes on. The finding that fear of the CS diminishes over the course of avoidance learning is well known. Solomon *et al.* (1953) first noticed that dogs well trained at avoiding shocks of traumatic intensity became rather nonchalant about the whole situation, and showed no overt signs of fear of the CS as they had at the outset of avoidance training. These anecdotal observations were later systematized and replicated by Kamin *et al.* (1963), who used an independent measure of fear of the CS, and explicitly compared rats at different stages of avoidance training. It was originally thought that this diminution in fear over the course of avoidance learning was simply a function of the fact that each successful avoidance trial is a Pavlovian fear extinction trial, i.e. a CS followed by no US. However, several experiments have now demonstrated that this account of the diminution in fear that occurs over the course of avoidance learning is not correct. Instead, as for escape learning, it appears to be the control and its correlated feedback, or the added predictability inherent in having an avoidance response available, that is responsible for the reduction in fear that occurs over the course of avoidance learning (Cook *et al.*, 1987; Starr and Mineka, 1977).

In brief, these experiments all replicated previous findings that master animals who were trained to avoid shock did show a reduction in fear as their avoidance responses became well-learned. However, unlike in prior experiments on this topic, each master group in these experiments had a group yoked to it that received the exact same pattern of CS–US pairings and non-reinforced CS trials. If the Pavlovian fear extinction account of the diminution in fear seen over the course of avoidance learning is correct, then groups yoked to very well-trained masters should show the same low levels of fear as the masters. Contrary to this hypothesis, results indicated that no such decline in fear occurred in the groups yoked to well-trained masters, thus implicating some aspect of the avoidance response contingency as an important factor in reducing fear. As in the escape experiments of Mineka *et al.*(1984) described above, however, it was not control *per se* that was important, but rather the added predictability inherent in having an avoidance response available. This conclusion derived from the finding that yoked subjects that received an exteroceptive feedback signal when the masters made their escape or avoidance response also showed the same low levels of fear as their masters, even though they did not have control over CS or US termination.

So again we see the importance of studying Pavlovian conditioning in more complex paradigms (that may better resemble the everyday life events where such conditioning often occurs) than those in which it has traditionally been studied. In particular, this experiment demonstrates that the reduction in fear that occurs as an avoidance response becomes well learned is not simply a result of the Pavlovian fear extinction trials that occur. Rather, the fear attenuation is more a function of the control and/or predictability and feedback that are inherent in having an avoidance response available. To the extent that parallel effects occur in humans, these results suggest that people who develop effective coping responses (such as flight) in the presence of feared objects or situations will experience less fear and distress than those who do not develop effective coping responses.

Cognitive-behavior therapies for anxiety disorders

Just as control and predictability have been strongly implicated in the reduction of fear seen over the course of avoidance learning in animals, so too are perceptions of increased control and predictability now implicated in mediating the effects of cognitive-behavioral therapies for anxiety disorders. As discussed above, several theorists have implicated the role of lack or loss of control, among other psychological factors, in the etiologies of the various anxiety disorders. To the extent that it is valid to conceptualize the anxiety disorders as products of feedback loops which include negative perceptions of control, then it is not too surprising that interventions targeted at increasing one's sense of control would affect the entire system in such a way as to decrease the resultant anxiety (Barlow, 1988). Although there is little research bearing directly on this topic, Barlow, a notable theorist in this area, stated in his comprehensive review of the cognitive-behavioral therapy literature that 'changing perceptions of helplessness is central to any therapeutic endeavor ... [Indeed] these therapeutic attempts will not be completely successful unless the patient begins to feel in control of potential upcoming events, whether environmental or somatic' (1988, pp. 313–314). Similarly, for over a decade, Bandura (1977) has advocated the importance of increasing patients' feelings of self-efficacy, which are related but not identical to perceptions of control, in order to decrease fear behavior.

It should be emphasized that initially Bandura considered perceived self-efficacy to be predictive only of *behavior*, and the research done to test the effect of increased self-efficacy on treatment outcome has generally supported his claim (e.g. Williams *et al.*, 1984). More recently, however, it has been suggested that the concept of self-efficacy be expanded to include not only one's perceptions of behavioral abilities but also the ability to cope with more internal phenomena, such as symptoms of anxiety or panic (Bandura, 1986; Barlow, 1988). Furthermore, the results of Sanderson *et al.* (1989) discussed above suggest that altering perceptions of control in patients has an impact on a variety of components of anxiety, including physiological, cognitive, affective and behavioral components. Such results are highly suggestive that altering perceptions of control during therapy and homework exercises will also have profound effects on all three fear-response systems. In the future, it would be important to more accurately delineate the causal mediating role that instilling a sense of control may play in fear/anxiety reduction. Finally, there are undoubtedly still many refinements of current cognitive-behavioral techniques yet to be discovered that may maximize the likelihood that these techniques will have the effect of increasing a sense of control.

CONCLUSIONS

In this chapter we have reviewed a considerable amount of research from both animal and human studies that implicates an important role for lack or loss of control in the etiology and maintenance of fear and anxiety. We have seen that having a prior history of control over important life events is thought to often protect the organism from the negative consequences of later experience with

environmental stressors. We also noted, however, that the immediate consequences of losing control for an organism that once had it may involve increased
arousal/stress, although the boundary conditions for producing these effects of
loss of control are not well understood at this point. In addition, we have seen
that having control (actual, perceived or potential) over aversive events substantially reduces the amount of fear/anxiety produced by those events, as evidenced
by cognitive, behavioral and physiological response measures. And for subjects
who have neutral stimuli paired with uncontrollable aversive events, considerably more fear is conditioned to those neutral stimuli than for subjects who have
neutral stimuli paired with controllable aversive events of the same intensity and
duration. We also discussed research and theory with human clinical anxiety
disorders which strongly implicates feelings of lack or loss of control in the origins
and maintenance of those disorders. This research demonstrates the importance
of control not only in the origins and maintenance of the 'normal' fears and
anxiety experienced by all animals and humans in certain circumstances, but also
in the more extreme pathological forms of fear and anxiety seen in the clinic.
Finally, we have also discussed the role played by control in reducing fear and
anxiety once it has been acquired. Although a good deal of research remains to be
done in this area before definitive conclusions can be drawn, an important,
perhaps crucial, element of cognitive-behavioral therapies for anxiety disorders
appears to be instilling a sense of control over environmental and/or somatic
events.

ACKNOWLEDGEMENTS

Preparation of this chapter was supported by grant BNS-8507340 from the
National Science Foundation to S. Mineka. The authors' research described in
the chapter has been generously supported by the following grants: grants BNS-
7823612, BNS-8119041, BNS-8216141, BNS-8507340 from the National Science
Foundation, and by grants from the Wisconsin Alumni Research Foundation.
The authors would especially like to thank Maribeth Champoux, Michael Cook
and Megan Gunnar for their help in conducting much of the research described
here.

REFERENCES

Abramson, L. Y., Seligman, M. E. P., and Teasdale, J. D. (1978). Learned helplessness in
humans: Critique and reformulation. *Journal of Abnormal Psychology*, **87**, 49–74.
Abramson, L. Y., Metalsky, G. I., and Alloy, L. B. (1989). Hopelessness depression: A
theory-based subtype of depression. *Psychological Review*, **96**, 358–372.
Adler, C. M., Craske, M. G., and Barlow, D. H. (1987). Relaxation-induced panic: When
resting isn't peaceful. *Integrative Psychiatry*, **5**, 94–112.

Ainsworth, M. D. S., Blehar, M., Waters, E., and Wall, S. (1978). *Patterns of Attachment.* Hillsdale, NJ: Erlbaum.

Alloy, L. B., Kelly, K. A., Mineka, S., and Clements, C. M. (in press). Comorbidity in anxiety and depressive disorders: A helplessness/hopelessness perspective. In: J. D. Maser and C. R. Cloninger (eds), *Comorbidity in Anxiety and Mood Disorders.* Washington, DC: American Psychiatric Press, Inc.

Averill, J. R. (1973). Personal control over aversive stimuli and its relationship to stress. *Psychological Bulletin*, **80**, 286–303.

Ball, T. S., and Vogler, R. E. (1971). Uncertain pain and the pain of uncertainty. *Perceptual Motor Skills*, **33**, 1195–1203.

Bandura, A. (1986). Social Foundations of Thought and Action: A Social Cognitive Theory. Englewood Cliffs, NJ: Prentice-Hall.

Barlow, D. H. (1985). The dimensions of anxiety disorders. In: A. H. Tuma and J. D. Maser (eds), *Anxiety and the Anxiety Disorders.* Hillsdale, NJ: Erlbaum.

Barlow, D. H. (1988). *Anxiety and its Disorders: The Nature and Treatment of Anxiety and Panic.* New York: Guilford Press.

Başoğlu, M., and Mineka, S. (in preparation). PTSD in torture victims: The role of unpredictability and uncontrollability.

Beck, A. T., and Emery, G. (1985). *Anxiety Disorders and Phobias: A Cognitive Perspective.* New York: Basic Books.

Björkstrand, P. (1973). Electrodermal responses as affected by subject—versus experimenter-controlled noxious stimulation. *Journal of Experimental Psychology*, **97**, 365–369.

Beck, A. T., and Emery, G. (1985). *Anxiety Disorders and Phobias: A Cognitive Perspective.* New York: Basic Books.

Björkstrand, P. (1973). Electrodermal responses as affected by subject—versus experimenter—controlled noxious stimulation. *Journal of Experimental Psychology*, **97**, 365–369.

Bowers, K. S. (1968). Pain, anxiety, and perceived control. *Journal of Consulting and Clinical Psychology*, **32**, 596–602.

Brennan, J. F., and Riccio, D. C. (1975). Stimulus generalization of suppression in rats following aversively motivated instrumental or Pavlovian training. *Journal of Comparative and Physiological Psychology*, **88**, 570–579.

Brier, A., Albus, M., Pickar, D., Zahn, T. P., Wolkowitz, O. M., and Paul, S. M. (1987). Controllable and uncontrollable stress in humans: Alterations in mood and neuroendocrine and psychophysiological function. *American Journal of Psychiatry*, **144**, 1419–1425.

Broadhurst, P. L. (1961). Abnormal animal behavior. In: H. J. Eysenck (ed.), *Handbook of Abnormal Psychology.* New York: Basic Books.

Broadhurst, P. L. (1973). Animal studies bearing on abnormal behavior. In: H. J. Eysenck (ed.), *Handbook of Abnormal Psychology* (2nd edn). New York: Basic Books.

Clarke-Stewart, K. A. (1973). Interactions between mothers and their young children: Characteristics and consequences. *Monograph of the Society for Research in Child Development*, **36** (6, Serial No. 153).

Cook, M., Mineka, S., and Trumble, D. (1987). The role of response-produced and exteroceptive feedback in the attenuation of fear over the course of avoidance learning. *Journal of Experimental Psychology: Animal Behavior Processes*, **13**, 239–249.

Corah, N. L., and Boffa, J. (1970). Perceived control, self-observation, and response to aversive stimulation. *Journal of Personality and Social Psychology*, **16**, 1–4.

Desiderato, O., and Newman, A. (1971). Conditioned suppression produced in rats by tones paired with escapable or inescapable shock. *Journal of Comparative and Physiological Psychology*, **77**, 427–431.

DiNardo, P. A., and Barlow, D. H. (in press). Syndrome and Symptom comorbidity in the anxiety disorders. In: J. D. Maser and C. R. Cloninger (eds), *Comorbidity in Anxiety and Mood Disorders*. Washington, DC: American Psychiatric Press, Inc.

Foa, E. B., Steketee, G., and Rothbaum, B. (1989). Behavioral/cognitive conceptualizations of post-traumatic stress disorder. *Behavior Therapy*, **20**, 155–176.

Garber, J., Miller, S. M., and Abramson, L. Y. (1980). On the distinction between anxiety states and depression: Perceived control, certainty, and probability of goal attainment. In: J. Garber and M. E. P. Seligman (eds), *Human Helplessness: Theory and Applications*. New York: Academic Press.

Gatchel, R. J., and Proctor, J. D. (1976). Physiological correlates of learned helplessness in man. *Journal of Abnormal Psychology*, **85**, 27–34.

Gatchel, R. J., Paulus, P. B., and Maples, C. W. (1975). Learned helplessness and self-reported affect. *Journal of Abnormal Psychology*, **84**, 732–734.

Geer, J., Davison, G. C., and Gatchel, R. J. (1970). Reduction of stress in humans through nonveridical perceived control of aversive stimulation. *Journal of Personality and Social Psychology*, **16**, 731–738.

Geer, J. H., and Maisel, E. (1972). Evaluating the effects of the prediction-control confound. *Journal of Personality and Social Psychology*, **23**, 314–319.

Glass, D. C., Singer, J. E., and Friedman, L. H. (1969). Psychic cost of adapation to an environmental stressor. *Journal of Personality and Social Psychology*, **12**, 200–210.

Glass, D. C., Reim, B., and Singer, J. R. (1971). Behavioral consequences of adaptation to controllable and uncontrollable noise. *Journal of Experimental Social Psychology*, **7**, 244–257.

Glass, D. C., Singer, J. E., Leonard, H. S., Krantz, D., Cohen, S., and Cummings, H. (1973). Perceived control of aversive stimulation and the reduction of stress responses. *Journal of Personality*, **41**, 577–595.

Haggard, E. A. (1943). Experimental studies in affective processes. I. Some effects of cognitive structure and active participation on certain autonomic reactions during and following experimentally induced stress. *Journal of Experimental Psychology*, **33**, 257–284.

Hanson, J. D., Larson, M. E., and Snowdon, C. T. (1976). The effects of control over high intensity noise on plasma cortisol levels in rhesus monkeys. *Behavioral Biology*, **16**, 333–340.

Heide, F. J., and Borkovec, T. D. (1983). Relaxation-induced anxiety: Paradoxical anxiety enhancement due to relaxation training. *Journal of Consulting and Clinical Psychology*, **51**, 171–182.

Hendersen, R. (1978). Forgetting of conditioned fear inhibition. *Learning and Motivation*, **8**, 16–30.

Kamin, L., Brimer, C., and Black, A. (1963). Conditioned suppression as a monitor of fear of the CS in the course of avoidance training. *Journal of Comparative and Physiological Psychology*, **56**, 497–501.

Klein, D. F. (1964). Delineation of two drug-responsive anxiety syndromes. *Psychopharmacologia*, **5**, 397–408.

Lang, P. J. (1968). Fear reduction and fear behavior: Problems in treating a construct. In: J. M. Shlien (ed.), *Research in Psychotherapy* (Vol. III). Washington, DC: American Psychological Association.

Lang, P. J. (1971). Application of psychophysiological methods to the study of psychotherapy and behavior modification. In: A. E. Bergin and S. L. Garfield (eds), *Handbook of Psychotherapy and Behavior Change*. New York: Wiley.

Lang, P. J. (1979). A bio-informational theory of emotional imagery. *Psychophysiology*, **16**, 495–512.

Lang, P. J. (1984). Cognition in emotion: Concept and action. In: C. Izard, J. Kagan, and R. Zajonc (eds), *Emotions, Cognition and Behavior*. New York: Cambridge University Press.

Lang, P. (1985). The cognitive psychophysiology of emotion: Fear and anxiety. In: A. H. Tuma and J. D. Maser (eds), *Anxiety and the Anxiety Disorders*. Hillsdale, NJ: Erlbaum.

Lewis, M., and Goldberg, S. (1969). Perceptual-cognitive development in infancy: A generalized expectancy model as a function of mother–infant interaction. *Merrill-Palmer Quarterly*, **15**, 81–85.

Maier, S., Seligman, M., and Solomon, R. (1969). Pavlovian fear conditioning and learned helplessness. In: B. A. Campbell and R. M. Church (eds), *Punishment and Aversive Behavior*. New York: Appleton-Century-Crofts.

Mandler, G. (1966). Anxiety. In: D. L. Sills (ed), *International Encyclopedia of the Social Sciences*. New York: Macmillan.

Mandler, G. (1972). Helplessness: Theory and research in anxiety. In: C. D. Spielberger (ed.), *Anxiety: Current Trends in Theory and Research III*. New York: Academic Press.

Margraf, J., Ehlers, A., and Roth, W. T. (1986). Biological models of panic disorder and agoraphobia: A review. *Behaviour Research and Therapy*, **24**, 553–567.

Marks, I. (1987). *Fears, Phobias, and Rituals: Panic, Anxiety and their Disorders*. New York: Oxford University Press.

Maser, J., and Cloninger, C. (eds) (in press). *Comorbidity in Anxiety and Mood Disorders*. Washington, DC: American Psychiatric Press, Inc.

Masserman, J. H. (1971). The principle of uncertainty in neurotogenesis. In: H. D. Kimmel (ed.), *Experimental Psychopathology: Recent Research and Theory*. New York: Academic Press.

Matthews, A., and MacLeod, C. (1985). Selective processing of threat cues in anxiety states. *Behaviour Research and Therapy*, **23**, 563–569.

Mavissakalian, M. R., and Barlow, D. H. (1981). Assessment of obsessive-compulsive disorders. In: D. H. Barlow (ed.), *Behavioral Assessment of Adult Disorders*. New York: Guilford Press.

Miller, S. M. (1979). Controllability and human stress: Method, evidence, and theory. *Behaviour Research and Therapy*, **17**, 287–306.

Miller, S. (1980). Why having control reduces stress: If I can stop the roller coaster, I don't want to get off. In: J. Garber and M. E. P. Seligman (eds), *Human Helplessness: Theory and Applications*. New York: Academic Press.

Miller, W. R., and Seligman, M. E. P. (1975). Depression and learned helplessness in man. *Journal of Abnormal Psychology*, **84**, 228–238.

Mineka, S. (1982). Depression and helplessness in primates. In: H. Fitzgerald, J. Mullins and P. Gage (eds), *Primate Behavior and Child Nurturance* (Child Nurturance Series, Vol. 3, pp. 197–242). New York: Plenum.

Mineka, S. (1985a). The frightful complexity of the origins of fears. In: F. Brush and J. Overmier (eds), *Affect, Conditioning, and Cognition: Essays on the Determinants of Behavior* Hillsdale, NJ: Erlbaum.

Mineka, S. (1985b). Animal models of anxiety-based disorders: Their usefulness and limitations. In: A. H. Tuma and J. D. Maser (eds), *Anxiety and the Anxiety Disorders*. Hillsdale, NJ: Erlbaum.

Mineka, S., and Hendersen, R. (1985). Controllability and predictability in acquired motivation. *Annual Review of Psychology*, **36**, 495–529.

Mineka, S., and Kihlstrom, J. (1978). Unpredictable and uncontrollable events: A new perspective on experimental neurosis. *Journal of Abnormal Psychology*, **87**, 256–271.

Mineka, S., and Tomarken, A. J. (1989). The role of cognitive biases in the origins and maintenance of fear and anxiety disorders. In: T. Archer and L. G. Nilsson (eds),

Aversion, Avoidance, and Anxiety: Perspectives on Aversively Motivated Behavior. Hillsdale, NJ: Erlbaum.

Mineka, S., Cook, M., and Miller, S. (1984). Fear conditioned with escapable and inescapable shock: The effects of a feedback stimulus. *Journal of Experimental Psychology: Animal Behavior Processes,* **10**, 307–323.

Mineka, S., Gunnar, M., and Champoux, M. (1986). Control and early socioemotional development: Infant rhesus monkeys reared in controllable versus uncontrollable environments. *Child Development,* **57**, 1241–1256.

Mowrer, D. H., and Viek, P. (1948). An experimental analogue of fear from a sense of helplessness. *Journal of Abnormal and Social Psychology,* **43**, 193–200.

Osborne, F., Mattingly, B., Redmond, W., and Osborne, J. (1975). Factors affecting the measurement of classically conditioned fear in rats following exposure to escapable versus inescapable signalled shock. *Journal of Experimental Psychology: Animal Behavior Processes,* **1**, 364–373.

Overmier, J. B., and Seligman, M. E. P. (1967). Effects of inescapable shock upon subsequent escape and avoidance learning. *Journal of Comparative and Physiological Psychology,* **63**, 23–33.

Pavlov, I. P. (1927). *Conditioned Reflexes: An Investigation of the Physiological Activity of the Cerebral Cortex.* London: Oxford University Press.

Pervin, L. A. (1963). The need to predict and control under conditions of threat. *Journal of Personality,* **31**, 570–587.

Rachman, S., Craske, M., Tallman, K., and Solyom, C. (1986). Does escape behavior strengthen agoraphobic avoidance? A replication. *Behavior Therapy,* **17**, 366–384.

Reim, B., Glass, D. C., and Singer, J. E. (1971). Behavioral consequences of exposure to uncontrollable and unpredictable noise. *Journal of Applied Social Psychology,* **1**, 44–56.

Sanderson, W. C., Rapee, R. M., and Barlow, D. H. (1989). The influence of an illusion of control on panic attacks induced via inhalation of 5.5% carbon-dioxide enriched air. *Archives of General Psychiatry,* **46**, 157–162.

Seligman, M. E. P. (1975). *Helplessness: On Depression, Development and Death.* San Francisco: W. H. Freeman.

Seligman, M. E. P., and Maier, S. F. (1967). Failure to escape traumatic shock. *Journal of Experimental Psychology,* **74**, 1–9.

Seligman, M., Maier, S., and Solomon, R. (1971). Unpredictable and uncontrollable aversive events. In: F. R. Brush (ed.), *Aversive Conditioning and Learning.* New York: Academic Press.

Solomon, R., Kamin, L., and Wynne, L. (1953). Traumatic avoidance learning: The outcomes of several extinction procedures with dogs. *Journal of Abnormal and Social Psychology,* **48**, 291–302.

Sroufe, A., Waters, E., and Matas, L. (1974). Contextual determinants of infant affective response. In: M. Lewis and L. Rosenblum (eds), *The Origins of Fear.* New York: Wiley.

Starr, M. D., and Mineka, S. (1977). Determinants of fear over the course of avoidance learning. *Learning and Motivation,* **8**, 332–350.

Staub, E., Tursky, B., and Schwartz, G. (1971). Self-control and predictability: Their effects on reaction to aversive stimulation. *Journal of Personality and Social Psychology,* **18**, 157–162.

Stroebel, C. F. (1969). Biologic rhythm correlates of disturbed behavior in the rhesus monkey. *Bibliotheca Primatologica,* **9**, 91–105.

Telch, M., Brouilard, M., Telch, C. F., Agras, W. S., and Taylor, C. B. (in press). Role of cognitive appraisal in panic-related avoidance. *Behaviour Research and Therapy.*

Warren, D., Rosellini, R., and Maier, S. (in press). Fear, stimulus feedback, and stressor controllability. In: G. Bower (ed.), *Advances in Learning and Motivation*. New York: Academic Press.

Watson, J. S. (1979). Perception of contingency as a determinant of social responsiveness. In: E. Thomas (ed.), *Origins of Infant's Social Responsiveness*. New York: Erlbaum.

White, R. W. (1959). Motivation reconsidered: The concept of competence. *Psychological Review*, **66**, 297–310.

Williams, S. L., and Watson, N. (1985). Perceived danger and perceived self-efficacy as cognitive determinants of acrophobic behavior. *Behavior Therapy*, **16**, 136–146.

Williams, S. L., Dooseman, G., and Kleifield, E. (1984). Comparative effectiveness of guided mastery and exposure treatments for intractable phobias. *Journal of Consulting and Clinical Psychology*, **52**, 505–518.

Zuckerman, M., and Lubin, B. (1965). *Manual for the Multiple Affect Adjective Checklist*. San Diego, CA: Educational and Industrial Testing Service.

CHAPTER 9

Life events, personal control and depression

Johan Ormel and Robbert Sanderman
Departments of Health Sciences and Psychiatry, University of Groningen, The Netherlands

INTRODUCTION

In recent years, depression has come increasingly to be viewed as an innate, reversible psychobiological response pattern, reflecting the breakdown of psychobiological regulatory mechanisms. This response pattern can be activated by a variety of psychological and biological factors, usually operating in complex interactions. In this chapter we will focus on a number of psychological and social factors and seek to identify the role played by life events and various notions of personal control in the aetiology of depression.

Our interest stems from psychiatric epidemiology, and this undoubtedly has coloured our selection and treatment of the many possible topics relevant to depression. The evidence regarding the aetiological significance of the main variables discussed, life events, general beliefs about control, self-esteem and social support, is largely collected from epidemiological studies. In addition, the focus is on studies of depressive disorder in the community, as it is now well established that depression is often unrecognized and even more frequently untreated, so studies of patient populations are biased by factors associated with detection and help-seeking behaviour. The meaning of this epidemiological evidence is evaluated in terms of pre-existing psychological and biological accounts of depression, and suggests that loss of control is somehow related to the most important aetiological factors.

The demonstration of a weak association between environmental stressors and a variety of psychiatric as well as physical disorders has become routine, and

Stress, Personal Control and Health.   Edited by A. Steptoe and A. Appels.
Published by John Wiley & Sons Ltd.
© ECSC–EEC–EAEC, Brussels–Luxembourg, 1989

efforts have moved to a number of fascinating and unresolved problems related to the elaboration of the 'crude link' between stress and ill health. These problems include the causal direction of the relationship, the role of moderators and intervening variables, the physiological and psychological mechanisms underlying this link, and the specificity issue, i.e. whether there are specific relationships between the nature of the stressor, the characteristics of the organism and the nature of the health disorder.

Although it is generally accepted that life events, in particular events involving loss, are capable of producing depression, a debate continues on the strengths and weaknesses of the major approaches to the assessment of depression and stress. At issue here is the conceptualization of depression and, more specifically, the separation of depression as a normal human psychobiological response from pathological, clinically relevant psychopathology, a problem generally denoted as the case-definition problem. In relation to life events, two major traditions have evolved. The event-list approach, which has gained unprecedented popularity (Cohen, 1988) and which is essentially a respondent-based method neglecting the context of the event; and the interview and rating procedure developed by Brown and Harris (1978), which leads to a common-sense, contextual severity rating of the event that takes into account the individual's biography. Because findings and theoretical implications have been shown to depend on the approach adopted, these issues will be addressed here in some detail.

The plan of this chapter is straightforward. It starts with a short discussion of major stress and coping models, followed by sections on the definition and measurement of depression, personal control and life events, respectively. Then a selective overview of research on the link between depression and life events, social support, self-esteem and related measures of control is presented. A theoretical integration closes the chapter.

BASIC STRESS AND COPING MODELS

The relationship between stress and ill health has generally been approached in the context of two paradigms: (1) the process-oriented, transactional model; and (2) the more traditional, global or structural model. In the latter model, the appraisal and coping processes are not explicitly examined.

The most influential transactional model has been developed by Lazarus and his collaborators. In their most recent formulation Lazarus and Folkman (1984) define stress in terms of the relationship between the person and his or her environment (in other words it is not uniquely stimulus- or response-bound). This relationship is seen as a reciprocal one that develops over time. Key variables within the transactional model are primary and secondary appraisal, problem-focused and emotion-focused coping. Primary appraisal refers to the assessment of the meaning of the situation for the person's well-being. Secondary appraisal refers to subjects' evaluation of the coping resources available to them and coping refers to problem-focused and emotion-focused strategies which can be used to overcome the problem and its aversive emotional effects.

A major exemplar of the structural approach is the influential work of Brown and Harris (1978, 1986) on the social origins of depression. In their vulnerability model Brown and Harris propose that the aetiologically significant factors can be partitioned into two groups: (1) vulnerability factors—these are conceptualized as relatively long-term attributes of individuals or their social environments which influence susceptibility to depression; (2) provoking factors—these are relatively short-term or medium-term aspects of the individual and his or her environment such as life events and difficulties which act to provoke, cause or exacerbate depressive symptoms. The defining feature of their model is that vulnerability and provoking factors are assumed to combine interactively so that symptoms develop only in subjects who are both vulnerable and exposed to provoking factors. Similar models have been proposed by, among others, Pearlin *et al.* (1981), Wheaton (1980) and Parkes (1986).

In these structural models no account is given of the time course of the person–environment transactions in terms of primary and secondary appraisal, and coping. This limits the potential insights in the stress and coping process that can be obtained in studies adopting the structural paradigm. However, in practice we do not have much choice. Owing to the lack of appropriate measurement and statistical methods there is not much research on life events or control and depression in which the complex processes linking appraisal and coping are taken into account.

CONCEPTUAL AND METHODOLOGICAL ISSUES

The construct of control has been incorporated into numerous psychological theories or theoretical conceptions. For example into: (1) locus of control theory (Rotter, 1966, 1975); (2) self-efficacy theory of Bandura (1977); (3) stress and coping theory of Lazarus and Folkman (Folkman, 1984; Lazarus and Folkman, 1984); (4) the mastery construct (Pearlin *et al.*, 1981); (5) hardiness (Kobasa *et al.*, 1982a); (6) the learned helplessness theory (Seligman, 1975; Abramson *et al.*, 1978); and (7) attributional research (Hammen *et al.*, 1981).

Since control is a seemingly clear construct, many authors do not feel obliged to give a definition of it. It will become clear that it is essential to define and operationalize what control exactly is. For, in fact, there is no thing like *the* construct of control. Lazarus and Folkman (1984) admittedly stated: 'There is no single construct of control; rather, it has many meanings and is used differently by different writers and even by the same writer at different times' (p. 20).

Three issues concerning the definition of personal control need here to be addressed: (1) control as coping versus control as belief or appraisal; (2) general versus situation-specific beliefs of control; and (3) control over what.

Some authors use the concept of control to describe the behavioural and cognitive efforts of the individual when dealing with stress (Averill, 1973). Most authors, however, view control as a belief or cognition, reflecting the extent to which people think they can influence the situation, either by altering it, by changing its meaning or by regulating their own behavioural and emotional reactions (Thompson, 1981; Lazarus and Folkman, 1984).

General concepts of personal control have dominated the traditional, structural research models of stress, control and depression. Among the best known is Rotter's (1966) external versus internal locus of control concept. An external locus of control represents the belief that situations are not contingent on a person's own behaviour; an internal locus of control refers to the belief that one in general can control events. Besides locus of control various related general concepts have been suggested, including sense of coherence (Antonowsky, 1987), sense of mastery or competence (Pearlin *et al.*, 1981), fatalism (Wheaton, 1980), hardiness (Kobasa *et al.*, 1982a) and self-esteem (Ingham *et al.*, 1986).

In addition to general beliefs about control a situation-specific version is often distinguished, referring to a person's attributions about control in a particular situation (e.g. Folkman, 1984).

A troubling aspect of the concept of situation-specific control is the question of control over what. In one of our studies (Ormel, 1980) we tried to assess controllability over the occurrence of life events and their consequences. Owing to lack of agreement among the raters we had to give up the rating on the consequences. Analysis revealed that the lack of agreement resulted from the multifacetedness of most events. Each consequence often had its own level of controllability. The raters appeared to have made their own selections and were unable to arrive at an overall judgment.

The conceptualization and measurement of depression

It is generally acknowledged that depression is not a single, clearly described syndrome but takes a variety of forms. The classification of depressive disorders is highly controversial, and remains a source of considerable research efforts. An authoritative classification is laid down in the *Diagnostic Statistical Manual* (DSM-III) of the American Psychiatric Association. The most prevalent single depressive disorder distinguished in the DSM-III is major depression. The essential feature of major depression is either a dysphoric mood, usually depression, or loss of interest or pleasure in all or almost all usual activities and pastimes. This disturbance is prominent, relatively persistent, and associated with other symptoms of the depressive syndrome. These symptoms include appetite disturbance, changes in weight, sleep disturbance, psychomotor agitation or retardation, decreased energy, feelings of worthlessness or guilt, difficulty concentrating or thinking, and thought of death or suicide or suicidal attempts. The empirical criteria for assignment to this category of major depression are the presence for at least two weeks of either dysphoric mood, or loss of interest or pleasure, plus four of the following eight symptoms: psychomotor agitation or retardation; feelings of worthlessness, self-reproach, or excessive or inappropriate guilt; decreased sex drive; sleep disturbance: appetite disturbance; suicidal ideation; decreased ability to concentrate; loss of energy.

DSM-III also proposes a number of dimensions in which major depressions may differ: the most important ones are the distinctions between unipolar and bipolar affective disorders and between depression with and without melancholia. The critical difference between the unipolar and bipolar forms of affective disorders concerns the presence of manic episodes. Patients with a history of manic episodes are classified as bipolars and patients who have only (recurrent) episodes of depression as unipolars. This is an important difference which has achieved considerable acceptance because of its implications for aetiology, treatment and prognosis. Most studies examining depression in the context of life events or control have used subjects with unipolar depressions. The DSM-III dimension of melancholia refers to the classical autonomous–reactive distinction. Conceptualized as two prototypical depressive disorders, the critical difference is their reactivity to psychosocial treatment. Autonomous or endogenomorphic depressions (Willner, 1985) follow a predetermined course and do not respond favourably to psychosocial interventions, whereas reactive depressions tend to respond. It should be noted that this distinction does not imply anything about the aetiology or severity of these prototypical disorders. On the symptom and sign level the defining characteristics of major depression with melancholia are the inability to experience pleasure, even when something good happens, plus three of the following symptoms: distinct quality of mood, excessive or inappropriate guilt, marked psychomotor change, anorexia, early morning awakening, or diurnal variation of mood. Although the autonomous–reactive dimension is not without problems, there is much evidence supporting it. Both factor- and cluster-analytical analyses as well as biological marker studies have demonstrated the validity of this prototypical distinction (Willner, 1985).

Regarding the measurement of depression two distinct methods have been used: standardized psychiatric interviews and self-report symptom scales. The interviews have been developed from clinical practice and are directly related to diagnostic classifications like the International Classification of Diseases (ICD-9) and the third edition of the *Diagnostic Statistical Manual* (DSM-III). As a result of their standardized structure and the use of glossaries, the assessment of caseness and the assignment to a diagnostic category have become reasonably reproducible. One of the most frequently used interviews is the Present State Examination (PSE; Wing *et al.*, 1978), which includes a schedule containing questions directed at eliciting information concerning 140 rateable items, most of them representing psychiatric symptoms defined in a glossary; and a computer program that produces an Index of Definition (ID) indicating the severity and diagnosability of the symptoms present; and, if a tentative classification is possible (ID 5 or more), an ICD diagnosis. The system arrives at a diagnosis by taking into account not only the number of symptoms but also their severity, duration and configuration. By now a small number of similar systems have been developed, among which the Diagnostic Interview Schedule (DIS) and DSM-III system are by far the most important. The use of these standardized procedures has dramatically reduced the traditionally large differences in depression rates found prior to their introduction. Unfortunately, the major prevailing systems do not coincide completely; there still remains some discrepancy in case identification and diagnostic allocation (Brink *et al.*, 1989; Surtees and Sashidharan, 1986). Prevalence rates of depression estimated with the PSE are in the region of 6% (one-month prevalence) and with the DIS/DSM-III approximately 3% for major depression and dysthymic disorder, respectively (six-month prevalence) (Myers *et al.*, 1984; Hodiamont *et al.*, 1987).

The symptom scales, embodying a more dimensional view of depression, are only indirectly related to diagnosable depressive disorder. Despite their very frequent use, there is still some uncertainty about what they exactly measure (Dohrenwend *et al.*, 1980; Bouman, 1987). Symptom scales such as the Center for Epidemiological Studies Depression Scale (CES-D), the Symptom Checklist of Derogatis (SCL-90) and Zung's Self-rating Depression Scale (SDS) consist of mood disturbances and the physiological, cognitive and motivational manifestations of depression, and produce information on the presence of symptoms according to the respondent's own thresholds. The problem is that various studies have demonstrated that these symptom patterns cannot be equated with depressive disorder as defined in psychiatric practice (Aneshensel, 1985; Bouman, 1987). Too many a 'symptom scale case' could not be assigned a psychiatric diagnosis. Therefore the findings on the event–depression relationship obtained using self-report symptom scales should be interpreted with care. Symptom scales can perhaps best be conceptualized as representing a continuum ranging from not depressed to severely depressed.

How should these symptoms of dysphoric mood, motivational and behavioural deficits and negative cognitions among people who currently have no diagnosable depression be interpreted? In a provocative paper Aneshensel (1985) has related these symptoms to the role they may play in the course of affective disorders, as precursors and sequelae, and as components of a continuing state of vulnerability to more severe impairment. Available evidence from longitudinal community studies on depression strongly suggests not only that some episodes of diagnosable depressive disorders run a recurrent and chronic course but that many episodes of subclinical depressive symptoms show a similar pattern. The course of depressive disorder and depressive symptoms appear to comprise both isolated-episode and recurrent-chronic types (Klerman, 1980; Aneshensel, 1985; Ormel and Schaufeli, submitted).

The existence of recurrent-chronic depressive episodes implies that individuals with these types of symptoms are over-represented in cross-sectional life event studies. This may seriously complicate the interpretation of the findings of these studies.

The definition and measurement of life events

Two distinct approaches to the measurement of life events have evolved during the past two decades. To some extent their differences run along the same lines as in the case of depression; the respondent-based checklist method versus the researcher-based interview and rating procedure (Katschnig, 1986). The checklist method consists of the presentation to the subjects under study of a predefined list of events, often including some long-term difficulties, thought to be relevant. The occurrence of these events is then endorsed by the subject (Holmes and Rahe, 1967; Henderson *et al.*, 1981). The use of such prepared lists does not guarantee complete standardization. Many events are not unambiguously described and as such give rise to multiple interpretations. For instance 'serious illness of a family member'. Exactly what is serious and who is a family member? It may well be that the interpretation depends on subject's mood, personality and mental health state.

The interview and rating procedure is substantially more time-consuming and requires extensive training. The interviewer elicits in detail from each subject what events have occurred during a given period of time, together with information about their contexts. In a second step this information is presented to a panel of raters, along with biographical information. The panel then rates the degree of undesirability posed by the event (or whatever dimension one is interested in), taking into account the context and biographical information (Brown and Harris, 1978). Precise rules have been laid down that determine what constitutes an event and what not.

There is substantial empirical and theoretical evidence suggesting that the interview and rating procedure is superior in terms of reliability and construct-validity (Tennant *et al.*, 1981; Brown and Harris, 1986; Katschnig, 1986).

A further important feature of the contextual rating method, which strongly enhances its construct validity, is that it constitutes an optimal trade-off between contamination by vulnerability factors and the loss of contextual detail. There is agreement that contextual detail is critical for a complete understanding of the demands posed by events. In general, it can be asserted that the subject's own assessment of the stressfulness of an event is the best measure since it reflects the influence of all contextual and biographical factors which make up its stressfulness in the particular case. Unfortunately, however, this subjective rating also includes the effects of vulnerability factors such as coping resources and the availability of social support which need to be examined separately. By presenting appropriate descriptions to the panel of raters, the contextual rating eliminates most of the contamination at least cost to contextual detail (Bebbington, 1986).

In spite of numerous life event studies, no generally accepted theory has evolved about which features of life events are stress-provoking. There are few theoretically based notions about mechanisms relating specific events or event features to specific types of ill health. In her discussion of this problem, Thoits (1983) contends that in the domain of psychopathology the features that appear most critical with respect to depression are undesirability, severity, time clustering and uncontrollability. The significance of uncontrollability for depression is also strongly emphasized by Brown and Harris (1986), who have presented compelling evidence that depression is related to loss events (which have by definition minimal controllability) and anxiety to events which entail suspending dangers. But with this we are already touching the subject of the following discussion.

LIFE EVENTS AND DEPRESSION

For the most part, research on life events and depression falls into three categories: (1) studies that employ the checklist method, do not rate and date events, and do not assess caseness, denoted here as checklist studies; (2) studies that use the panel method for the severity rating of events, date events and assess caseness and onset, further denoted as rating studies; and (3) studies that examine the consequences of a particular life crisis such as rape, job loss and widowhood for psychological health, denoted here as life crisis studies. Recently a number of excellent reviews have been published (Brown and Harris, 1978; Cohen, 1988; Paykel, 1978; Kessler *et al.*, 1985; Silver and Wortman, 1980; Thoits, 1983; Sanderman, 1988). Much of the following is based on these reports.

The checklist and rating studies also differ in the methods of analysis. Two issues should be distinguished here: (a) how the global stress exposure indices for a certain time interval are established on the basis of the life events occurring in the interval; and (b) how the effects of these indices on the onset of depression are determined. Two models have typically been used in the construction of indices. In the threshold model, each subject is assessed on whether or not they have been exposed to an a priori defined level of life event stress, usually at least one severe event. In the additive model a quantitative measure of stress exposure is calculated for each subject. This measure is usually based on the number of events and the severity of the experienced events as assessed by subjects themselves or a priori by the investigator. Checklist life event studies have typically adopted the additive model whereas the rating studies have employed the threshold model. A variety of statistical approaches can be found to the analysis of life event effects. For the most part, checklist studies have used regression methods, while rating studies have in general been analysed with two by two tables using such measures as relative risk and attributional proportion.

In the early phases of life event research the focus was on demonstrating a link between event exposure and illness. The findings of checklist studies suggested the existence of a rather weak relationship of at most 10% explained variance in illness measures. To some extent this weak relation was attributed to methodological weaknesses. But in spite of a number of improvements (more specific and valid event and depression measures, elimination of ambiguous events, prospective designs) the predictive power was not substantially increased. As far as the checklist studies are concerned, three factors may be responsible for this weak predictive power. First, chronicity may play a deflating role. It is nowadays well accepted that a major proportion of the (sub)clinical depressive distress in the community is more or less chronic (Aneshensel, 1985; Surtees *et al.*, 1986; Ormel, 1980; Ormel and Schaufeli, submitted), and this chronic distress may well be independent of acute life stress. A probably more significant problem is event and onset timing. Not dating event occurrence and symptom onset not only seriously hampers causal inference, it may also dilute the effects of events preceding onset. The third factor lies in the relatively low reliability and validity of the checklist approach. In particular the fact that no contextually specific information is collected and used for the severity rating may be critical.

From a methodological point of view the rating studies are considerably more appropriate for assessing the effects of life events. In this type of research, most problems affecting the checklist studies are taken into account: events and onset are dated, diagnostic criteria are employed, chronic cases are omitted and events are rated on contextual severity dimensions and, in some studies, an independence rating is made. The latter indicates the extent to which subjects themselves were responsible for the occurrence and/or severity of the event. Some studies have even used a longitudinal design that enables chronic cases to be excluded more reliably, and estimations of the risk of depressive disorder associated with event exposure to be made (Brown *et al.*, 1986; Surtees *et al.*, 1986).

The results consistently document a substantial relationship between the occurrence of at least one severely undesirable event and the onset of depressive symptoms and disorder. There is also strong evidence that events representing the loss of attachment figures, significant peers, physical health, major possessions and cherished ideas about oneself or significant others, are particularly capable of producing depression (Finlay-Jones and Brown, 1981; Miller and Ingham, 1989; Brown *et al.*, 1986). However, it should be stressed that highly undesirable events and even major losses are neither a sufficient nor necessary condition for the onset of depression. Some depressions are not preceded by a major (loss) event, and most severely undesirable events are not followed by depression.

The third type of study distinguished earlier involves exploring the psychological consequences of various life crises (Silver and Wortman, 1980). Compared with the life event studies using the rating method, the value of most life crisis research is difficult to assess owing to a lack of methodological rigour. The few studies that have employed valid psychopathology measures and control groups show significant differences in long-term psychiatric symptoms between controls and index groups (Kessler *et al.*, 1985).

Although the weight of evidence suggests that events are causally implicated in depression, there is still some debate about a number of issues, including the importance of the effects of events and their significance (Brown and Harris, 1986; Tennant *et al.*, 1981). Brown and Harris have shown that this is largely due to the use of two different classes of effect measures—one based on the notion of explained variance and the other on the notion of relative and attributable risk. The amount of explained variance in checklist studies usually does not exceed 10%, whereas relative risks and attributable percentages in rating studies suggest much stronger relationships. We have calculated relative risk and attributable percentage on the basis of the pooled findings of eight studies using the rating method (Brown and Harris, 1978; Campbell, 1982; Brown and Prudo, 1981; Bebbington *et al.*, 1984; Costello, 1982; Surtees *et al.*, 1986; Brown *et al.*, 1986; Sanderman, 1988). Some of these studies also include major difficulties. The relative risk amounted to 5.3 and Levin's attributable risk percentage to 56.4%.

There are at least two other controversial issues that should be mentioned here, without exploring them in detail. One is the separation of depressive illness from more or less normal emotional responses to adversity. Some argue that even if community cases reach severity levels that seem to justify a label of caseness, major qualitative differences between most community cases and depressive patients may remain (Bebbington, 1986; Brown and Harris, 1986). A second issue of continuing concern is the possible contamination of the contextual severity rating by buffering or modifier effects. In order to obtain a severity rating that is close to the meaning the event has for the respondent, in such a way that no information on the subject's reaction is used, objective contextual information is collected. The reporting of the context of the event might still be influenced to some degree by the subject's vulnerability to stress, current mental health state and mood (Kessler *et al.*, 1985). This reporting effect might bias upwardly estimates of the contribution of life events in the aetiology, and also renders the contribution of vulnerability factors more difficult to detect.

Social support and depression

One of the most popular modifiers studied is social support. The buffering hypothesis of social support asserts that social support buffers or ameliorates the impact of stress on health and has nearly attracted as much research as the life event hypothesis has done. Unfortunately there has been and still is much confusion and debate on the nature, the components and measurement of social support. In spite of this confusion, major reviews agree that social support is involved in the aetiology of affective disorder and probably has significant buffering potential (Kessler and Mcleod, 1985; Cohen and Syme, 1985; Sarason and Sarason, 1984). What appears especially critical is having someone close to whom one can and actually does confide, together with receiving active emotional support from significant others when facing adversity (Thoits, 1982;

Brown *et al.*, 1986). These components may well derive their buffering properties from their potential to restore damaged self-esteem and prevent the development of feelings of abandonment and helplessness.

SELF-ESTEEM

The existence of a strong relationship between self-esteem or negative self-appraisal and depression is well known and documented. Self-esteem is substantially lowered among depressives. What is not clear to date is the nature of the link. The traditional view is that self-esteem is intimately linked with affective illness, i.e. change in affect is primary and the altered self-concept secondary. In this view low self-esteem is considered to be just one of the symptoms making up the depressive syndrome (Ingham *et al.*, 1986; Lewinsohn *et al.*, 1981; Koeter *et al.*, in press). An alternative position states that low self-esteem has aetiological significance and thus increases the risk for negative changes in affect.

The view of self-esteem as a symptom is supported by a large body of evidence showing that recovered depressives generally regain normal levels of self-esteem (Ingham *et al.*, 1986). This, however, does not completely rule out the alternative; only prospective studies can do this. Unfortunately, the rare prospective studies into this problem show contradictory findings. Negative or miniscule results (low self-esteem did not predict future onset of affective disorder) have been reported by Lewinsohn *et al.* (1981) and Ingham *et al.* (1986), each using respondent-based self-report scales. Positive findings have been published by Brown *et al.* (1986), using the Negative Evaluation of Self index from the Self Evaluation and Social Support (SESS) schedule. This rating measure was based almost entirely on the presence of negative comments subjects made largely spontaneously about themselves during 3- to 5-hour interviews covering many personal topics.

For two reasons we tend to attach most weight to the findings of Brown and colleagues. First, although the urgent need for replication of their findings and for more convincing reliability data needs to be acknowledged, we feel the investigator-based interview and rating procedure may have greater validity. The second reason lies in some preliminary findings of our own longitudinal study with three measurements over a period of ten years into the change and stability of negative affect (Ormel and Schaufeli, submitted). Using structural modelling it was found that somewhat more than 60% of the between-subject differences in negative affect could be attributed to a common factor. This common factor was strongly correlated with a variable representing low self-esteem. In addition, changes in negative affect levels were reflected in temporarily lowered levels of self-esteem. These findings suggest that both aforementioned views may be correct: low self-esteem predisposes to depressive symptoms, but beside that it is also temporarily further lowered during an episode of depressive mood.

LOCUS OF CONTROL, HARDINESS AND MASTERY

The locus of control construct stems from Rotter's social learning theory. The model proposes that people learn to relate their own behaviour with its outcome, and consequently learn to increase their feelings of control over outcome expectancies. In addition, behaviour is dependent upon the expectancy of obtaining reinforcement contingencies (and the value of the reinforcer to the subject). Internals therefore anticipate that their own behaviours will help to determine outcome, whereas externals feel that outcome depends on chance or luck.

The theory may be very helpful in evaluating the relationship between stressors and depression. It would be expected that subjects with an internal locus of control would be less vulnerable to stress, for they consider various stressors as controllable, whereas externals have lower beliefs in personal control, and may anticipate stress with feelings of hopelessness. They will consequently be less capable of influencing the situation.

Various studies have investigated locus of control and stress. Johnson and Sarason (1978) found a correlation between negative life-stress and depression and trait-anxiety only among externals. Hence the effects of life-stress might be mediated by the (locus of) control over the events. Schill *et al.* (1982) divided externals into 'congruent' and 'defensive' groups. It is supposed that congruent externals have internalized this cognitive style, whereas defensive externals use it as a verbal technique without internalizing the style. Results indicated that defensive externals were particularly vulnerable to stress. An explanation given by the authors was that defensive externals do not seek or obtain social support.

Sarason *et al.* (1978) reported a significant correlation ($r = 0.24$) between negative life-stress and depression and between negative life-stress and locus of control ($r = 0.32$), thus indicating that an external locus of control and life-stress are associated. It was further hypothesized that externals are less capable in controlling reinforcement contingencies. Parker (1980), however, found no evidence to support this contention.

Ormel *et al.* (1988) studied the modifier effects of locus of control in a prospective design. The outcomes of the LISREL analysis suggested that locus of control did not modify the response to adversity, although locus of control *did* somewhat modify the impact of *desirable events* on symptom level (by a small reduction in symptom level among the externals).

McFarlane *et al.* (1983) reported that locus of control was associated with baseline distress but showed no relation to change in distress over time. They stated: 'Presumably, individuals who do not perceive themselves in control of their environment are more likely to experience distress both in the presence and the absence of stressful life-events'.

Sanderman (1988) also studied the effects of locus of control in psychological distress and the interaction effects with life-events in a prospective design. Life-events were assessed and rated with a procedure similar to the Brown and Harris method. Interestingly, neither a main effect for locus of control nor an interaction effect of control and stress was found. In other words, locus of control seems not to influence subsequent distress and had no buffering effect on the stress–distress relationship. It is apparent that the prospective design which was used provides a more rigorous test of the role of these variables than retrospective or cross-sectional studies. For—as was also found by McFarlane *et al.* (1983)—locus of control correlated significantly with the symptomatology when assessed simultaneously ($r = -0.23$ at time 1 and $r = -0.25$ at time 2) but it did not predict symptomatology longitudinally ($r = -0.10$) (Sanderman, 1988). Hence, a cross-sectional analysis would have overestimated the role of locus of control. Furthermore, it was found that locus of control correlated 0.95 (after correction for attenuation) with itself over an 18-month period, supporting the contention that it is a trait-like characteristic.

Almost synonymous with locus of control is the concept of mastery (Pearlin *et al.*, 1981). In a two-wave study on stress and health Pearlin *et al.* studied, among other variables, the role of mastery. An analysis on a subsample of their material specifically related to job-disruptive events and depression revealed that the impact of these events are mediated by mastery. Pearlin *et al.* (1981) further argued that threatened mastery is not a mere symptom of stress but that it is a source of it.

The concept of hardiness developed by Kobasa *et al.* (1982a) also relates to locus of control. Hardiness is a composite score of challenge, control and commitment. Several research findings support the contention that hardiness is negatively related to depression and distress, and that it buffers the stress–illness relationship. Rhodewalt and Agustsdottir (1984) found that hardy individuals perceive events as more controllable and that they report fewer symptoms than others. However, personality did *not* influence the exposure to events. Kobasa *et al.* (1982a) reported main effects of stress and hardiness on illness (physical and mental symptoms), and an interaction effect of stress and hardiness on illness. Contrary to this finding are the results reported by Schmied and Lawler (1986), who found neither a main effect nor an interaction effect for hardiness. Kobasa *et al.* (1982b) reported evidence for the buffering role of hardiness. Interestingly, they also found that the buffering effect of hardiness and exercise (sport activities) were additive. Persons both high in hardiness and high in exercise were the healthiest. They reason that hardiness has a buffering effect 'through activities which directly transform events, thereby decreasing their stressfulness, whereas exercise buffers by decreasing the organismic strain produced by stressful events' (Kobasa *et al.*, 1982b, p. 401). Finally, Kuo and Tsai (1986) studied Asian immigrants in Seattle and found evidence for the hypothesis that hardy immigrants show lesser depressive symptoms in the presence of stress. In addition, a hardy personality seems to inhibit the occurrence of stress.

A few remarks should be made at this point concerning the usefulness of the locus of control construct in stress research:

(1) A general feeling of control might be related to a specific feeling of control (e.g. health locus of control) but the relationship is not necessary linear (Lefcourt, 1980). Although it is likely that such constructs are related it is obvious that—if the relationship is not perfect—a decrease in explanatory power must be anticipated when a general locus of control measure is used in combination with a specific stressor.

(2) Rotter (1975) stressed the particular significance of locus of control in ambiguous situations. When a situation is *not* ambiguous, externals and internals may very well not differ in their behaviour, and situational characteristics may become more significant. In fact, experimental research has substantiated this contention.

(3) Frequently research is cross-sectional; both McFarlane *et al.* (1983) and Sanderman (1988) found a significant correlation between baseline symptoms and locus of control but no significant relationship between the two prospectively. Hence, prospective research is essential in order to obtain a clear view of locus of control in long-term adaptational processes.

(4) An internal locus of control is not necessarily a positive facet in the process of coping with stressful encounters (Lefcourt, 1980), for a feeling of control may very well be counterproductive in certain situations.

(5) Locus of control may predict a favourable outcome with one event while being not predictive with another. Consequently, the specific role of locus of control cannot be effectively documented by correlating it with an aggregated life-event index.

(6) Although locus of control has been studied extensively, there is still some doubt about the reliability and validity of the scales (Coombs and Schroeder, 1988). Future research must be conducted with reliable and valid assessments of locus of control. In addition, it would be interesting to develop an interview-based procedure of locus of control. Brown and Harris have produced such assessment procedures for social support and self-esteem (see above), and research findings with these measures are promising.

In sum, people who consider life-events and their consequences beyond personal control (externals) are supposed to be more vulnerable to life-stress (mediating effect). The fact that there is only sparse evidence to support this view has, in our opinion, to do with methodological flaws in existing research. It would therefore be premature to eliminate the construct of locus of control from further research on the relationships between stress and health outcomes.

THEORETICAL INTEGRATION

We are now in a position to draw a few preliminary conclusions. The major risk factors of depression are reasonably well known. The available evidence reviewed above suggests that an important provoking role can be attributed to severe events and long-term difficulties, in particular events and difficulties involving loss, failure or disappointment. Meticulous analysis of the provoking factors which seem to be most strongly associated with the onset of depressive symptoms reveals that, for many, these concern: (a) loss of attachment figures, significant others, or social status-providing activities such as employment and child caring, and disappointment; or (b) disappointment in the sense of loss of cherished ideas of beliefs; or (c) failures which might be interpreted as loss of self-efficacy cognitions. However, many individuals exposed to these provoking factors do not develop depression. Two major factors that seem to buffer against the negative consequences of loss are social support and high self-esteem. Jointly, measures of provoking factors, personality (dependency, emotional instability and introversion), social support and self-esteem are able to account for the majority of onsets of depressions found in the community (Brown *et al.*, 1986; Aneshensel and Stone, 1982; Akiskal, 1984).

In addition it has been demonstrated that various neurophysiological disturbances are involved in depression (Gilbert, 1984; Willner, 1985). Consequently, the question arises whether there is a relationship between the risk factors and the neurophysiological disturbances found among depressives, and how this relationship should be conceptualized. Recently a number of comprehensive and provocative accounts have been published which address this very issue (Akiskal, 1984; Gilbert, 1984; Willner, 1985).

The content of thinking of depressives and the nature of their coping difficulties centre on interpersonal relationship concerns. Gilbert (1984) has linked these concerns to perceived loss of what might be labelled 'personal social significance', encompassing social embeddedness, social status and self-esteem. He goes on to argue that these loss appraisals have evolutionary significance and, because of this, that the psychobiological response patterns to these losses are innately determined. The significance of psychological and social factors lies in their ability to activate, amplify and modify these response patterns.

How does the argument outlined above relate to the empirical data on life events, social support and general beliefs about control presented above? We feel that these findings can be interpreted in terms of the psychobiological argument. The concepts of the stress and coping theory as described by Lazarus and Folkman (1984) can perhaps best be used to carry out this task.

The type of events and long-term difficulties which appear to be most strongly associated with the onset of depression are situations involving loss of either physical abilities, attachment figures, significant peers, social status or a major source of social reinforcement, failures and disappointments (Brown and Harris, 1986; Sanderman, 1988). Such situations may be relatively potent in triggering primary appraisals in terms of loss of 'personal social significance'. Vulnerable individuals, for instance, due to low self-esteem or a self-esteem that is easily shattered in the face of adversity may see themselves as unable to change the situation (problem-focused coping) or to tolerate the emotional consequences (emotion-focused coping). Various psychological, social and biological characteristics of the individual may interact with the properties of the situation in producing these secondary appraisals. The individual characteristics making up his or her vulnerability include, among others, sensitivity to loss through early object loss, low self-esteem, dependency, other sources of stress, impaired interpersonal skills, and high biological reactivity to stress and loss of control, either learned or genetically determined. Hence, what seems particularly important in the aetiology of depression are: (1) situations involving loss of personal social significance; and (2) personal resources related to social skills and sources of social support.

The critical role of social support in the appraisal process is supported by the literature on its buffering potential. In particular, the evidence concerning 'let-down behaviour' in the face of a crisis is illustrative. The risk of depression among people exposed to major stresses appears to be markedly raised when their call for support is turned down by significant others, generally the spouse or confidant, on whom they thought they could count. It is not unreasonable to suggest that experience of being let down in the face of a major crisis deals a final blow to the person's already weakened feelings of social personal significance.

General beliefs about personal control may also affect the situation-specific secondary appraisals. The impact of general beliefs about personal control probably depends on two factors: the extent to which they refer to values and coping abilities relevant to the interpersonal domain, and the degree to which the loss situation or its consequences can be transformed. Coping behaviour in situations which are completely controllable or uncontrollable is probably not much affected by beliefs about personal control.

The neurophysiological changes and cognitive distortions involved in depression do not, of themselves, produce depression. These changes seem to be secondary to psychological or neurophysiological processes. The crucial question that then arises is, secondary to what? Several authors have stressed the similarities between the psychobiological consequences of uncontrollable stress and neurochemical and cognitive correlates of depression (Weiss *et al.*, 1976; Anisman, 1978; Willner, 1985). The paradigm of the learned helplessness model (Garber and Seligman, 1980) suggests that a similar approach to depression may be rewarding: examining the cognitive and neurophysiological functioning of persons exposed to events involving potential and actual loss of personal social significance. These individuals can perhaps best be identified in naturalistic settings, as it is unlikely that strong and enduring feelings of loss can be induced under laboratory conditions. If such a combined effort of epidemiologists, cognitive psychologists and biological psychiatrists could be developed in a way that included measures of presumed vulnerability factors, fascinating options for theory testing would arise.

Anxiety and depressive symptoms often occur simultaneously, and episodes of both disorders follow each other in the course of time (Dobson, 1985; Tyrer, 1985). The explanation of this state of affairs has been addressed from various perspectives. One explanation is based on the notion that the nature of the provoking agent largely determines the nature of the symptom pattern. To examine this relationship Finlay-Jones and Brown (1981) introduced the notions of loss and danger. Loss events would relate to depression whereas danger would trigger anxiety. The findings clearly corroborated their hypothesis. Finlay-Jones and Brown's notions of loss and depression show remarkable similarity with the concepts used by Garber *et al.* (1980) to characterize uncontrollable outcomes. According to their position, depression would result from outcomes perceived as uncontrollable but highly likely, whereas anxiety would be produced by uncontrollable and uncertain outcomes. Thus the critical difference lies in the perceived uncertainty with respect to the outcome. Garber *et al.* (1980) argued that many depressives display symptoms of anxiety, because in real life many undesirable and often largely uncontrollable events involve both actual loss and the threat of loss, particularly when they are assessed over time. In our own ratings of events on the dimensions of loss and danger, the two have tended to be moderately correlated.

Finally some comments should be made about the status of the argument presented here. First, it is not intended to be an outline of a comprehensive psychobiological theory of depression. We have only presented some elements of a possible approach to the way in which findings from various scientific fields might be integrated and used to formulate suggestions about future research. We have stressed the importance of a combined approach using epidemiological, cognitive-psychological and neurobiological methods. It should be recognized that other approaches are possible. In addition, it is important to note that, although the evidence on loss events and depression is strong, the possibility that the relationship is confounded by severity of events and changes in social support cannot be ruled out. After all, loss events might simply be more severe than other events, and they often involve disruption of confiding relationships. To our knowledge, no study has as yet explicitly examined these issues.

CONCLUDING REMARKS

In this chapter we have presented an overview of the assessment of depression and life-events, and have provided a selective review on notions of control and their significance in the onset of depressive disorders. Clearly, recent advances in various disciplines have produced a number of improvements in the assessment of depressive disorders and life-events. Many issues remain unresolved, but as a whole the 'state of the art' seems to be very promising. One of the interesting developments in stress research is the recognition of the role of control in the onset of depressive disorders. However, at present it is difficult convincingly to establish the role of control in aetiology. There is a pressing need to improve the conceptualizations of control and to develop clear operationalizations of the distinct properties of control. Finally, it appears valuable to propose specific models of social stress, vulnerability factors and disorders, so as to attempt to predict the onset of disorders most reliably. Notions of control should certainly be integrated into these models.

REFERENCES

Abramson, L. Y., Seligman, M. E. P., and Teasdale, J. D. (1978). Learned helplessness in humans: Critique and reformulation. *Journal of Abnormal Psychology*, **87**, 49–74.
Akiskal, H. S. (1984). An integrative view of the aetiology and treatment of depression. In: J. Korf and L. Pepplinkhuizen (eds), *Depression: Molecular and Psychologically Based Therapies*. Drachten, Netherlands: TGO Foundation.
Aneshensel, C. S. (1985). The natural history of depressive symptoms: Implications for psychiatric epidemiology. In: J. R. Greenley (ed.), *Research in Community and Mental Health* (Vol. 5). Greenwich, CT: JAI Press.
Aneshensel, C. S., and Stone, J. D. (1982). Stress and depression: A test of the buffering model of social support. *Archives of General Psychiatry*, **39**, 1392–1396.
Anisman, H. (1978). Neurochemical changes elicited by stress: Behavioral correlates. In: H. Anisman and G. Bignami (eds), *Psychopharmacology of Aversively Motivated Behavior*. New York: Plenum Press.
Antonovsky, A. (1987). *Unraveling the Mystery of Health: How People Manage Stress and Stay Well*. San Francisco: Jossey-Bass.
Averill, J. R. (1973). Personal control over aversive stimuli and its relationship to stress. *Psychological Bulletin*, **80**, 286–303.
Bandura, A. (1977). Self-efficacy: Toward a unifying theory of behavioral change. *Psychological Review*, **84**, 191–215.
Bebbington, P. E. (1986). Establishing causal links: Recent controversies. In: H. Katschnig (ed.), *Life Events and Psychiatric Disorders*. Cambridge: Cambridge University Press.
Bebbington, P. E., Tennant, C., Sturt, E., and Hurry, J. (1984). The domain of life events: A comparison of two techniques of description. *Psychological Medicine*, **14**, 219–222.
Bouman, T. K. (1987). *The measurement of depression with questionnaires*. PhD thesis, University of Groningen.
Brink, W., vanden, Koeter, M., Ormel, J., Dijkstra, W., Giel, R., Slooff, C. J., and Wolfarth, T. (1989). Psychiatric diagnosis in an outpatient population. A comparative study of PSE-Catego and DSM-III. *Archives of General Psychiatry*, **46**, 369–372.
Brown, G. W., and Harris, T. (1978). *Social Origins of Depression*. London: Tavistock.
Brown, G. W., and Harris, T. O. (1986). Establishing causal links: The Bedford College Studies of Depression. In: H. Katschnig (ed.), *Life Events and Psychiatric Disorders*. Cambridge: Cambridge University Press.
Brown, G. W., Andrews, B., Harris, T. A., Alder, Z., and Bridge, L. (1986). Social support, self-esteem and depression. *Psychological Medicine*, **16**, 813–831.
Brown, G. W., and Prudo, R. (1981). Psychiatric disorder in a rural and an urban population. 1. Aetiology of depression. *Psychological Medicine*, **11**, 581–599.

Campbell, E. (1982). *Vulnerability to depression and cognitive predisposition: Psychosocial correlates of Brown and Harris's vulnerability factors.* Paper presented at British Psychological Society Annual Conference, April 1982.

Cohen, L. H. (ed.) (1988). *Life Events and Psychological Functioning: Theoretical and Methodological Issues.* Beverly Hills: Sage Publications.

Cohen, S., and Syme, S. L. (eds) (1985). *Social Support and Health.* New York: Academic Press.

Coombs, W. N., and Schroeder, H. E. (1988). Generalized locus of control: An analysis of factor analytic data. *Personality and Individual Differences*, **9**, 79–85.

Costello, C. G. (1982). Social factors associated with depression: A retrospective community study. *Psychological Medicine*, **12**, 329–339.

Dobson, K. S. (1985). The relationship between anxiety and depression. *Clinical Psychological Review*, **5**, 307–324.

Dohrenwend, B. P., Shrout, P. E., Egri, G., and Mendelsohn, F. S. (1980). Nonspecific psychological distress and other dimensions of psychopathology: Measures for use in the general population. *Archives of General Psychiatry*, **37**, 1229–1236.

Finlay-Jones, R., and Brown, G. W. (1981). Types of stressful life event and the onset of anxiety and depressive disorders. *Psychological Medicine*, **11**, 803–815.

Folkman, S. (1984). Personal control and stress and coping processes: A theoretical analysis. *Journal of Personality and Social Psychology*, **46**, 839–852.

Garber, J., and Seligman, M. E. P. (eds) (1980). *Human Helplessness: Theory and Applications.* New York: Academic Press.

Garber, J., Miller, S. M., and Abramson, L. Y. (1980). On the distinction between anxiety and depression: Perceived control, certainty, and probability of goal attainment. In: J. Garber and M. E. P. Seligman (eds), *Human Helplessness: Theory and Applications.* New York: Academic Press.

Gilbert, P. (1984). *Depression: From Psychology to Brain State.* London: Lawrence Erlbaum.

Hammen, C., Krantz, S. E., and Cochran, S. D. (1981). Relationships between depression and causal attributions about stressful life events. *Cognitive Therapy and Research*, **5**, 351–358.

Henderson, S., Byrne, D. G., and Duncan-Jones, P. (1981). *Neurosis and the Social Environment.* London: Academic Press.

Hodiamont, P., Peer, N. and Syben, N. (1987). Epidemiological aspects of psychiatric disorder in a Dutch health area. *Psychological Medicine*, **17**, 495–505.

Holmes, T. H., and Rahe, R. H. (1967). The Social Readjustment Rating Scale. *Journal of Psychosomatic Research*, **11**, 213–218.

Ingham, J. G., Kreitman, N. B., Miller, P.McC., Sashidharan, S. P., and Surtees, P. G. (1986). Self-esteem, vulnerability and psychiatric disorder in the community. *British Journal of Psychiatry*, **148**, 375–385.

Johnson, J. H., and Sarason, I. G. (1978). Life stress, depression and anxiety: Internal–external control as a moderator variable. *Journal of Psychosomatic Research*, **27**, 205–208.

Katschnig, H. (1986). Measuring life stress: A comparison of the checklist and panel technique. In: H. Katschnig (ed.), *Life Events and Psychiatric Disorders.* Cambridge: Cambridge University Press.

Kessler, R. C., and McLeod, J. (1985). Social support and psychological distress in community surveys. In: S. Cohen and S. L. Syme (eds), *Social Support and Health.* New York: Academic Press.

Kessler, R. C., Price, R. H., and Wortman, C. B. (1985). Social factors in psychopathology: Stress, social support, and coping processes. *Annual Review of Psychology*, **36**, 531–572.

Klerman, G. L. (1980). Affective disorders. In: A. M. Nicholi (ed.), *Harvard Guide to Modern Psychiatry*. Cambridge, MA: Harvard University Press.

Kobasa, S. C., Maddi, S. R., and Kahn, S. (1982a). Hardiness and health: A prospective study. *Journal of Personality and Social Psychology*, **42**, 168–177.

Kobasa, S. C., Maddi, S. R., and Puccetti, M. C. (1982b). Personality and exercise as buffers in the stress–illness relationship. *Journal of Behavioral Medicine*, **5**, 391–404.

Koeter, M. W. J., Ormel, J., Brink, W. van den and Dijkstra, W. (in press). Mental health state and personality assessment. *Nederlands Tijdschrift voor de Psychologie*.

Kuo, W. H., and Tsai, Y.-M. (1986). Social networking, hardiness and immigrants' mental health. *Journal of Health and Social Behavior*, **27**, 133–149.

Lazarus, R. S., and Folkman, S. (1984). *Stress, Appraisal and Coping*. New York: Springer.

Lefcourt, H. M. (1980). Locus of control and coping with life events. In: F. Staub (ed.), *Personality*. Englewood Cliffs, NJ: Prentice-Hall.

Lewinsohn, P. M., Steinmetz, J. L., Larson, D. W., and Franklin, J. (1981). Depression-related cognitions: Antecedent or consequent? *Journal of Abnormal Psychology*, **90**, 213–219.

McFarlane, A. H., Norman, G. R., Streiner, D. L., and Roy, R. G. (1983). The process of social stress: Stable, reciprocal and mediating relationships. *Journal of Health and Social Behavior*, **24**, 160–173.

Miller, P.McC. and Ingham, J. G. (1989). Dimensions of experience and symptomatology. *Journal of Psychosomatic Research* (in press).

Myers, J. K., Weissman, M. M., Tischler, G. L., Holzer, C. E., Leaf, P. J., Orvaschel, H., Anthony, J. C., Boyd, J. H., Burke, J. D., Kramer, M., and Stoltzman, R. (1984). Six-month prevalence of psychiatric disorders in three communities. *Archives of General Psychiatry*, **41**, 959–967.

Ormel, J. (1989). *Moeite met leven of een moeilijk leven* (Problems with life or a stressful life). Groningen: Konstapel.

Ormel, J., Sanderman, R., and Stewart, R. (1988). Personality as modifier of the life-events–distress relationship: A longitudinal structural equation model. *Personality and Individual Differences*, **9**, 973–982.

Ormel, J., and Schaufeli, W. (submitted). Stability and change in negative affect: A structural longitudinal model fitted on two data sets on distress, self-esteem and locus of control.

Parker, G. (1980). Vulnerability factors to normal depression. *Journal of Psychosomatic Research*, **24**, 67–74.

Parkes, K. R. (1986). Coping in stressful episodes: The role of individual differences, environmental factors, and situational characteristics. *Journal of Personality and Social Psychology*, **51**, 1277–1292.

Paykel, E. S. (1978). Contribution of life events to causation of psychiatric illness. *Psychological Medicine*, **8**, 245–253.

Pearlin, L. I., Menaghan, E. G., Lieberman, M. A., and Mullan, J. T. (1981). The stress process. *Journal of Health and Social Behavior*, **22**, 337–356.

Rhodewalt, F., and Agustsdottir, S. (1984). On the relationship of hardiness to the type A behavior pattern: Perception of life events versus coping with life events. *Journal of Research in Personality*, **18**, 212–223.

Rotter, J. B. (1966). Generalized expectancies for internal versus external control of reinforcement. *Psychological Monographs*, **80**, 1–28.

Rotter, J. B. (1975). Some problems and misconceptions related to the construct of internal versus external control of reinforcement. *Journal of Consulting and Clinical Psychology*, **43**, 56–67.

Sanderman, R. (1988). *Life events, mediating variables and psychological functioning: a longitudinal study.* PhD thesis, University of Groningen.

Sarason, I. G. and Sarason, B. R. (eds) (1984). *Social Support: Theory, Research and Applications.* Dordrecht: Martinus Nijhoff.

Sarason, I. G., Johnson, J. H., and Siegel, J. M. (1978). Assessing the impact of life changes: Development of the life experiences survey. *Journal of Consulting and Clinical Psychology,* **46**, 932–946.

Schill, T., Ramanaiak, N., and Toves, C. (1982). Defensive externality and vulnerability to life stress. *Psychological Reports,* **51**, 878.

Schmied, L. A., and Lawler, K. A. (1986). Hardiness, type A behavior, and stress–illness relations in working women. *Journal of Personality and Social Psychology,* **51**, 1218–1223.

Seligman, M. E. P. (1975). *Helplessness: On Depression, Development and Death.* San Francisco: Freeman.

Silver, R. L., and Wortman, C. B. (1980). Coping with undesirable life events. In: J. Garber and M. E. P. Seligman (eds), *Human Helplessness: Theory and Applications.* New York: Academic Press.

Surtees, P. G., Miller, P.McC., Ingham, J. G., Kreitman, N. B., Rennie, D., and Sashidharan, S. P. (1986). Life events and the onset of affective disorder: A longitudinal general population study. *Journal of Affective Disorders,* **10**, 37–50.

Surtees, P.G., and Sashidharan, S. P. (1986). Psychiatric morbidity in two matched community samples: A comparison of rates and risks in Edinburgh and St. Louis. *Journal of Affective Disorders,* **10**, 101–113.

Tennant, C., Bebbington, P., and Hurry, J. (1981). The role of life events in depressive illness: Is there a substantial causal relation? *Psychological Medicine,* **11**, 379–389.

Thoits, P. A. (1982). Conceptual, methodological and theoretical problems in studying social support as a buffer against life stress. *Journal of Health and Social Behavior,* **23**, 145–159.

Thoits, P. A. (1983). Dimensions of life events that influence psychological distress: An evaluation and synthesis of the literature. In: H. B. Kaplan (ed.), *Psychosocial Stress: Trends in Theory and Research.* New York: Academic Press.

Thompson, S. C. (1981). Will it hurt less if I can control it? A complex answer to a simple question. *Psychological Bulletin,* **90**, 89–101.

Tyrer, P. (1985). Neurosis divisible? Lancet, March 23, 685–688.

Weiss, J. M., Glazer, H. I., and Pohorecky, L. A. (1976). Coping behaviour and neurochemical changes: An alternative explanation for the original 'learned helplessness' experiments. In: G. Serban and A. Kling (eds), *Animal Models in Human Psychobiology.* New York: Plenum Press.

Wheaton, B. (1980). The sociogenesis of psychological disorder: An attributional theory. *Journal of Health and Social Behavior,* **21**, 100–124.

Willner, P. (1985). *Depression: A Psychobiological Synthesis.* New York: Wiley.

Wing, J. K., Mann, S., Leff, J. P., and Nixon, J. M. (1978). The concept of a 'case' in psychiatric population surveys. *Psychological Medicine,* **8**, 203–217.

CHAPTER 10

Loss of control, vital exhaustion and coronary heart disease

AD APPELS
Department of Medical Psychology, University of Limburg, Maastricht, The Netherlands

INTRODUCTION

The notion that a challenged need for control or loss of control is involved in the aetiology of coronary heart disease has been present in the field of cardiovascular research for many years. However, no epidemiological study has directly addressed the question of whether or not those who are high in need for control as a personality characteristic, or those who lose control over their environment, are at increased risk for myocardial infarction. Generally speaking, need for control or loss of control are only mentioned in the discussion sections of empirical papers. Rosenman, for example, makes use of the control concept in an attempt to achieve greater insight into the origins of type A behaviour. 'The Type A behavior pattern (TABP) may be a characteristic style of response to environmental stressors that threaten an individual's sense of control over his or her environment. Thus, Type A behavior appears to be an enhanced performance to assert and maintain control over the environment whenever this control is challenged or threatened. The high drive and pace of Type A persons reflect their need for mastery over their environment' (Rosenman, 1986, p. 23).

David Glass should be credited as being the first author explicitly to draw attention to loss of control as a possible determinant of myocardial infarction and sudden cardiac death. His basic assertion is 'that Type A individuals exert greater efforts than their Type B counterparts to control stressful events that are perceived as threats to their sense of control. These active coping attempts

Stress, Personal Control and Health. Edited by A. Steptoe and A. Appels.
Published by John Wiley & Sons Ltd.
© ECSC–EEC–EAEC, Brussels–Luxembourg, 1989

eventually extinguish, for without reward, the relentless striving of the Type A individual leads to frustration and psychic exhaustion, which culminates in a reduction of efforts at control' (Glass, 1977). This description illustrates the notion that type A individuals who suffer from coronary heart disease (CHD) have passed through a state of frustration and exhaustion prior to myocardial infarction. Glass described this state as a 'prodromal depression'. He suggested that this state is characterized by a change from initial hyper-responsiveness into subsequent hypo-responsiveness:

> If the Type A individual concludes that little can be done to rectify the situation, we may expect him to experience more intense feelings of helplessness than are experienced by a Type B in similar circumstances. This prediction is derived from the assumption that Type A's probably try harder than Type B's to avoid losing their jobs when that possibility first becomes apparent. Exerting greater initial efforts at control, Type A's experience greater helplessness when they become convinced that nothing can be done about being fired. The precise role of initial hyper-responsiveness and subsequent hypo-responsiveness (helplessness) in the development of cardiovascular pathology remains unclear . . . we should first determine whether the interaction of Pattern A and helplessness is indeed prodromal to clinical CHD. (Glass, 1977)

This hypothesis needs to be tested directly in prospective epidemiological studies. Such a test was not done by Glass, but his book provides some indications that exposure to uncontrollable stress results in hypo-responsive behavior in type A individuals.

We agree with Glass's view, because the clinical examination of infarction patients not only reveals the presence of type A behaviour in most cases, but also a history of frustration, demoralization and psychic exhaustion. Such a history seems to characterize the year before myocardial infarction. We therefore hypothesized that a successful type A individual is not at increased risk for myocardial infarction but that the type A person who has lost control over his or her environment is at elevated risk. An additional hypothesis was that type A individuals are at increased risk of losing control because their deep commitment to their vocation (both in relation to occupation and family life) makes them rather vulnerable when negative events occur in their immediate environment.

The question of whether the year before myocardial infaction is characterized by a state of 'loss of control' was investigated in several stages. Loss of control is not itself a measurable concept. Therefore, the first question we addressed was: how is loss of control experienced by potential coronary victims? The second question was: are the feelings reported by coronary patients precursors of myocardial infarction, or should they be interpreted as consequences of the disease or of hospitalization? The related questions we examined were: are type A individuals at increased risk of entering a state of demoralization and psychological exhaustion? What life events or situations provoke this state? What can be said about the biological correlates of this state? The research programme addressing these issues is not yet finished. This chapter describes the history of this work, some major findings and some unresolved problems. It is preceded by a brief review of the literature concerning premonitory symptoms of myocardial infarction. The chapter concludes with an attempt to locate these findings within the framework of theories concerning loss of control.

PREMONITORY SYMPTOMS OF MYOCARDIAL INFARCTION

The identification of impending heart attacks before they occur is one of the major challenges confronting clinical and preventive cardiology. Several cardiologists have therefore studied the symptoms that are experienced by coronary victims shortly before myocardial infarction or cardiac death. These retrospective studies indicate that the premonitory symptoms generally include the following: unstable angina pectoris, dyspnea and excessive fatigue. Estimates of the prevalence of excessive fatigue differ between studies and vary from 30% to 60%, a rate that is equal to or larger than the prevalence of other prodromal symptoms (Stowers and Short, 1970; Romo, 1973; Feinleib *et al.*, 1975; Alonzo *et al.*, 1975; Kuller, 1978; Rissanen *et al.*, 1978; Fraser, 1978; Klaeboe *et al.*, 1987). These cardiological studies not only indicate that exhaustion precedes myocardial infarction, but that it is mainly experienced as a 'lack of energy' or 'excess tiredness'. Table 1 illustrates results from three of these studies. Cardiologists have generally avoided making any interpretation of these feelings of excessive fatigue or lack of energy, but those who pay attention to these symptoms are inclined to attribute them to angina pectoris, medication or aging.

The mental precursors of myocardial infarction have also been studied by several psychiatrists. In general, the complaints of cardiac patients have been viewed in the context of breakdown of defence mechanisms before or after myocardial infarction. Descriptions of patients' experiences have much in common, although they differ in the terminology used to summarize findings. The psychiatric labels that have been used include 'hidden withdrawal and masked depression' (Fischer *et al.*, 1964), 'a combination of depression and arousal effects' (Greene *et al.*, 1972), 'pseudo-neurasthenic syndrome' (Polzien and Walter, 1971), and 'emotional drain' (Bruhn *et al.*, 1968). The first quantitative study on short-term precursors of myocardial infarction was published by Hahn (1971), who observed that coronary patients were significantly more compulsive counters of trivial things (like houses and trees) than were controls. Hahn interpreted this compulsive behavior as a defence mechanism directed against depressive ambivalence conflicts. Following decompensation of this defence through conflicts or stress, the underlying anxieties and depressive way of coping with conflicts became manifest. By means of a questionnaire, Hahn looked into the ways in which decompensation was experienced by coronary patients. The vast majority reported having experienced increasing irritability, strong mood changes and the general feeling of not being well.

TABLE 1. Premonitory symptoms of myocardial infarction and sudden death in three studies (percentages)

	Alonzo		Rissanen	Kuller
	Myocardial infarction	Sudden death	Sudden death	Sudden death
Chest pain	67	35		37
Discomfort in the chest			24	
Changed angina pectoris			15	
Recent angina pectoris			6	
Dyspnoea	36	39	15	42
Dizziness–syncope fainting	10	8		14
Heaviness of arms	14	10	3	
Fatigue–weakness	38	42	32	56
Emotional changes	14	20		
Nervousness–depression			3	
Difficulty sleeping				28
General malaise	16	17	5	
Anorexia–nausea	14	17	4	
Dysrhythmia			5	
Sweating			3	
Coughing				31
Palpitation				11
Ankle oedema–ascites	1	7		

The first prospective psychiatric study on the mental precursors of myocardial infarction was published by Crisp et al. (1984). The database for this study comprised patients aged 40–65 who were registered with a group general practice in London. The cohort was screened in 1969, 1971 and 1973. Nearly all participants completed the Crown–Crisp Experiential Index (CCEI) on each occasion. During the five-year observation period, 26 men were admitted to hospital with a confirmed diagnosis of severe myocardial infarction. Scores on the CCEI were compared with those of the remainder of the male study population. Differences between groups in scores on the individual items of the CCEI were assessed, and a discriminant analysis was carried out in order to devise a linear combination of variables that discriminated the groups most accurately. Twelve items were found to discriminate between individuals destined and those not destined for myocardial infarction. The authors interpret this item subset as reflecting 'a state of sadness, coupled with loss of libido and exhaustion'. Although the study has advantages stemming from the longitudinal design, it cannot be taken as definitive since the final results are based on an a posteriori analysis. Chance fluctuations may have influenced the observed associations (Thompson, 1984).

When we initiated our research programme in this area, we felt strongly that premature item selection should be avoided because the phenomenology of mental decompensation before myocardial infarction was still not well documented. Therefore, we began by interviewing coronary patients and by formulating items that came as close as possible to the wording and labels used by patients to describe the feelings that were dominant in the months preceding infarction. Nearly all coronary patients reported that loss of energy was their core feeling. They often used metaphors like 'the well was drying out', or 'my body was like a battery which was losing its power' to summarize their feelings. Therefore we decided to label this state as 'vital exhaustion'.

THE DEVELOPMENT OF FORM A
OF THE MAASTRICHT QUESTIONNAIRE

The first opportunity to test the hypothesis that a state of vital exhaustion precedes the onset of myocardial infarction was provided by the Imminent Myocardial Infarction Rotterdam study. This involved 415 men (mean age 49) who visited their general practitioner with complaints of a possible cardiac origin, who were followed up over ten months. On entry to the study, all subjects completed a newly designed questionnaire of 63 items. These items were derived from clinical interviews, the cardiological literature, stress theory and the description of the given up–giving up complex formulated by Engel and Schmale (Engel, 1962, 1968; Schmale, 1972). During the follow-up period, 37 subjects suffered from a 'new coronary event' (new angina, myocardial infarction or cardiac death). Five items were found to be predictive of a new coronary event within this highly selected group. Forty items, including the five just mentioned, discriminated between future cases and a healthy control group (Appels, 1980). As a consequence of the design of the study, the data did not prove that feelings of vital exhaustion are predictive of myocardial infarction. Nevertheless, they strengthened the belief that this domain merited further exploration. Following this study the item pool was reduced to 37 by removing three redundant questions. We called this 'Form A' of the questionnaire, which was labelled as the Maastricht Questionnaire (MQ) so as to give it a neutral name. A case–control study by Verhagen *et al.* (1980) found that the MQ discriminated between a group of myocardial infarction patients and a healthy control group. However, the final proof that those who have elevated scores on Form A of the MQ are at increased risk for myocardial infarction required a prospective study.

Test of the hypothesis: the Rotterdam civil servants study

The municipal health authority of the city of Rotterdam began a periodic health check for city employees in 1979. Between January 1979 and December 1980, 3877 male employees aged 39–65 participated. The medical examination included measurements of blood pressure, cholesterol, glucose tolerance, relative weight, smoking and an assessment of angina pectoris using the Rose Questionnaire. A resting electrocardiogram completed the cardiovascular assessment. Feelings of vital exhaustion were assessed using Form A of the Maastricht Questionnaire. Twenty-one new items derived from clinical interviews were added to the existing item set.

The cohort was followed up for an average of 4.2 years. During this period, 59 men free of coronary heart disease at screening suffered from a well-documented myocardial infarction. Vital exhaustion was found to be predictive of future infarction when adjusted for somatic risk factors separately in stratified analyses. Table 2 shows that a score above the median of the MQ increased the risk by 150%. Table 3 summarizes the association between Form A of the MQ and future infarction, controlling simultaneously for the somatic risk factors in a multiple logistic regression. In this analysis the MQ was introduced as a continuous score. It indicates that feelings of exhaustion are predictive of future myocardial infarction. No interactions between MQ scores and any of the somatic risk factors was found. Nor were any associations observed between MQ scores and future cancer or duodenal ulcer. This suggests that vital exhaustion is specifically related to coronary heart disease. Of the 21 items added to Form A of the questionnaire, 8 items were found to be associated with future infarction or cardiac death when adjusted for age. Based upon an analysis of the predictive power of each item separately, the total pool was reduced to a short scale consisting of 21 items. This scale (Form B of the Maastricht Questionnaire) is presented in the Appendix (Appels *et al.*, 1987).

It is our hypothesis that the feelings measured by Form A of the MQ are short-term risk factors for coronary heart disease. Consequently, we studied the relative risk associated with a score above the median of Form A of the MQ for each year of follow-up and observed a sharp decline from 10.05 for the first year of follow-up to 2.23, 3.04 and 0.68 for the second, third and fourth years of follow-up, respectively. This strongly suggests that the predictive power of the scale over the total follow-up time is based mainly upon its predictive power in the first year of follow-up. A close inspection of the predictive power of each single item as a

TABLE 2. Relative risk for future myocardial infarction associated with a score above the median of Form A of the Maastricht Questionnaire, adjusted for somatic risk factors separately

Adjusted for	Relative risk	95% confidence interval	χ^2mh
Age	2.45	1.41–4.26	10.11*
Systolic blood pressure	2.84	1.65–4.90	14.14*
Diastolic blood pressure	2.91	1.68–4.85	14.90*
Cholesterol	2.88	1.67–4.92	14.67*
Smoking	2.80	1.68–4.87	14.59*

$*p = 0.01$.

TABLE 3. Maximum likelihood estimates of logistic parameters relating age, smoking, systolic blood pressure, cholesterol and exhaustion to the risk of myocardial infarction during the 4.2 years follow-up

Variable	Coefficient	St. error	Coefficient/SE	p
Constant	−9.1800	1.2100	−7.59	
Cholesterol	0.0341	0.0111	3.09	0.01
Systol. blood pressure	0.0131	0.0063	2.08	0.04
Smoking (yes/no)	1.0700	0.3106	3.45	0.01
Age (54–58)	0.2593	0.1910	1.36	0.17
(59–65)	0.5739	0.1934	2.97	0.01
Exhaustion	0.0227	0.0085	2.68	0.01

function of duration of follow-up showed that most items had rather stable relative risks, averaging around 2.00. However, the risk ratios for some items decreased markedly over time, as is illustrated in Table 4. These items which have a short-term predictive power express a loss of vitality and strong feelings of irritation or demoralization. Most other items reached statistical significance when the power of the test was increased by the number of cases (i.e. in the second or third year of follow-up). This may indicate either that they are only modestly associated with infarction, or that they form the beginning of a process of decompensation.

The relative importance of vital exhaustion in comparison with somatic risk factors was estimated by multiplying the coefficient of each variable as generated in the multiple logistic regression analysis by the standard deviation of the corresponding variable. The standardized regression coefficients (SRC) showed that age and smoking were the most important parameters (SRC = 0.63 and 0.54, respectively). Cholesterol came next (SRC = 0.36), followed by vital exhaustion (SRC = 0.31) and systolic blood pressure (SRC = 0.26) (Appels *et al.*, 1987; Appels and Mulder, 1988).

TABLE 4. Age-adjusted relative risk for myocardial infarction associated with five complaints during four years of follow-up

Items	Year of follow-up			
	1	2	3	4
Not accomplishing much	4.53**	2.80**	1.89*	1.37
Easily irritated	5.88**	1.90*	1.53	1.40
Want to be dead	7.65**	4.32**	3.60**	2.90**
Strange bodily sensations	3.30**	1.04	0.91	1.04
Shrink from work	3.01**	1.49	1.39	1.33

* $p < 0.05$; ** $p < 0.01$.

The data from the Rotterdam civil servants study support the hypothesis that feelings of exhaustion precede the onset of fatal or non-fatal myocardial infarction. They enable us to specify the feelings or complaints which have prognostic significance. A direct comparison of the relative importance of vital exhaustion compared with the major somatic risk factors showed that the predictive value of this complex of symptoms was of about the same magnitude as that of cholesterol and blood pressure. Because of operational limitations, no other psychosocial factors could be assessed in the Rotterdam study. A case–control study by Falger, however, provides some evidence on which to test the hypothesis that type A individuals are at increased risk of becoming exhausted, together with the hypothesis that exhausted type A individuals are at increased risk for myocardial infarction compared with vital type A individuals. This study also provides some information about the links between vital exhaustion and exposure to objective environmental stress.

Vital exhaustion, type A behaviour and myocardial infarction

Falger (1989) compared 133 men hospitalized for a first myocardial infarction with 192 hospital controls and 133 neighbourhood controls matched for age in a case–control study. This study included an assessment of vital exhaustion as experienced in the months preceding the coronary event using Form B of the MQ, together with assessments of type A behaviour by the structured interview technique, and an interview about major life events experienced over the whole life span.

The mean MQ score for type A men was found to be significantly higher than the mean MQ score of type Bs ($t = 3.51$, $p < 0.01$). This provides some support for the hypothesis that type A individuals have an increased risk of becoming exhausted. Because the positive association observed by Falger was concurrent, it does not prove that type A behaviour precedes a state of vital exhaustion. Recently, Gostautas observed that type A men as measured by the Jenkins Activity Survey in 1972 had elevated MQ scores at rescreening after fifteen years, in comparison with type Bs (Gostautas, personal communication). These data were collected within the framework of the Kaunas–Rotterdam Intervention Study (Glasunov *et al.*, 1981). Because vital exhaustion was not measured on the initial screening, even Gostautas' follow-up data do not prove that type A behaviour increases the risk of becoming exhausted. It might be that the type A individuals had similar MQ scores at screening as they had fifteen years later. Although possible, this is rather unlikely because the test–retest stability of the MQ was found to be rather low in the Rotterdam civil servants study, namely 0.30 when retesting was done after four years among a random subsample of 92 participants.

The hypothesis that exhausted type A people are at increased risk compared to vital type A individuals was tested by dividing cases and controls into vital or exhausted type As and type Bs, according to the assessments on the structured interview and a score below or above the median of the MQ. The results of this classification are shown in Table 5. These data indicate that 109 of the 133 coronary patients (82%) scored above the median of the MQ. Seventy-five coronary cases (56%) were classified as exhausted type As. Table 5 also shows a synergism between type A behaviour pattern and vital exhaustion. Compared to vital type B individuals, the exhausted type As had a fivefold increase in estimated risk in the hospital series, and an elevenfold increase in estimated risk in the neighbourhood series. When exhausted type A individuals are compared with vital type As, the estimated relative risk is 2.67 in the hospital series and 5.52 in the neighbourhood series.

Multivariate analysis of the same data shows that vital exhaustion and type A behaviour were both independently associated with myocardial infarction, after controlling for age, smoking and angina pectoris. This indicates that type A behaviour is not a risk factor solely because it often results in a state of vital exhaustion. Consequently, we cannot conclude that Falger's data support our original hypothesis that only type As who lose control over their environment are at increased risk for myocardial infarction.

Feelings of vital exhaustion were found to be positively associated with a number of life events or more chronic aversive conditions, namely 'prolonged family conflicts' and 'prolonged financial problems of the parents during childhood'; 'past or present unemployment', 'serious conflicts at work with supervisor(s)', 'serious conflicts at work with subordinates' and 'prolonged overtime work'; 'serious educational problems with children', 'serious marital conflicts', 'prolonged conflicts with family members' and 'prolonged financial problems'. These findings are based upon the combined group of cases and controls. This makes it unlikely that the association is influenced by a gloomy recall of past events by coronary patients when they are searching for an explanation of why they are afflicted by a myocardial infarction.

TABLE 5. Standardized relative risk for myocardial infarction of vital and exhausted type B and type A individuals

	Vital B	Vital A	Exhausted B	Exhausted A	Total
Coronary cases	10	14	34	75	133
Hospital referents	43	31	56	62	192
SRR[a]	1.00	1.96	2.61	5.20	
Coronary cases	10	14	34	75	133
Neighbourhood referents	47	33	21	32	133
SRR[b]	1.00	1.99	7.61	11.02	

[a] χ^2 ext = 4.78; $p < 0.01$.
[b] χ^2 ext = 7.05; $p < 0.01$.

The strongest association between any of these conditions and vital exhaustion was that between the MQ and 'prolonged overtime work'. This item discriminated significantly between cases and controls, but lost its discriminatory power when controlled for vital exhaustion. Thus overwork is a risk factor for coronary heart disease when it leads to exhaustion. This finding also indicates that feelings of exhaustion are not only caused by uncontrollable events or other forms of mental stress, but also may be caused by more physical factors like double jobs or too many hours of work, which leave people devoid of sufficient time to spend in rest or relaxation. In other words, it may not be only the experience of helplessness which accounts for the presence of vital exhaustion.

WHY IS VITAL EXHAUSTION ASSOCIATED WITH AN INCREASED RISK FOR MYOCARDIAL INFARCTION?

The possibility that the association between vital exhaustion and future coronary heart disease can be attributed to clinically manifest heart disease can be ruled out, since those who suffered from past or present heart disease at screening were not included in the analysis of the Rotterdam civil servants study data. This does not, however, prove that perceived loss of control, as reflected in feelings of vital exhaustion, causes coronary heart disease. Hypertensive medication may result in increased feelings of tiredness. Participants in the Rotterdam study who were treated for hypertension reported significantly more symptoms of exhaustion than both normotensives and unmedicated hypertensives. Nevertheless, inclusion of a variable 'treated for hypertension' did not alter the results of the multiple logistic regression.

Is the association between vital exhaustion and future infarctions spurious because subclinical levels of atherosclerosis or cardiac degeneration result in elevated scores on the Maastricht Questionnaire? We do not know. A study is currently in progress to evaluate the association between findings obtained at angiography and Maastricht Questionnaire scores. If the outcome of this study shows that the degree of coronary atherosclerosis does not predict MQ scores, it is rather unlikely that subclinical levels of atherosclerosis explain the association observed in the Rotterdam study. If, on the other hand, we find a positive association, no firm conclusion can be drawn, because a concurrent association does not prove that a disease leads to a psychological change or vice versa. Any positive association may be a function of the fact that people who are at increased risk for infarction in the near future are also likely to have high levels of coronary atherosclerosis. Studies of this kind are, however, the furthest that we can go at present in considering possible confounding factors. Given the possibility that other factors such as early unrecognized ischaemia may underlie the observed association, any suggestion that vital exhaustion is a cause of heart disease should be avoided. What we do know is that only a minority of individuals with elevated MQ scores are destined for myocardial infarction in the near future. Only 5% of those scoring in the upper tertile of the MQ suffered from a hard (documented myocardial infarction; cardiac death) or soft (documented angina pectoris; bypass surgery) coronary event during follow-up. The MQ shares its low sensitivity with other risk factors. A state of exhaustion is clearly not a sufficient cause of coronary arterial disease. Unless the heart is already vulnerable, an exhausted individual is most likely to go through a period of mental strain but not to fall ill. We think of vital exhaustion as a strong wind which may stir up an already existing fire. But what is the 'oxygen'?

When attempting to answer this question, we enter a virtually unexplored territory. Some clues have been provided in a study by Van Doornen (1988). In search of a real life stressor he selected the defence of the PhD thesis. In the Netherlands a PhD thesis concludes with a public defence of the thesis in front of a large audience. The professors and the candidate dress officially, the audience is made up of family members and colleagues and discussions are held at a high academic level. All of the ingredients of a real-life stressor are present although people never actually fail.

Van Doornen measured catecholamines, heart rate, serum cholesterol and blood pressure on the morning of the day of the thesis defence and again several weeks later, the latter serving as the control day. Psychological variables included type A behaviour assessed by a Dutch adaptation of the Jenkins Activity Survey, vital exhaustion and a self-developed state anxiety and state depression scale each comprising ten items. Thirty-three men with a mean age of 35.7 years (SD = 7.5) took part in the experiment. Heart rate, systolic and diastolic blood pressure, adrenaline and noradrenaline were significantly higher on the day of the thesis defence compared with the control day. Mean cholesterol levels were also higher on the stress day but the difference was not significant. State anxiety and depression measures were also higher on the stress day. Vital exhaustion was associated with higher serum cholesterol levels on the control day ($r = 0.37$; $p < 0.05$), and with an increase in cholesterol and adrenaline on the stress compared with control day. The positive association between vital exhaustion and increase in cholesterol was independent of the increase in adrenaline. On the stress day, vital exhaustion was strongly related to cholesterol ($r = 0.60$) and noradrenaline ($r = 0.32$). Type A behaviour was found to be associated with an increase in diastolic blood pressure and adrenaline on the stress day.

In an effort to integrate these findings into a tentative model, principal components analyses were performed both for the change scores and the physiological measures of the stress day. Two reasonably consistent factors emerged for both variables. In both analyses type A behaviour and vital exhaustion loaded on separate dimensions. On the vital exhaustion dimension, cholesterol and noradrenaline showed the highest loadings. Type A appeared consistently on a second factor, together with heart rate, systolic blood pressure and adrenaline. This suggests that type A behaviour and vital exhaustion exert their influence on CHD risk by way of different intervening mechanisms; type A behaviour may operate by way of exaggerated cardiovascular dynamics and vital exhaustion by way of lipid metabolism, especially noradrenaline-induced free fatty acid (FFA) mobilization. These data offer excellent suggestions for further exploration, although results are difficult to interpret in the absence of comparable data. In the Rotterdam civil servants study, no association was found between cholesterol and vital exhaustion. However, the samples and situations in the two studies were not at all similar.

A second exploration of the mechanisms which can possibly explain the association between vital exhaustion and myocardial infarction has been done by Lulofs (in preparation). In this study, 24 male volunteers with a mean age of 40 years (SD = 0.81), and free of cardiovascular disease and medication, were tested in three sessions, one control session and two experimental sessions. During the control or baseline session subjects watched TV documentaries on a walking tour of the Madeira islands and on water pollution. The task assigned to the subjects during the experimental session was an auditory vigilance task. The subjects had to pay attention to a series of clicks presented at two different noise levels. They had to respond whenever a click was weak. The four versions of this task differed in terms of event rate and signal rate. Event rate was either one click every 2 seconds or one every 6 seconds. Signal rate was on average either one weak click in every 5 or one weak click in every 15 clicks. Within each experimental session, event rate was kept constant and signal rate was balanced for order. For each subject the three sessions were held a week apart and at the same time of day. At each session venous blood samples were drawn to assess levels of catecholamines and of platelet aggregation. Vital exhaustion was assessed by Form A of the Maastricht Questionnaire.

According to ratings made of experienced distress and effort during the baseline and experimental conditions, only the high event–high signal condition was experienced as stressful. The rank order correlation between vital exhaustion and noradrenaline was 0.24 ($p = 0.20$) during the rest conditions and 0.51 ($p < 0.01$) during the high event–high signal condition. No associations between adrenaline and vital exhaustion were observed.

Spearman rank correlations were also calculated between the MQ scores, the change in freely circulating platelets, and the number of platelets that had formed reversible aggregates. Those correlations showed an interesting pattern: with increasing levels of stress the association between vital exhaustion and change in the number of platelets that had formed reversible aggregates increased, and (conversely) the association with changes in freely circulating platelets decreased.

The common finding of the studies of van Doornen and of Lulofs is that vital exhaustion is associated with the absolute level of noradrenaline during a high stress situation. Van Doornen's data suggest that this reaction is associated with a mobilization of FFA, and Lulofs' data suggest that during a high-stress situation thrombogenic properties of blood change unfavourably in the exhausted group.

As mentioned in the Introduction, these studies are the first investigations of virtually unexplored territory. The observed data were not predicted. These pioneering studies enable us to formulate three specific hypotheses: (1) the level of noradrenaline secreted during high-stress situations is positively correlated with a state of vital exhaustion; (2) during high-stress situations the aggregability of blood platelets increases to a greater extent in those who are vitally exhausted; (3) during high-stress situations, vitally exhausted subjects in particular will react with lipid mobilization.

Some unresolved questions

Vital exhaustion and depression

Over the years we have worked on the specification of mental precursors of myocardial infarction, we have always had, and still have, doubts as to whether it was worth while to label a new personality characteristic and devise a test to measure it, because the concept seems very closely related to depression. Are we contributing to the eternal pest of psychology, where each psychologist formulates a new concept and a new scale to measure it, instead of deriving a hypothesis from established personality theories and testing it by a well-documented scale? It is the aim of science to present facts in the simplest and most economical conceptual form. New concepts rarely contribute to economical formulation. Would the Zung test, the Minnesota Multiphasic Personality Inventory or one of its subscales have done the same job? Are we falling into a semantic trap when coronary victims answer the question whether they felt depressed before myocardial infarction with: 'No, but I was deadly tired and sad'? The same answer has been heard by all those cardiologists and epidemiologists who have studied the prodromata of myocardial infarction and sudden death. Maybe they were naive listeners and did not choose the word 'depression' to label what they heard, because of psychiatric ignorance. There is no reason, however, to believe that cardiologists are not familiar with the concept of depression. We felt that a conceptualization derived from general psychology would not be sufficiently specific. After all, the development of concepts which are as close to reality as possible is also among the aims of science. Therefore we decided to remain naive and to develop a questionnaire which was as close as possible to the self-reports of coronary victims, trusting that this approach would reveal important things which would have been left unnoticed if a more parsimonious strategy had been adopted.

Now that the prospective study has been completed, the question of whether the advantages of our strategy outweigh the disadvantages of making new

constructs and scales should be addressed. When we apply DSM-III criteria to
our findings we probably have to conclude that the MQ measures depression.
Consequently, we would not object to those who say that the Rotterdam civil
servants study has provided some evidence that the onset of myocardial infarction
is preceded by depressive feelings. We would, however, add that such a statement
remains too crude. It is known that depression is reliably associated with
coronary heart disease (Booth-Kewley and Friedman, 1987). However, we are
not sure what type of depression is involved in the aetiology of myocardial
infarction or sudden cardiac death. Our efforts enable us to make some
specifications.

Depression commonly has five sets of characteristics: (1) a sad, apathetic
mood; (2) a negative self-concept involving self-reproach, self-blame and so on;
(3) a desire to avoid other people; (4) a loss of sleep, appetite and sexual desire;
(5) 'a change in activity level, which may take the form of agitation, but more
usually involves lethargy' (Strongman, 1987). The Maastricht Questionnaire
includes items which correspond to the first, fourth and fifth characteristics.
These aspects of the mental state before myocardial infarction indicate some
similarities with depression. However, two other elements—a negative self-
concept involving self-reproach and a desire to avoid other people—are not
among the precursors of myocardial infarction. None of the items about lowered
self-esteem or guilt feelings were found to be predictive in the Rotterdam civil
servants study. Typically, coronary patients blame others for the occurrence of
negative life events (Byrne, 1980). Self-reproach is rare among coronary victims.
Coronary patients may report that they tended to avoid other people in the
months preceding myocardial infarction and disliked parties or meetings. This
behaviour should be understood as an energy-saving behaviour, a heightening of
thresholds for being stimulated. The item 'I have often withdrawn from company
lately' was not found to be predictive of future myocardial infarction in the
Rotterdam study.

Loss of appetite is rarely mentioned by coronary patients as a feature of the
emotional climate before myocardial infarction. Sleep problems are often mentioned as having occurred more frequently in the year before myocardial
infarction. Items asking for trouble falling asleep or staying asleep had a modest
but statistically significant predictive power in the Rotterdam study. The
strongest risk was found to be associated with an affirmation of the question: 'Do
you ever wake up with a feeling of exhaustion and fatigue?' This item remained
predictive when controlling for other sleep complaints or when the analysis was
restricted to those who wake up exhausted but had no problems in falling or
staying asleep. 'Trouble falling asleep' or 'staying asleep' lost their predictive
power when controlled for 'wake up exhausted'. These findings support the
notion that the loss of a vital component of sleep, namely its restoring anabolic
quality, is a risk factor for coronary heart disease.

We did not observe an increase in agitation but an increase in irritability. This
aspect of the prodromal state is especially stressed by the family members of a

coronary victim, when they are asked which behavioural changes took place in the months preceding the coronary event. In Falger's case–control study, items reflecting irritability had the strongest discriminative power of all MQ items. In the prospective study, the item having the strongest predictive power was 'Do you want to be dead at times?' When formulating this item we believed that it expressed depression. Discussions with coronary heart patients who had endorsed that item taught us that a positive answer did not express a wish to be dead but very strong feelings of annoyance or irritation. We therefore believe that agitation in the sense of restlessness does not belong to the precursors of myocardial infarction, but agitation in the sense of increased irritability forms a major component of the precursors.

We still believe that vital exhaustion is an appropriate description because guilt feelings and lowered self-esteem were not found to belong to the precursors of myocardial infarction, and because the emotional climate before a coronary event is mainly characterized by unusual fatigue, lack of energy and irritation. This label has the advantage that it fits well into the description of premonitory symptoms given by cardiologists.

Another concept which might be close to vital exhaustion is 'burnout'. Maslach and Jackson (1982) have defined burnout as

> a syndrome of emotional exhaustion, depersonalization, and reduced personal accomplishment. Emotional exhaustion refers to a depletion of one's emotional resources and the feeling that one has nothing left to give to others at a psychological level. The depersonalization phase of burnout is the development of negative and callous attitudes about the people one works with. This depersonalized perception of others can lead one to judge them as somehow deserving of their troubles. A third aspect of burnout is the perception that one's accomplishments on the job fall short of personal expectations, and thus it involves a negative self evaluation.

The concept of burnout was developed in studies of social and situational sources of job-related stress, especially of stress among health professionals. The concept of vital exhaustion was developed to provide an accurate description of a state preceding myocardial infarction. The origin of the two concepts may have resulted in their varying operationalization. Burnout reflects job-related stress and consequently the Maslach Burnout Inventory has many job-related items. Form A of the Maastricht Questionnaire has only one job-related question. Both the burnout syndrome and vital exhaustion appear to be responses to chronic stress. In practice these concepts differ widely. A close comparison could certainly reveal some of the sources of vital exhaustion and/or contribute to a fuller description of the burnout syndrome. Such a study has yet to be done.

Vital exhaustion and other somatic conditions

As mentioned briefly in the description of the Rotterdam study results, future cases of cancer or duodenal ulcer did not have elevated scores on the MQ at screening. This suggests that vital exhaustion is specifically related to coronary heart disease. Any firm conclusion, however, would be premature because a diagnosis of duodenal ulcer was accepted in the absence of roentgenological evidence, and because some participants who died from cancer during follow-up may have had cancer at screening without knowing it. In the absence of any other empirical data we can only say that we do not know whether vital exhaustion precedes other diseases also.

Vital exhaustion and other heart diseases

Roll and Theorell (1987) observed that patients attending the emergency care unit because of chest pain, without obvious organic causes, had highly elevated vital exhaustion scores compared to randomly sampled healthy subjects matched for age and sex. This result corresponds to some extent with the findings of the Rotterdam civil servants study that nearly all who suffered from unstable angina at entrance scored in the upper tertile of the MQ (odds ratio = 17.21). However, concurrent associations between variables that are dependent on self-reports do not prove very much.

Another untested and unresolved question is whether vital exhaustion increases the risk of sudden death among those who suffer from cardiac rhythm disturbances. Lown (1987) has put forward the hypothesis that a psychological state, which he describes as a long-standing condition frequently manifested by depression or a no-exit life situation, psychological triggers with their higher neural activation of the heart and myocardial electrical instability, are the three factors mainly responsible for susceptibility to ventricular fibrillation. When electrical instability is marked, even slight perturbations will trigger arrythmia. This hypothesis can be easily translated into the hypothesis that vital exhaustion increases the risk of cardiac death among those with a moderate or severe electrical instability of the myocardium. A study on this issue remains to be carried out.

Can vital exhaustion be treated?

The final unresolved question is whether some form of psychological help could reduce feelings of exhaustion, and whether such a reduction would result in a decreased incidence of coronary heart disease in a treated group compared to a non-treated group. We still lack insight into many mechanisms underlying this state, and tend to believe that it is still premature to think about interventions. However, there is much truth in an old Marxist saying that to understand the world one should try to change the world. Therefore we started an experimental programme for patients who are treated by percutaneous transluminal coronary angioplasty (PTCA) because of an imminent myocardial infarction. This cardiological intervention, also known as dottering, removes the stenoses in the coronary vessels but not their determinants. About 20–25% of those treated with PTCA suffer from a restenosis within one year. The determinants of restenoses are unknown. If vital exhaustion is associated with the risk for restenoses (a question currently being studied) and if an intervention could restore vitality, some interesting controlled intervention trials might be carried out. These types of studies are still far away. Nevertheless, the procedure in the current investigation is as follows.

Patients are invited to cooperate in a research programme in which we want to find out how they can protect their health. If they agree, MQ score is assessed by interview to estimate level of exhaustion and to gain insight into its causes as seen by the patient. This information is used to discuss the following points, if relevant:

(1) Sleep patterns: exhausted people do not sleep well, therefore they often go to bed too early or too late and take rests or naps at the wrong times. They often drink alcohol to help them sleep. We try to restore normal sleep patterns and, if necessary, refer them to a special programme.
(2) Physical exercise: exhausted people often feel too tired to do any physical exercise. Strenuous physical exercise is one of the best ways of improving both physical and mental condition. We therefore devise programmes of physical exercise tailored to each individual's needs.
(3) Smoking: although the association between vital exhaustion and smoking is weak we try to influence this behaviour.
(4) Daily schedule: we discuss the number of hours rest a patient takes during the working week and the weekend. Should the number of hours worked exceed 40, we strongly recommend that this number be reduced.
(5) Work or family problems: many of these patients are strong type As who rigidly and aggressively try to find one and only one solution to the problems they encounter or conflicts in which they become involved. Not only is the conflict itself discussed but also the way in which they cope with it. Together we try to find some alternative solutions or to accept an unavoidable or unchangeable situation.

The experiences we have with this programme are still very limited. We have achieved some success but are aware of how deeply seated the loss of energy can be. Several patients have said that they could not 'recharge the battery'. However, the philosophical discussions of the situation may help them to accept an unavoidable decision or situation.

LOSS OF CONTROL AND CORONARY HEART DISEASE: SOME HYPOTHESES

As mentioned in the Introduction to this chapter, the concepts of need for control or loss of control are usually mentioned only in the discussion sections of research papers. Nearly all concepts used in cardiovascular research—social mobility, social support, decision latitude, stressful life events, type A behaviour or vital exhaustion—refer to the need for control as a personality characteristic, or to devices used to maintain control. Something which can be said about everything does not give much information about specific issues. Is the concept of control as vague as the concept of stress? Or is it a parsimonious concept with great potential for integrating separate findings and for the development of new hypotheses? The proof of the pudding is in the eating. If the following attempt to integrate a diversity of observations made in cardiovascular research remains vague, it is at least intellectually enjoyable.

Looking at the global picture of the incidence of coronary heart disease, we see a belt around the world which largely overlaps the industrialized parts of the world. In these countries coronary heart disease is the leading cause of death. Japan is the only exception, and it is exceptional epidemiologically in many respects. Within this belt, a decline in the Western countries and an increase in Eastern European countries can be observed. Ioannidis has found that international trends of arterial disease mortality show an increase during decades of increasing per capita national income until a certain point of economical welfare has been achieved. The incidence rate then tends to decrease (Ioannidis and Efthyniopoulou, 1982). Increasing industrialization seems to be accompanied by an increase in coronary heart disease mortality until a certain point is reached. The process of industrialization disturbs an existing culture, increases the tempo of life, causes geographical and social mobility and may destroy cultural niches which provide people with the social support they need. In other words, the onset of the process of industrialization is a massive threat to control. It takes two or more decades for a society to adapt (for example by legislation) and for individuals to adapt by learning new behaviour and coping styles (for example by anticipation of changes). The notion that the process of industrialization is accompanied by loss of control and that an increase in coronary heart disease mortality is one of the results of modernization leads to some testable hypotheses. If true, coronary heart disease mortality is going to increase in those regions which have only recently joined the European Community.

Within populations the incidence of coronary heart disease varies across social–economical strata. It seems that the increase in coronary heart disease mortality starts in the upper strata and is followed by an increase in the lower strata. Major behavioural changes seem to start in the upper strata; unfortunately, there is little evidence at present concerning these patterns. Marmot *et al.* (1978) have demonstrated that such a process took place in the UK; however, there is no information available about other countries. Mortality statistics, especially before 1950, are unreliable. There is evidence that the actual decline of coronary heart disease in Western countries is mainly due to a decline in the higher socio-economic strata. There are many conflicting explanations to account for these findings; differences in the ability to keep control over one's situation might be one. If this is true, coronary patients might be characterized by a relative inability to anticipate social and cultural changes, for example religious changes or changes with regard to marriage. It is a testable hypothesis that coronary patients rigidly try to keep control over events which are unavoidable because of economic developments (for example, the shop owner confronted with a new supermarket in his or her neighbourhood) or cultural changes (say, the way in which children behave).

Within societies or economic strata, some people are more vulnerable to losing control than others. Psychoanalysts have noted that aggressive tendencies and striving for achievement and dominance are the prominent traits of 'coronary-prone' individuals and that these tendencies are caused by a strongly repressed feeling of uncertainty and doubts about personal value. This insecurity results in a constant striving to obtain symbols of recognition and respect. This behaviour is easily reinforced because hard work is rewarded. It is hard to test psychodynamic views empirically, but I believe they are true. Most coronary patients have very high moral standards. They often praise their sense of responsibility and are easily annoyed by others who, in their eyes, behave irresponsibly. Because of fear that their behaviour does not match their own moral standards, they direct their aggression both inwardly and outwardly. This aggression and hostility reflects a constantly challenged need for control. The feeling that one can never fulfil the demands of conscience is projected outwardly as aggression or hostility. If this notion is true, a positive correlation should be observed between outwardly and inwardly directed aggression among coronary patients.

Vital exhaustion reflects a state after a loss of control has occurred. It is a testable hypothesis that this state mainly occurs after events which were perceived as threats to the symbols of high moral standards or as moral injustice.

REFERENCES

Alonzo, A., Simon, A., and Feinleib, M. (1975). Prodromata of myocardial infarction and sudden death. *Circulation*, **52**, 1056–1062.

Appels, A. (1980). Psychological prodromata of myocardial infarction and sudden death. *Psychotherapy and Psychosomatics*, **34**, 187–195.

Appels, A., and Mulder, P. (1988). Excess fatigue as a precursor of myocardial infarction. *European Heart Journal*, **9**, 758–764.

Appels, A., Höppener, P., and Mulder, P. (1987). A questionnaire to assess premonitory symptoms of myocardial infarction. *International Journal of Cardiology*, **17**, 15–24.

Booth-Kewley, S., and Friedman, H. (1987). Psychological predictors of heart-disease: A quantitative review. *Psychological Bulletin*, **101**, 343–362.

Bruhn, J. G., McCrady, K. E., and Plessis, A. (1968). Evidence of 'emotional drain' preceding death from myocardial infarction. *Psychiatry Digest*, **29**, 34–40.

Byrne, D. G. (1980). Attributed responsibility for life events in survivors of myocardial infarction. *Psychotherapy and Psychosomatics*, **33**, 7–13.

Crisp, A., Queenan, M., and D'Souza, M. F. (1984). Myocardial infarction and the emotional climate. *Lancet*, **i**, 616–619.

Engel, G. L. (1962). Anxiety and depression withdrawal: The primary affects of unpleasure. *International Journal of Psychoanalysis*, **43**, 89–97.

Engel, G. L. (1968). A life setting conducive to illness. *Bulletin Menninger Clinics*, **32**, 355–365.

Falger, P. (1989). *Life Span Development and Myocardial Infarction: An Epidemiologic Study*. PhD dissertation, Maastricht.

Feinleib, M., Simon, A., Gillum, R., and Marjolis, J. (1975). Prodromal symptoms and signs of sudden death. *Circulation* (suppl. vols **51** and **52**), 155–159.

Fischer, H. K., Dlin, B., Winter, W. H., Hagners, S. B., Russel, G. W., and Weiss, E. (1964). Emotional factors in coronary occlusion. II: Time patterns and factors related to onset. *Psychosomatics*, **5**, 280–291.

Fraser, G. E. (1978). Sudden death in Auckland. *Australian and New Zealand Journal of Medicine*, **8**, 490–499.

Glass, D. C. (1977). *Behavior Patterns, Stress and Coronary Disease*. Hillsdale: Lawrence Erlbaum.

Glasunov, I., Dowd, E., Baubiniene, A., Grabauskas, V., Sturmans, F., and Schuurman, J. (eds) (1981). *The Kaunas Rotterdam Intervention Study*. Amsterdam: Elsevier.

Greene, W. A., Goldstein, S., and Moss, A. J. (1972). Psychological aspects of sudden death. *Archives of Internal Medicine*, **129**, 725–731.

Hahn, P. (1971). *Der Herzinfarkt in psychosomatischer Sicht*. Göttingen: Verlag für Medizinische Psychologie im Verlag Vandenhoeck und Ruprecht.

Ioannidis, P., and Efthyniopoulou, G. D. (1982). International transeconomic trends of arterial diseases in the mid 1970's. *American Journal of Epidemiology*, **115**, 278–299.

Klaeboe, G., Otterstad, J. E., Winsness, T., and Espeland, N. (1987). Predictive value of prodromal symptoms in myocardial infarction. *Acta Medica Scandinavica*, **222**, 27–30.

Kuller, L. (1978). Prodromata of sudden death and myocardial infarction. *Advances in Cardiology*, **25**, 61–72.

Lown, B. (1987). Sudden cardiac death: Biobehavioral perspective. *Circulation*, **76** (Suppl. I), 186–196.

Lulofs, R. Stress reactions of persons at psychological risk for myocardial infarction (in preparation).

Marmot, M. G., Adelstein, A. M., Robinson, N., and Rose, G. (1978). Changing social-class distribution of heart disease. *British Medical Journal*, **2**, 1109–1112.

Maslach, C., and Jackson, S. E. (1982). Burnout in health professions: A social psychological analysis. In: G. Sanders and J. Suls (eds), *Social Psychology of Health and Illness*. Hillsdale: Lawrence Erlbaum.

Polzien, P., and Walter, J. (1971). Das pseunoneurasthenische Syndrom im Frühstadium der Koronarsklerose. *Münchener Medizinische Wochenschrift*, **44**, 1453–1456.

Rissanen, V., Romo, M., and Sittanen, P. (1978). Premonitory symptoms and stress-factors preceding sudden death from ischaemic heart disease. *Acta Medica Scandinavia*, **20**, 389–396.

Roll, M., and Theorell, T. (1987). Acute chest pain without obvious organic cause before age 40: Personality and recent life events. *Journal of Psychosomatic Research*, **31**, 215–222.

Romo, M. (1973). Factors related to sudden death in acute ischaemic heart disease. A community study in Helsinki. *Acta Medica Scandinavia*, **547**, 5–92.

Rosenman, R. H. (1986). Current and past history of type A behavior pattern. In: Th. Schmidt, T. Dembroski and G. Blümchen (eds), *Biological and Psychological Factors in Cardiovascular Disease*. Berlin: Springer Verlag.

Schmale, A. H. (1972). Giving up as a final common pathway to change in health. *Advances in Psychosomatic Medicine*, **8**, 20–40.

Stowers, M., and Short, D. (1970). Warning symptoms before myocardial infarction. *British Heart Journal*, **32**, 833–838.

Strongman, K. T. (1987). *The Psychology of Emotion*. Chichester: Wiley.

Thompson, S. G. (1984). Predicting myocardial infarction. *Lancet*, **i**, 1021–1022.
van Doornen, L. (1988). *Physiological stress reactivity*. PhD dissertation, Amsterdam.
Verhagen, F., Nass, C., Appels, A., van Bastelaer, A., and Winnubst, J. (1980). Cross
    validation of the A/B typology in the Netherlands. *Psychotherapy and Psychosomatics*, **34**,
    178–186.

APPENDIX: FORM B OF THE MAASTRICHT QUESTIONNAIRE

Medical research is constantly trying to track down the causes of disease. You
would help this research by answering the following questions about how you
have been feeling lately. Please mark the answers that are true for you. If you
don't know or cannot decide circle the ?. There are no 'right' or 'wrong'
answers.

1.	Do you often feel tired?	yes ? no
2.	Do you often have trouble falling asleep?	yes ? no
3.	Do you wake up repeatedly during the night?	yes ? no
4.	Do you feel weak all over?	yes ? no
5.	Do you have the feeling that you haven't been accomplishing much lately?	yes ? no
6.	Do you have the feeling that you can't cope with everyday problems as well as you used to?	yes ? no
7.	Do you believe that you have come to a 'dead end'?	yes ? no
8.	Do you lately feel more listless than before?	yes ? no
9.	I enjoy sex as much as ever	yes ? no
10.	Have you experienced a feeling of hopelessness recently?	yes ? no
11.	Does it take more time to grasp a difficult problem than it did a year ago?	yes ? no
12.	Do little things irritate you more lately than they used to?	yes ? no
13.	Do you feel you want to give up trying?	yes ? no
14.	I feel fine	yes ? no
15.	Do you sometimes feel that your body is like a battery that is losing its power?	yes ? no
16.	Would you want to be dead at times?	yes ? no
17.	Do you have the feeling these days that you just don't have what it takes anymore?	yes ? no
18.	Do you feel dejected?	yes ? no
19.	Do you feel like crying sometimes?	yes ? no
20.	Do you ever wake up with a feeling of exhaustion and fatigue?	yes ? no
21.	Do you have increasing difficulty in concentrating on a single subject for long?	yes ? no

Scoring: Each confirmation of a complaint is coded as 2. All question marks are coded as
    1. A negative answer is coded as 0. Note that questions 9 and 14 are reversed
    (no = 2; ? = 1; yes = 0). The scale score is obtained by summing the answers.
From Appels *et al.* (1987). Reprinted with permission of the *International Journal of
Cardiology* and Elsevier Science Publishers.

Section III

Mechanisms relating stress with control

CHAPTER 11

Psychophysiological consequences of behavioural choice in aversive situations

KEITH PHILLIPS
Department of Psychology, Polytechnic of East London, London, UK

INTRODUCTION

Increasingly theorists are making use of the construct 'control' to explain the impact of environmental and psychosocial variables upon the physical and mental health of individuals and populations. It is a beguiling construct since it can be utilized at several levels of analysis and across a broad spectrum of situations: epidemiological studies, e.g. the relationship between socio-economic factors and cardiovascular disease (Syme, 1985); performance and health in occupational settings (Karasek *et al.*, 1981); life events and psychopathologies (e.g. Seligman, 1975); conditioning contingencies and health pathologies (Abbott *et al.*, 1984); individual responses to threatened events (e.g. Phillips *et al.*, 1985). Despite the promise of parsimony offered by this construct we should not be blind to the complexities of the relationships it seeks to summarize. Nor should it mislead us into believing that the mediating mechanisms between control and health are simple. As the contributions to this volume show, elaborate and sophisticated analyses are involved in understanding the relationships between personal control and individual well-being. There is a danger, I believe, that just as the construct 'stress' has proven difficult to justify (Steptoe, 1983), 'control' may also disguise the complexities and problems that it is supposed to explain. For example, control might be seen as the critical variable mediating the effects of environmental demands upon health, where absence or loss of control is viewed as being stressful and conversely that availability of control is stress-reducing. Evidence from psychophysiological studies with humans and other animals

Stress, Personal Control and Health.   Edited by A. Steptoe and A. Appels.
Published by John Wiley & Sons Ltd.

involving several different tasks and situations indicate that such conclusions would be naive and largely unsupportable: their acceptance would be at best premature and probably entirely misguided.

One of the difficulties of the construct 'control' is the absence of unanimity about its definition. Recent analyses (Averill, 1973; Miller, 1979a; Thompson, 1981) that have sought to classify meanings of control as evidenced by studies of response to aversive events in different behavioural contexts have produced quite different typologies, as Table 1 shows. As Fisher (1986) has remarked, 'The differences in typology provide some indication of how difficult adequate conceptualisation of control is; its form may vary according to time and circumstance as well as with the nature of the subjects—human or animal' (p. 29). Indeed, if one accepts each of the types shown in Table 1, it becomes difficult to imagine any behavioural context where control of some kind would not be available to an organism.

A further difficulty is that studies that have tried to manipulate the controllability of some event are inevitably confounded by changes in the predictability of that event. Someone having control of an event must be able to predict the occurrence of the event in order for the control to be exercised. If 'control' is

TABLE 1. Classifications of 'control'

		Control	
	Type	Description	
Averill (1973)	Behavioural	Direct action upon environment that terminates, avoids or modifies an aversive stimulus	
	Cognitive	Imposition of meaning upon or interpretation of aversive events	
	Decisional	Availability of choice or response options open to individual	
Miller (1979a)	Instrumental	Possession (real or believed) of a behavioural response that modifies the aversive event	
	Self-administered	Predicted occurrence of the aversive event by self-delivery	
	Potential	Availability (real or believed) of a controlling response for use in future at the discretion of the individual	
Thompson (1981)	Behavioural	Belief that there exists a behavioural response that will modify the aversiveness of the situation	
	Cognitive	Belief that there exists a cognitive strategy that will modify the aversiveness of the situation	
	Information	Knowledge (predictability, effects, causes) about a forthcoming aversive event	
	Retrospective	Imposition of meaning and attribution of cause upon past aversive event	

intrinsically beneficial, as the prevailing view would have us believe, then in aversive situations predictability should be preferred if control is possible or even potentially possible. If control is not possible then it is less obvious what benefits might be offered by predictability alone. Could it be that any benefits that supposedly derive from availability of control over an aversive event are in reality simply a function of the predictability of the event?

PREFERENCE FOR PREDICTABILITY

Laboratory studies of preference for predictability of aversive events in choice situations using animals have been consistent in the finding that where animals may choose behaviourally between either receipt of predictable electric shock (i.e. shock preceded by a warning signal or shocks delivered at fixed temporal intervals) or unpredictable shock (i.e. non-signalled or variable interval presentation) then the predictable option is preferred (Badia *et al.*, 1979). Indeed, titration of predictability associated with greater intensity or duration of the shock delivered against lower intensity or duration of unpredictable shock indicates that, for rats at least, the benefit derived from predictability is sufficient to outweigh the punishing effect of greater shock severity in this situation (Badia *et al.*, 1973).

Animals' preferences for predictable over unpredictable shock conditions require explanation. The reliability of the finding points to an explanation in terms of some biological advantage that ensues from predictability. This view is strengthened by reports that, in aversive situations, unpredictability may have debilitating physiological consequences such as plasma corticosterone release or loss of body weight, and may result in severe pathological end-points such as gastric ulceration. Since predictable conditions are preferred it has been assumed that their influence is less stressful than unpredictable conditions. A recent review of a complex and inconsistent literature, however, finds that it is by no means clear that behavioural choice for predictability is accompanied by either fewer or less severe indicators of physiological harm (Abbott *et al.*, 1984). Weight loss, gastric lesions or corticosterone release may be greater following predictable rather than unpredictable shock. Some of the inconsistencies in this literature upon the advantages of predictability, including the apparently conflicting evidence from behavioural versus physiological measures, may be explained by the diversity of physiological indicators used as dependent measures of stress effects, and of experimental variables such as the severity of electric shock and its method of delivery. Abbott *et al.* suggest that the most significant variable is the distinction between chronic versus acute exposure to the aversive situation. During chronic exposure predictable shock is more stressful than unpredictable; but in acute situations the reverse is true—unpredictable shock is more stressful than predictable. This interpretation has been challenged by Arthur (1986), who argues that predictable shock, defined by the presence of a warning signal, is more stressful in *both* acute and chronic duration studies. It is clear from the reply (Abbott and Badia, 1986) to Arthur's critique that, despite the consistency of behavioural findings showing preference for predictability, there remains considerable uncertainty about the *physiological* advantages to be accrued from behavioural choice of predictable shock conditions.

The issue of whether or not stressful or debilitating consequences follow exposure to predictable aversive situations has also been examined in laboratory studies with volunteer human subjects. Although concerned with similar issues it should be noted that they bear only superficial resemblance to the animal studies. It is true that they typically involve threat of delivery of electric shock, but unlike the animal studies they use infrequent or even non-existent shocks of mild severity, during acute and relatively brief sessions. Obviously it is of interest to know how human subjects behave in aversive situations, and studies of preference for predictability in human subjects have been conducted using a paradigmatic task pioneered by Averill and his colleagues (Averill and Rosenn, 1972), and which may be regarded as a laboratory analogue of the real-life threats encountered by everyone throughout their lives; threats such as anticipation of pain, facing forthcoming surgery or awaiting threatening news. Averill's task involves challenging individuals with the threat of an aversive event that is preceded by a warning signal. Subjects are offered a behavioural choice between seeking information about the warning signal which predicts the occurrence of the aversive event or avoiding information about it by distracting themselves from the task. It is inevitable that seeking information (vigilance) about the warning signal makes the occurrence of the aversive event predictable, whereas the choice for distraction effectively makes the event an unpredictable one, since the warning signal will not be perceived.

Criticisms of laboratory studies such as these are that they are inevitably artificial and contrived, that they use selected samples, usually volunteer undergraduates, and that their findings should not be generalized, since although they have high internal validity their external validity is low: in brief they lack ecological validity. Despite the merit of these criticisms, laboratory studies have a vital role in identifying significant variables, and these studies utilize designs that allow parametric measurement of the independent influence of variables such as predictability and controllability (for further discussion of the merits of acute laboratory tasks see Steptoe, 1985). In real-life situations, it is often impossible to manipulate independently these and other variables, and their consequences may be more usefully assessed by other techniques, including quasi-experimental designs and multivariate analyses.

Relatively few laboratory studies have examined preference for predictability of aversive events in humans. Averill *et al.* (1977) threatened volunteer male subjects with electric shock, and offered them the choice of responding by pressing a button to gain access to a signal that warned of the delivery of the shock, or to distract themselves from information about the shock by listening to music. They found that in general predictability was preferred *if* subjects had the opportunity of making an instrumental response to avoid imminent shock. Some subjects, however, preferred to distract themselves by listening to music, ignoring the opportunity to observe a warning signal even when it was the cue for the instrumental response that would avoid the shock. Subjects choosing the former strategy of monitoring the warning signal may be thought of as preferring a vigilant, information-seeking strategy and their behaviour may be described as 'vigilant coping' or monitoring. The alternative strategy which may also be described as coping behaviour is distraction or non-vigilance, and this is regarded as a passive information-avoidance strategy.

Using the same paradigm although with rather different parameters of threat and with female subjects, Miller (1979b) also found individual differences in preference for predictability. Again it was found that offering subjects the opportunity of making an avoidance response increased the proportion of time spent monitoring for the presence of the warning signal, i.e. increased preferences for predictability. Despite the procedural differences between these two studies, both confirmed that on average human subjects monitor a warning signal more if some degree of instrumental control is available.

To clarify further the role of factors that influence choice for monitoring, i.e. choice for predictability, Evans *et al.* (1984) carried out a study that systematically examined preferences for predictability using the Averill paradigm under different levels of controllability, using both male and female subjects, and different levels of probability of shock on different trials. Some subjects had prior experience of the shock to be used on experimental trials whilst others faced the prospect of unknown, i.e. non-experienced, shock. The experiment attempted to maintain subjects' involvement in the task at similar levels whether they were monitoring or distracting. To achieve this, subjects participated in a computer-controlled version of the Averill task, where pressing a button selected a channel displayed on a monitor showing randomly generated playing cards with reselection of a new card every 10 seconds throughout 3-minute trials. The subjects were told that the appearance of the ace of spades would be followed after 4 seconds by an electric shock delivered through electrodes attached to the subject's ankle. Selection of this channel, i.e. monitoring for the warning signal, represents choice for predictability and is an active coping strategy. Subjects were free to select the alternative channel by pressing another key which eliminated the cards display and instead presented subjects with a display of 'interesting facts' taken from the *Guinness Book of Records*, with each item displayed for 10 seconds. Choice of this distraction channel prevented subjects from detecting the warning signal cueing the delivery of electric shock.

It was found that monitoring (choosing predictability) was significantly influenced by the nature of the threat. Threat of unexperienced shock produced significantly greater monitoring than unexperienced aversive noise, which in turn produced significantly greater monitoring than previously experienced electric shock. Female subjects monitored more than did males, and female subjects were more likely to monitor when offered control over the threatened shock. The behavioural choices of males in this study were anomalous in that they distracted when offered control over the shock. Over all subjects, provision of behavioural control was preferred but the effect was of marginal significance. The probability of the threatened event, i.e. its likelihood of occurrence, also influenced monitoring to some degree. Three levels of probability were used in association with different trials. The highest level of probability (one in two chance of shock) produced significantly greater monitoring than either moderate (one in five chance) or low (one in twenty chance) which did not differ. This indicates perhaps that there may be a threshold below which the level of threat is so remote as to not promote active control strategies. These behavioural findings clearly indicate that situational variables singly and in combination determine choice behaviour or preference for predictability. It is only by quantifying their influences that individual differences in coping strategy will be understood (Phillips, 1986). A meta-analysis by Patterson and Neufeld (1987) of the effects of situational factors upon individuals' appraisal of threat identifies the significance of several of the variables manipulated in the experimental studies upon behavioural choice including the severity, imminence and probability of threat. They argue that future research should '... examine each factor further ... dissecting their influences in more detail.' I concur, but would go further and ask that their influences be measured in relation to individuals' *behaviours* when facing threat rather than simply to their appraisals, i.e. as correlates of different coping strategies.

PSYCHOPHYSIOLOGICAL CORRELATES
OF MONITORING AND DISTRACTION

Studies of preference for predictability have examined not only the behavioural choices made by human subjects but also some psychophysiological correlates of those choices. The reason that psychophysiological measures have been recorded arises from the belief that maladaptive psychophysiological responses or patterns of response are implicated in the aetiology of stress-related disorders. In particular, there is an implicit belief that excessive physiological reactivity is harmful and may have pathological consequences. This belief is sustained by findings of research using laboratory tasks involving a variety of stressors such as cognitive tasks, cold pressor test as well as threat of electric shock or shock avoidance, which have implicated exaggerated cardiovascular reactivity with coronary heart disease and hypertension (Krantz and Manuck, 1984; Rose and Chesney, 1986; Steptoe *et al.*, 1984). The aversive choice paradigm has proven useful for examining individual differences in both behavioural choices and physiological responsivity—differences that might be of critical significance for the identification of individuals at risk for particular disorders.

Where individual differences are shown to exist it is of course important to determine whether they can be attributed to trait characteristics of the subjects, or to situational factors or more probably to interactions between these variables. In studies that examine both behavioural and physiological dependent measures it should not be forgotten that the relationships between these measures, although usually assessed by correlational analyses, *may* be causal. It is not inconceivable that a pattern of physiological reactivity is the consequence of adoption of a particular behavioural strategy by an individual. Preliminary data reported by Phillips *et al.* (1986), for example, indicate that the monitoring strategy results in significantly greater elevations of heart rate than does distraction and that this effect is a direct consequence of monitoring. If these results are confirmed and it is found that psychophysiological reactivity is a direct effect caused by particular behavioural choices, they would have significant implications for the treatment or management of stress-related disorders. It would mean that interventions aimed at modifying individuals' physiological responses to aversive or threatening situations could be based upon adjustment or retraining of their behavioural strategies adopted in that situation (see Jacob and Chesney, 1986).

The empirical studies of choice for predictability cited above (Averill and Rosenn, 1972; Miller, 1979b; Evans *et al.*, 1984) measured some psychophysiological correlates of individuals' choice of coping strategy—monitoring or distraction—in an attempt to understand whether predictability is stress-reducing. In these studies prior experience of the aversive event, probability of the event and level of controllability have been used as independent variables with behavioural choice—extent of monitoring and distraction—used as the primary dependent variable. The psychophysiological measures—heart rate and skin conductance—have been examined as correlates of subjects' behavioural choices.

Both Miller (1979b) and Phillips *et al.* (1985) found that greater physiological responsiveness was associated with monitoring than with distraction. It can be argued, therefore, that choice for predictability causes greater physiological activation than unpredictability in aversive situations. This finding might seem counter-intuitive given the observed behavioural preference for predictability, but it is in accord with many other studies that find predictable shock is associated with greater physiological activation than unpredictable shock (see Miller, 1979a). A contrary result reported by Averill and Rosenn (1972) that greater physiological arousal was associated with unpredictability, i.e. the distraction strategy, is difficult to explain but may be attributable to the much greater level of threat presented by the Averill study compared to that posed by either Miller or Phillips *et al.*

It seems that, in general, predictability is associated with greater physiological responsiveness than unpredictability in this choice situation. The level of controllability offered by the situation interacts with predictability, however, and might play a significant role in determining the subject's behaviour and pattern of physiological response. In the study by Evans *et al.* (1984) subjects were offered different levels of potential control over the threatened shock. Three different groups of subjects were told respectively that the warning signal (ace of spades) would be followed after a 4-second interval by delivery of electric shock (no control condition), that pressing a key during the 4-second interval between warning signal and subsequent shock would avoid the shock (full control condition), or that pressing the key within 4 seconds of the appearance of the warning signal would give a 50% opportunity of avoiding the shock (uncertain control). Skin conductance level was not responsive to this manipulation of the controllability of the situation, although it was associated with the probability of shock, which might be interpreted as an index of aversiveness of the situation. The pattern of heart rate changes, however, showed that the greatest heart rate elevations, measured as change from base level, occurred during the condition of moderate or uncertain control and that they were absent under conditions of either full or no control. This is of interest because it suggests, first, that controllability may interact with predictability in aversive situations and, second that in terms of their physiological correlates, what may be of importance is not whether or not control is possible but whether *the consequences of executive control* are predictable.

This interpretation is given some credence by the findings from Obrist's laboratory which led to the distinction between active and passive coping (Obrist, 1981).

Active versus passive coping

The active versus passive coping distinction was based originally upon the extent of subjects' behavioural involvement in an aversive task. The protypical task for active coping is a signalled shock avoidance reaction time task where subjects are provided with an instrumental avoidance response. Passive coping is elicited by tasks that involve exposure of subjects to an aversive situation but without an instrumental avoidance response being available. Appropriate tasks are the cold pressor test or viewing a pornographic movie whilst being observed by others. Obrist's studies have shown that the active coping demanded by the shock-avoidance task results in much greater cardiovascular reactivity, indexed by increases in heart rate and carotid blood pressure and decreases in pulse transit time, than either the cold pressor test or exposure to unavoidable electric shocks. The use of β-adrenergic blocking agents eliminated the effect, indicating that this reactivity depended upon sympathetic (noradrenergic) mediation (Obrist *et al.*, 1978; Light and Obrist, 1980). A more recent study has indicated that myocardial contractility assessed by left ventricular pre-ejection time also differentiates between active and passive coping demands, with the active task causing a greater decrease of pre-ejection time (Obrist *et al.*, 1987). It seems therefore that the opportunity to exercise instrumental control will elicit large myocardial responses that are sympathetically mediated. Manuck *et al.* (1978) have demonstrated that in a similar aversive task *perceived* control, in the absence of actual behavioural control, is itself sufficient to produce elevation of systolic pressure. Light and Obrist (1983) have reported similar cardiovascular responses in an appetitive reaction time task in which reward was both uncertain and dependent upon instrumental performance, which suggests that the β-adrenergic reaction is a consequence of perceived behavioural demands rather than a reaction to aversiveness.

It is not only the nature of the strategy demanded by the task (active or passive) but also situational variables that influence psychophysiological responses in aversive tasks. Two significant influences are the level of difficulty of the task and the novelty of either the task itself or of the aversive stimulus presented.

Level of difficulty

Several studies (described elsewhere in this volume) have found that cardiac reactions to a task may be manipulated by adjusting the level of task difficulty. During active coping Obrist *et al.* (1978) assigned groups of subjects to three levels of difficulty—easy, difficult and impossible. Greater elevations of heart rate and systolic pressure were found during the difficult condition than either the easy or impossible conditions. Light *et al.* (1983) demonstrated a parallel result using an appetitive reaction time task. These findings are consistent with those of Evans *et al.* (1984), which showed that, when threatened with electric shock, subjects offered behavioural control with uncertain outcome showed greater heart rate increases than subjects offered either total control or absence of control. Cognitive tasks, mental arithmetic and Raven's matrices, structured to offer easy, difficult and impossible levels of difficulty, have also been found to produce cardiac reactions that reflect task difficulty (Carroll *et al.*, 1986a,b). Additional heart rates, a measure of suprametabolic physiological activation (Blix *et al.*, 1974), were significantly greater during the difficult and impossible conditions and reflected subjects' self-reported levels of active engagement and arousal.

Novelty

In a series of studies with rats involving wheel turn shock avoidance conditioning, Brener *et al.* (1977, 1980) consistently found that tonic elevations of heart rate in excess of somatomotor effort were greatest during initial conditioning sessions. Similarly Phillips *et al.* (1985) reported that human subjects offered choice for predictable versus unpredictable electric shock show significantly greater heart rate elevations if the threatened shock has not been previously experienced than if subjects have been given prior exposure. This effect has also been reported by Elliott (1966) and Light and Obrist (1980).

Explanations of an organism's pattern of responding in aversive situations will need to take account of both choice of response strategy and the influences of situational variables. One general dimension that has biological significance for the organism that may account for the psychophysiological effects of these different variables is *behavioural uncertainty*.

Behavioural uncertainty as an explanatory construct

The findings from studies of preference for predictability suggest that in aversive choice situations different physiological responses reflect different behavioural processes. Changes in electrodermal measures are indicative of generalized affective activation including anticipation of aversiveness (Sosnowski, 1983). Heart rate changes, however, are sensitive to the degree of behavioural uncertainty engendered by the situation. In the choice between monitoring and distraction, what is of prime importance is not the occurrence or otherwise of the shock but the uncertainty surrounding the warning signal. Selection of the monitoring channel causes uncertainty about observation of the warning signal: Will it appear? If so when? Will an appropriate response be made? Those uncertainties produce autonomic sympathetic activation which in the long term could be harmful, but which in the short term are tolerable *if* instrumental control is available when the threatened event is delivered. Choice of distraction, however, eliminates stimulus uncertainty; the warning signal will not be seen. This may be an effective strategy where the threat is of limited harm, such that the aversive event even when experienced is not damaging; when its potential harm is greater then distraction becomes less favoured. This interpretation implies that the warning signal should not be regarded as incidental but rather as a key factor for the interpretation of the psychophysiological responses in choice situations. This interpretation is consistent with the findings from animal studies upon signalled shock avoidance. A warning signal itself may be stressful but by indicating through its absence periods of safety its presence may still be preferred (Abbott and Badia, 1986).

Were this the only consideration then monitoring an aversive event would inevitably be associated with both greater electrodermal responsiveness due to anticipation of the event and greater cardiac responsiveness due to the uncertainty surrounding its occurrence. However, uncertainty extends beyond the occurrence or otherwise of the warning signal and concerns also the consequences of responding. If control is available then will execution of the controlling response be successful? Taking these effects together it can be argued that an aversive situation and particularly one involving behavioural choice may be coped with by different behavioural strategies: the behavioural objective is to lessen or eliminate behavioural uncertainty, and that is achieved by executing 'a prepared response', which is defined as a behavioural response that leads to a known or previously experienced outcome. Execution of a prepared response will be associated with less physiological activation than for unprepared responses since the metabolic demands of a prepared response are more predictable than of more diffuse unprepared responses.

RESPONDING IN AVERSIVE SITUATIONS: A GENERAL MODEL

I have proposed that behavioural choices in aversive situations have psychophysiological consequences that are interpretable in terms of the extent to which behavioural uncertainty is resolved by the predictability of the threatened event and the outcome of instrumental responses made. This viewpoint offers a general model which may resolve some apparent paradoxes within studies of preference for predictability in humans and other animals (Phillips, 1986).

The model is shown in Figure 1 and has as its basis the assumption that coping behaviours are directed towards the resolution of behavioural uncertainty. It can be seen that the model equates uncertainty with response inefficiency which in turn is accompanied by exaggerated sympathetic autonomic activation. Resolution of uncertainty not only increases behavioural efficiency; it also produces autonomic–behavioural integration and eliminates inappropriate sympathetic reactions. Similar ideas were expressed by Germana (1972), who provided empirical evidence in support of the notion that the differential autonomic activation that accompanies somatic–behavioural events depends upon response uncertainty. In this context resolution of uncertainty means that the organism recognizes regularities of contingency between response and outcome. Although I use the term 'recognizes', I do not mean to imply that this involves conscious awareness; recognition may occur simply at a mechanical level elicited by appropriate discriminative cues. Of course, human subjects may seek to impose self-conscious awareness upon this process and may actively seek to recognize these contingencies ('cognitive control')—even where they may not exist. Moreover, it is possible for human subjects by their verbal reports to inform us of retrospective rationalization and recognition of regularities based upon attributions of causal relationships between stimulus events and their behaviours ('retrospective control'). We cannot know whether equivalent processes are occurring in infrahuman animals; we can simply observe their patterns of responding in the face of contingency regularities.

Predictability, then, is preferred because organisms seek to resolve behavioural uncertainty. Why should this be so? What advantages follow? These questions are fundamental and the answers will be found, I believe, in studies that analyse behaviour in terms of the metabolic economy of organisms. Behavioural uncertainty must be resolved because it causes inefficient behavioural responding that is metabolically expensive and inappropriate. In novel situations or other

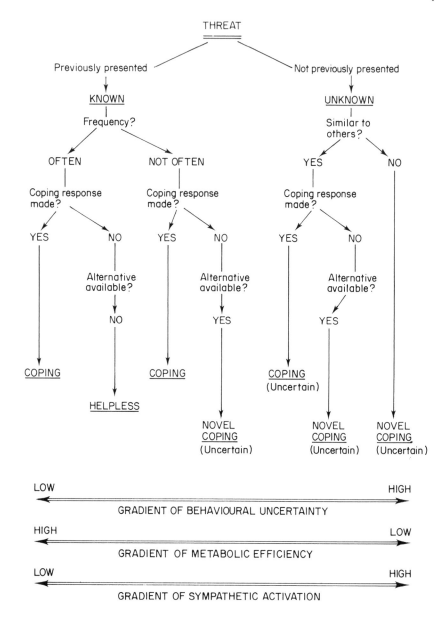

FIGURE 1. Behavioural, metabolic and physiological consequences of responding to threatening aversive events.

situations where behavioural uncertainty exists, then, an organism responds by making a range of behavioural responses of varying intensity and duration. As uncertainty is resolved the responses become more finely tuned or more skilled and any unnecessary or inappropriate components of the original response pattern are abandoned, i.e. there is a refining of behavioural response. Predictability aids this refining process because it allows discriminative selectivity of the appropriate coping response and temporal control of its execution. Microanalyses of operant responding by rats have demonstrated empirically these metabolic advantages that follow from the resolution of behavioural uncertainty (Brener, 1987).

Studies by Weiss (1970, 1971) are of interest here because they show how for rats this refinement of coping behaviour does occur in aversive situations with predictable shock but not with unpredictable shock conditions. Continued exposure to unpredictable and inescapable shock leads to a resolution of behavioural uncertainty by non-responding, a pattern of behaviour referred to as helplessness (Seligman *et al.*, 1971). The adoption of helplessness as a strategy for resolving uncertainty about response outcome does not prevent the debilitating effects of the shock, but non-responding does eliminate the metabolically costly alternative of engaging in escape behaviours that continued punishment shows to be ineffective.

According to this model the concept of behavioural uncertainty is of paramount significance. Its definition is dependent upon ideas of energetic efficiency of behaviour and it may best be understood as responding in the absence of an established contingency. Behavioural certainty is present when an organism is able to emit a behavioural response that *in the past* has led to a successful outcome. That response may then be described as 'a prepared response'; it exists as a behavioural unit that may be emitted at known energetic cost to an appropriate discriminative cue. Coping behaviour is defined as the execution of a behavioural response to eliminate behavioural uncertainty. Coping is defined as the successful elimination of behavioural uncertainty. Coping behaviours that do not successfully eliminate behavioural uncertainty will be modified, e.g. repeated at greater intensity or with different temporal characteristics (see Brener, 1987) or replaced by some alternative response. Response certainty may even be achieved by patterns of coping behaviours that *appear* pathologically inappropriate if no other means of resolving uncertainty can be established, e.g. learned helplessness. Even in this instance, however, the consequences of continued striving to escape or cope with unavoidable stressors or punishment may be far costlier than passive acceptance of the situation accompanied by behavioural immobility, which according to the model is seen as one strategy for the resolution of behavioural uncertainty.

Within this model a stressor becomes identified as stimulus conditions that produce behavioural uncertainty, and stress may be regarded as ineffective or

unsuccessful coping that fails to resolve behavioural uncertainty. Coping behaviours comprise response patterns that may become 'prepared responses' if
they are successful in reducing or eliminating behavioural uncertainty.

Studies of conditioning in rats based upon ambulatory wheel turning as the
specified instrumental response have clearly shown that novel experience of the
aversive situation leads to elevations of heart rate that are in excess of the
organism's motor demands (Brener *et al.*, 1977, 1980). Brener (1986) has
proposed that such 'metabolically excessive elevations' in heart rate are mediated by central feed-forward mechanisms that promote cardiovascular activation for generalized motor preparation. If behavioural uncertainty can be
resolved a more specific motor pattern emerges and the heart rate becomes
synchronized to that pattern. If, however, adaptation does not occur, i.e. the
coping response does not achieve successful resolution of uncertainty, or if the
experimental contingency demands a state of sustained motor preparation, then
tonic elevation of heart rate will persist (Sherwood *et al.*, 1983). If such sustained
metabolically excessive elevations of heart rate are mediated by sympathetic
activation—and there is evidence from drug studies that they are in part—then
they might be regarded as maladaptive. This would be entirely consistent with
Obrist's view that sympathetically mediated and excessive cardiac output (which
is highly correlated with heart rate under most conditions) is implicated in the
aetiology of hypertension and coronary heart disease (Obrist, 1981).

There is equivalent evidence from studies with human subjects that demanding challenges, including shock avoidance, mental arithmetic and video game
playing, produce metabolically excessive cardiac responses (Carroll *et al.* 1986a;
Sherwood *et al.*, 1986). Carroll has argued that the key situational determinant of
such suprametabolic activity is task difficulty since the shared attribute of
conditions producing this activity is that success is 'neither assured nor unrealiz-
able' (Carroll *et al.*, 1986b). An equally compelling interpretation, however,
would be that the suprametabolic activity results from conditions of *uncertainty*.
The merit of utilizing 'uncertainty' rather than 'difficulty' is that it has wider
applicability. It can be used for levels of difficulty within a particular type of task
such as mental arithmetic but it can also summarize the effects of different types
of task, including perceptual tasks where discriminability rather than difficulty is
manipulated.

This chapter began with a consideration of the construct 'control' and I return
to this now. Experimental studies of control have utilized the construct as an
environmental variable that may be manipulated by an experimenter to
influence behavioural and physiological dependent measures. The model I have
outlined above treats control as a dependent variable; it is measured by
observation of an organism's response to uncertainty. If the organism responds
by making prepared responses that are energetically efficient then it may be said
to be exercising control in that its behaviour evidences an effective adaptation to
its environment. I believe that this model provides a framework for integrating

the findings from animal and human studies of responding in aversive situations. It clearly depends upon an assumption that behaviour is directed by biological utility. It also challenges the popular view of 'control' and sees it not as a determinant of behaviour but instead as an outcome of an organism's behavioural response to conditions of uncertainty.

Although this interpretation is derived from studies of responding in aversive situations, it may have wider appeal since it is consistent with models of stress that emphasize the importance of the relationship between task demands such as stimulus complexity, time pressure and feedback, and an individual's capacity (e.g. Schönpflug, 1983). Using this model Schönpflug has argued that stress may be prevented by improving the 'demand–capacity ratio' through the exercise of control by 'planning' response strategies. He proposes that formulation of plans allows individuals to control task demands and to optimize capacity allocation by implementing strategies that are based upon the utilization of skills already available to an individual through past experiences. In a simulation task involving planning the daily appointments of a travelling store supervisor, Schönpflug and Battmann (1982) found that planning does aid task performance and reduces the psychophysiological effort involved in performance. However, the data also showed that, although planning is an investment for future efficiency of behaviour, it has associated with it immediate costs. If the costs of planning are too expensive, either because the individual has insufficient abilities or resources to justify the plan, or because the plan proves to be non-effective, then the investment in planning may be counter-productive. If control is achieved, however, then planning is both efficient and stress-reducing.

The cognitive problem-solving approach is not incompatible with a more general biological model of the type that I am proposing and which is based upon adaptation as its guiding principle. Adaptation may be viewed as successful solution of task demands presented to an organism by its interaction with its environment or as the resolution of behavioural uncertainty. Control is indicated by the observation that an organism's behaviour comprises prepared responses executed to meet a specific set of task demands. Human subjects may be able, in some situations, although not all, to indicate their prepared responses, i.e. their plans, in advance. However, the existence of plans may also be inferred from the regularities of observed goal-directed behaviours of animals, including humans. In these terms, control may be equated with neural realization of an effective plan for behaviour by the elimination of behavioural uncertainty. Once realized, that neural entity will be recalled whenever the task demands or stimulus conditions are appropriate, i.e. descriminable, and response *allocation* will be effortless. The various classifications of control shown in Table 1 all view control as something that is imposed upon a situation by an individual. The interpretation that I have outlined views control as a consequence of responding within a situation. Control cannot exist independently of the behaviours that define it. Its presence or absence may be indicated by the pattern of psychophysiological responses that accompany coping behaviours and in particular by the integration of autonomic and somatic components of a response.

REFERENCES

Abbott, B. A., and Badia, P. (1986). Predictable versus unpredictable shock conditions and physiological measures of stress: A reply to Arthur. *Psychological Bulletin*, **100**, 384–387.

Abbott, B. A., Schoen, L. S., and Badia, P. (1984). Predictable and unpredictable shock: Behavioral measures of aversion and physiological measures of stress. *Psychological Bulletin*, **96**, 45–71.

Arthur, A. Z. (1986). Stress of predictable and unpredictable shock. *Psychological Bulletin*, **100**, 379–383.

Averill, J. R. (1973). Personal control of aversive stimulation and its relationship to stress. *Psychological Bulletin*, **80**, 286–303.

Averill, J. R., and Rosenn, M. (1972). Vigilant and nonvigilant coping strategies and psychophysiological stress reactions during the anticipation of electric shock. *Journal of Personality and Social Psychology*, **23**, 128–141.

Averill, J. R., O'Brien, L., and Dewitt, G. W. (1977). The influence of response effectiveness on the preference for warning and on psychophysiological stress reactions. *Journal of Personality*, **45**, 395–418.

Badia, P., Culbertson, S., and Harsh, J. (1973). Choice of longer or stronger signalled shock over shorter or weaker unsignalled shock. *Journal of the Experimental Analysis of Behavior*, **19**, 25–33.

Badia, P., Harsh, J., and Abbott, B. A. (1979). Choosing between predictable and unpredictable shock conditions: Data and theory. *Psychological Bulletin*, **86**, 1107–1131.

Blix, A. S., Stromme, S. B., and Ursin, H. (1974). Additional heart rate: An indication of psychological activation. *Journal of Applied Physiology*, **53**, 1583–1589.

Brener, J. (1986). Behavioural efficiency: A biological link between informational and energetic processes. In: G. J. R. Hockey, A. W. K. Gaillard and M. G. H. Coles (eds), *Energetics and Human Information Processing*. Dordrecht: Martinus Nijhoff.

Brener, J. (1987). Behavioral energetics: Some effects of uncertainty on the mobilisation and distribution of energy. *Psychophysiology*, **24**, 499–512.

Brener, J., Phillips, K. C., and Connally, S. (1977). Oxygen consumption and ambulation during operant conditioning of heart rate increases and decreases in rates. *Psychophysiology*, **14**, 483–491.

Brener, J., Phillips, K. C., and Connally, S. (1980). Energy expenditure, heart rate, and ambulation during shock avoidance conditioning of heart rate increases and ambulation in freely-moving rats. *Psychophysiology*, **17**, 64–74.

Carroll, D., Turner, J. R., and Hellawell, J. C. (1986a). Heart rate and oxygen consumption during active psychological challenge: The effects of level of difficulty. *Psychophysiology*, **23**, 174–181.

Carroll, D., Turner, J. R., and Prasad, R. (1986b). The effects of level of difficulty of mental arithmetic challenge on heart rate and oxygen consumption. *International Journal of Psychophysiology*, **4**, 167–173.

Elliott, R. (1966). Effects of uncertainty about the nature and advent of a noxious stimulus (shock) upon heart rate. *Journal of Personality and Social Psychology*, **3**, 353–356.

Evans, P. D., Phillips, K. C., and Fearn, J. (1984). On choosing to make aversive events predictable or unpredictable: Some behavioural and psychophysiological findings. *British Journal of Psychology*, **75**, 377–391.

Fisher, S. (1986). *Stress and Strategy*. London: Lawrence Erlbaum.

Germana, J. (1972). Response uncertainty and autonomic–behavioral integration. *Annals of the New York Academy of Sciences*, **193**, 185–188.

Jacob, R. G., and Chesney, M. A. (1986). Psychological and behavioral methods to reduce cardiovascular reactivity. In: K. A. Matthews, S. M. Weiss, T. Detre, T. Dembroski, B. Falker *et al.* (eds), *Stress, Reactivity and Cardiovascular Disease: Status and Prospects*. New York: Wiley.

Karasek, R., Baker, D., Marxer, F., Ahlbom, A., and Theorell, T. (1981). Job decision latitude, job demands and cardiovascular disease: A prospective study of Swedish men. *American Journal of Public Health*, **71**, 694–705.

Krantz, D. S., and Manuck, S. B. (1984). Acute psychophysiologic reactivity and risk of cardiovascular disease: a review and methodologic critique. *Psychological Bulletin*, **96**, 435–464.

Light, K. C., and Obrist, P. A. (1980). Cardiovascular response to stress: Effects of opportunity to avoid, shock experience and performance feedback. *Psychophysiology*, **17**, 243–252.

Light, K. C., and Obrist, P. A. (1983). Task difficulty, heart rate reactivity and cardiovascular response to an appetitive reaction time task. *Psychophysiology*, **20**, 301–312.

Manuck, S. B., Harvey, A. E., Lechleiter, S. L., and Neal, K. S. (1978). Effects of coping on blood pressure responses to threat of aversive stimulation. *Psychophysiology*, **15**, 544–549.

Miller, S. M. (1979a). Controllability and human stress: Method, evidence and theory. *Behaviour Research and Therapy*, **17**, 287–304.

Miller, S. M. (1979b). Coping with impending stress: Psychological and cognitive correlates of choice. *Psychophysiology*, **16**, 572–581.

Obrist, P. A. (1981). *Cardiovascular Psychophysiology: A Perspective*. New York: Plenum.

Obrist, P. A., Gaebelein, C. J., Teller, E. S., Langer, A .W., Grignololo, A., Light, K. C., and McCubbin, J. A. (1978). The relationship among heart rate, carotid dp/dt and blood pressure in humans as a function of the type of stress. *Psychophysiology*, **15**, 102–115.

Obrist, P. A., Light, K. C., James, S. A., and Strogatz, D. S. (1987). Cardiovascular responses to stress. I. Measures of myocardial response and relationship to high resting systolic pressure and parental hypertension. *Psychophysiology*, **24**, 65–78.

Patterson, R. J., and Neufeld, R. W. J. (1987). Clear danger: Situational determinants of the appraisal of threat. *Psychological Bulletin*, **101**, 404–416.

Phillips, K. C. (1986). *Facing threats: Uncertainty and its consequences*. Paper presented at Commission of the European Communities Medical and Public Health Research Programme: Meeting upon Personal Control and Health. University of Limburg, Netherlands, November, 1986.

Phillips, K. C., Evans, P. D., and Fearn, J. M. (1985). Heart rate and skin conductance correlates of monitoring or distraction as strategies for 'coping'. In: D. Papakostopoulos, S. Butler and I. Martin (eds), *Clinical and Experimental Neuropsychophysiology*. London: Croom Helm.

Phillips, K. C., Evans, P. D., Moran, P., and Price, J. (1986). *Psychophysiological consequences of vigilant coping style*. Paper presented at the Annual Conference of the British Psychological Society, Sheffield 1986. Abstract in *Bulletin of the British Psychological Society*, **39**, A84.

Rose, R. J., and Chesney, M. A. (1986). Cardiovascular stress reactivity: A behavior-genetic perspective. *Behavior Therapy*, **17**, 314–323.

Schönpflug, W. (1983). Coping efficiency and situational demands. In: G. J. R. Hockey (ed.), *Stress and Fatigue in Human Performance*. New York: Wiley.

Schönpflug, W., and Battmann, W. (1982). *Psychologische Effekte bei Langzeiteinwirkung uon Verkehrslarm*. Berlin: Umweltbundeamt Bericht 82-10501304.

Seligman, M. E. P. (1975). *Helplessness: On Depression, Development and Death*. San Francisco: Freeman.

Seligman, M. E. P., Maier, S. D., and Solomon, R. L. (1971). Unpredictable and uncontrollable aversive events. In: F. R. Brush (ed.), *Aversive Conditioning and Learning*. New York: Academic Press.

Sherwood, A., Brener, J., and Moncur, D. (1983). Information and states of motor readiness: Their effects on the covariation of heart rate and energy expenditure. *Psychophysiology*, **20**, 513–529.

Sherwood, A., Allen, M. T., Obrist, P. A., and Langer, A. W. (1986). Evaluation of beta-adrenergic influences on cardiovascular and metabolic adjustments to physical and psychological stress. *Psychophysiology*, **23**, 89–104.

Sosnowski, T. (1983). Sources of uncertainty and psychophysiological state changes under conditions of noxious stimulus anticipation. *Biological Psychology*, **17**, 297–309.

Steptoe, A. (1983). Stress, helplessness and control: The implications of laboratory studies. *Journal of Psychosomatic Research*, **27**, 361–367.

Steptoe, A. (1985). Theoretical bases for task selection in cardiovascular psychophysiology. In: A. Steptoe, H. Rüddel and H. Neus (eds), *Clinical and Methodological Issues in Cardiovascular Psychophysiology*. Berlin: Springer-Verlag.

Steptoe, A., Melville, D., and Ross, A. (1984). Behavioral response demands, cardiovascular reactivity, and essential hypertension. *Psychosomatic Medicine*, **46**, 33–47.

Syme, L. S. (1985). Socioeconomic factors: Content discussion. In: A. M. Ostfeld and E. D. Eaker (eds), *Measuring Psychosocial Variables in Epidemiologic Studies of Cardiovascular Disease. Proceedings of a Workshop*. US Department of Health and Human Services: NIH Publication No. 85-2270.

Thompson, S. C. (1981). Will it hurt less if I can control it? A complex answer to a simple question. *Psychological Bulletin*, **90**, 89–101.

Weiss, J. M. (1970). Somatic effects of predictable and unpredictable shock. *Psychosomatic Medicine*, **32**, 397–408.

Weiss, J. M. (1971). Effects of coping behaviour in different warning signal conditions on stress pathology in rats. *Journal of Comparative and Physiological Psychology*, **77**, 1–13.

CHAPTER 12

The role of controllability in cardiovascular activation and cardiovascular disease: help or hindrance?

ARNE ÖHMAN AND GUNILLA BOHLIN
Department of Clinical Psychology, University of Uppsala, Sweden

INTRODUCTION

Striving for control provides an essential ingredient in human existence. Making the environment controllable by our own actions provides a necessary condition for freedom of choice. Yet such control can never be perfect. Although humankind through its cultural evolution has achieved an impressive mastery of its environment, nature remains capricious and may suddenly take back the control it has yielded. Furthermore, in the social domain, where striving for control essentially becomes equivalent to striving for dominance, humans have to accept many contexts where the control they can exert is quite modest. In particular, they are part of a production system and a working life which limits the freedom that is afforded to individuals.

Work environment and cardiovascular disease

The effects on individuals of a work environment lacking in controllability were graphically illustrated in a recent study by Ragland *et al.* (1987). They examined the prevalence of hypertension among San Francisco bus drivers, and reported that more than three-quarters of those over 50 years and all of those over 60 years either took antihypertension medication or had pressures above 140/90 mmHg.

Stress, Personal Control and Health. Edited by A. Steptoe and A. Appels.
Published by John Wiley & Sons Ltd.
© ECSC–EEC–EAEC, Brussels–Luxembourg, 1989

This contrasts markedly to the approximately 50% prevalence that was reported before employment or in random population samples of the same ages. The elevated rate of hypertension was attributed to characteristics of the work environment which may be summarized as lack of control. Thus, driving a bus (or a cable car) in metropolitan areas involves performing a complex task with high social responsibility in a context of time pressure and unpredictable interferences from other traffic. This finding illustrates a general principle brought home by Alfredsson *et al.* (1982) in an analysis of the male Swedish work force. They reported elevated rates of myocardial infarctions in occupations such as cooks, truck drivers, assembly-line workers or head waiters, whose working situations can be described in terms of a combination of rushed tempo and low decision latitudes, i.e. as low in controllability. Theorell *et al.* (1985) brought the analysis a significant step further in a more detailed psychophysiological study. They compared self-recorded blood pressures taken at work and at home in subjects selected for high, medium and low pressures ten years earlier when they, as 18-year-olds, took a medical examination before entering military service. The subjects were further subdivided according to whether they now had high- or low-control occupations. The results showed that the group which was hypertensive at age 18 tended to remain high in systolic blood pressure (SBP), that it showed a larger difference than the other groups between SBP at work and SBP at home and, most importantly, that this latter effect was significantly greater among those with a low-control (or high-strain) occupation. Thus, as predicted by influential theories (e.g. Folkow, 1987), hypertension appeared to be the interactive result of an individual predisposition (as revealed by early pressure elevations) and psychosocial stress factors such as work environments affording little control over important events.

The importance of controllability to cardiovascular disease was incorporated into an interesting model of work environment and cardiovascular disease by Karasek *et al.* (1982), described in more detail elsewhere in this volume. They argued that work environments can be ordered along two independent dimensions: one ranging from low to high frequency of stressors and the other from low to high potential control of these stressors. Psychophysiological strain was then defined as low when the stressors were few and controllable and as high when they were frequent and hard or impossible to control.

Controllability, ill health and cardiovascular reactivity

The considerations presented above suggest a consensus that cardiovascular disease provides just another example of the generally documented relationship between lack of control and illness (see reviews by Anisman and Zacharko, 1982; Garber and Seligman, 1980; Rodin, 1980; Sklar and Anisman, 1981; Weiss, 1977). Such a consensus, however, dissipates when results from laboratory studies of cardiovascular reactivity are entered into the equation. As pointed out by

Steptoe (1983), such studies appear to support the opposite contention, namely that control, and particularly control that requires effort to exert, is associated with cardiovascular reaction patterns which may predispose to hypertension and coronary heart disease (see Krantz and Manuck, 1984). Thus, studies of haemodynamics in early (or borderline) hypertension show that the elevated pressure in most patients is related primarily to increased cardiac output with unchanged peripheral resistance. Similarly β-adrenergically mediated increases in heart rate, contractility and systolic blood pressure can be seen in young normotensives engaged in laboratory tasks that can only be mastered with effort (Light, 1987; Obrist, 1981). Although fraught with potential difficulties (e.g. Weder and Julius, 1985), it seems a small step to take to suggest that such reactions, if repeated and sustained, may form the beginning of a path leading to hypertension.

The present chapter is an attempt to reconcile the seemingly opposite suppositions of the role of controllability in hypertension, which flow from epidemiological–naturalistic studies on the one hand, and laboratory studies of cardiovascular reactivity on the other. To achieve this, we performed a conceptual analysis of control and associated constructs, and then we proceeded to examine primarily the literature on laboratory studies in people with normal blood pressure in order to pinpoint the effects of controllability on cardiovascular responses. After briefly considering laboratory studies of hypertensives, we conclude the chapter with an interpretative discussion where we argue that the seeming contradiction between the two sources of data is more apparent than real. If carefully considered, it appears that controllability has the same kind of attenuating effects on cardiovascular reactions that have been documented for other types of stress response.

CONCEPTUAL ASPECTS OF CONTROLLABILITY

Objective controllability

Controllability pertains to a particular type of relation between organism and environment. More specifically, it refers to a contingency between the organism's behaviour and potentially significant environmental events such as reinforcing stimuli or, more loosely, 'stressors'. An event is uncontrollable by a particular behaviour when its occurrence is no more likely in the presence than in the absence of this behaviour (see Seligman, 1975; Seligman *et al.*, 1971). If the likelihood of an event is modified either by the emitting or withholding of a response, then the event is controllable by this response. If a stressor cannot be controlled by any response in the organism's repertoire, then the organism is helpless with regard to that stressor (Seligman, 1975).

While controllability is defined by a relation between environment and behaviour, a related construct, *predictability*, is defined solely in terms of relations between environmental events. Thus, an event is predictable from another event when the likelihood of its occurrence is related to the presence or the absence of another event (Seligman *et al.*, 1971). Predictability should not be confused with controllability. Predictability affords a weak kind of control in the sense that it allows the organism to know when something is going to happen. Some authors actually include cognitive control as one type of control of a stressor, which then includes predictability as an essential component (Averill, 1973). However, like Steptoe (1983) we wish to reserve the term 'control' for instances of 'behavioural control'.

Events may be completely predictable yet impossible to affect by behavioural means. Thus, predictability and controllability are independent constructs, although they may be partly overlapping. For example, predictability may facilitate controllability by providing crucial information for the timing of coping responses.

Objective control as here defined typically refers to control of the occurrence or duration of stressors such as aversive stimuli. However, control may also pertain not directly to such stressors but to some associated parameter of the situation. For example, DeGood (1975; see also Hokanson *et al.*, 1971) gave his subjects control over time-out periods from aversive stimulation so that they could decide when to rest. Similarly, Bohlin *et al.* (1986a,b) examined the effects of personal control of work-pace in a problem-solving task.

Subjective controllability

Even if a situation can be objectively defined as uncontrollable, one cannot unequivocally infer that it will be so perceived by experimental participants. Indeed, humans seem to be inherently optimistic in the sense that they tend to judge events as somewhat controllable even if they are objectively uncontrollable (Alloy and Abramson, 1979). Similarly, people seem to perceive illusory correlations between events bearing no predictive relationship to each other. For example, college students exposed to series of slides and electric shock judged shock as occurring more often after slides depicting potentially phobic objects such as snakes and spiders than after neutral pictures (Mineka and Tomarken, 1989). Alloy and Tabachnik (1984) developed a theoretical framework to account for judgements of event covariation in humans and animals in terms of two interacting factors: (a) prior expectations of covariation; and (b) current situational information about covariation. The important point for the present context is that objective controllability is not necessarily isomorphic with subjective judgements of controllability.

Generalized expectations of controllability

If expectations of controllability/uncontrollability become generalized over many situational contexts they can be described as beliefs about controllability. Essentially such beliefs constitute prior expectancies of covariation between events. Some persons may believe that the world is structured to be controllable, that control is just a question of effort and skill. Other persons, on the other hand, may believe that the world is basically uncontrollable, that humans are victims of merciless external circumstances or blind fate. The former are said to have an internal locus of control, and the latter may be said to have an external locus of control (see Rotter, 1966; Lefcourt, 1976). This dimension of individual differences has been found to be relevant in very diverse psychological contexts (see Lefcourt, 1976). However, even though persons may have extremely external loci of control, they cannot automatically be taken to perceive events as uncontrollable in a particlar context. As pointed out by Alloy and Tabachnik (1984), such judgements are jointly determined by beliefs and the actual situation. If the situational information of controllability is salient enough, it may override the generalized belief.

Outcome and efficacy expectations

Persons may correctly perceive that events are controllable, yet completely disregard the implications of this perception because they judge the relevant coping response as lacking from their behavioural repertoire. In response to this problem Bandura (1977) introduced a distinction between outcome expectancy and efficacy expectancy. The former refers to a perception of a relationship between response and outcome (e.g. avoidance of an aversive event), and the latter to whether the person is able to perform the relevant response or not.

When the importance of efficacy expectations is recognized, task difficulty is inevitably introduced as a potentially troublesome confounding variable in many controllability contexts. Even though tasks may be objectively possible to solve, they may be so difficult under the particular task parameters that they essentially become, or are perceived as, impossible. Because of this state of affairs, the rewards in the situation become unavailable to the person. However, an impossibly difficult task does not automatically fulfil the definition of being uncontrollable. This is because it is required for an uncontrollable event that it is completely uncorrelated with particular coping responses. In an impossible task, however, there is a correlation between coping responses (attempts to solve the task) and failure. Thus, formally, the situation is rather one of punishment than of uncontrollability. At least for free operant situations where the subjects freely initiate their responses, they are able to minimize punishment (i.e. failure) in an impossible task merely by refraining from trying. For example, if subjects are required to solve as many problems as possible within a defined time period and are punished for errors, they can reduce punishment by giving up the task. In an uncontrollable situation, on the other hand, aversive stimuli are presented even in the absence of coping responses. This may occur in an avoidance task where successful coping responses salvage the subject from aversive stimulation. If the coping response becomes exceedingly difficult, such a situation is turned into an uncontrollable one, because the subjects now are punished regardless of what they are doing. Depending on the way that task difficulty is manipulated, therefore, impossible tasks may or may not fulfil criteria of uncontrollability.

Thus, although task difficulty and uncontrollability are obviously related in many situations, it is important that their distinctiveness is not blurred. As task difficulty increases to very hard or impossible, uncontrollability may or may not be introduced. At any level of task difficulty, the control afforded to the subject may differ depending on several task parameters, such as control over work-pace or the spacing of resting periods. Thus, controllability may well have effects beyond those of difficulty. In fact, it becomes a theoretical priority to sort out which effects can be attributed to difficulty and which to controllability.

Conclusion

The present discussion has highlighted the complexities encountered with the concept of controllability. It is easy enough to define the concept in terms of objective contingencies between behavioural responses and potentially stress-producing environmental events. Such objectively observable contingencies immediately produce a sequence of psychological events, including perception of the contingency, activation of beliefs about controllability, and efficacy expectations, which in concert influence the outcome of the person–situation interaction. The ubiquity of the psychological side has prompted some authors to favour subjective definitions of controllability in terms of perceived contingency (e.g. Thompson, 1981). In particular, it is often complicated to separate the effects of controllability from difficulty of the particular experimental task. However, depending on the purpose of the particular analysis, one needs to take account of these psychological complexities to a greater or lesser extent. While it is imperative and important to be cognizant of potentially confounding psychological processes, it nonetheless has important practical advantages to be able to stick to an objective definition of control. This is particularly true if part of the focus is on work environments, because if one loses sight of the objective contingencies in this context then one's position with regard to suggestions about potential reforms is seriously undermined. Given the conceptual complexities and our present aim to discuss effects of response–outcome contingencies in terms of physiological responses, it is necessary to rely on laboratory studies in order to clarify the effects of controllability on any given dependent variable. Of course, the theoretical statements, which provide the goal of the activity, eventually must incorporate the various psychological processes enumerated in the discussion above as they apply to work environments. In our view, however, it is clearly preferable to have these psychological processes anchored, not only at the dependent variable side, but also in terms of objectively manipulable independent variables. If this prerequisite can be met, then much is gained in terms of theoretical specificity and precision.

CONTROLLABILTY AND CARDIOVASCULAR ACTIVATION

Control over aversive stimulation

Early studies by DeGood and co-workers (DeGood, 1975; Hokanson *et al.*, 1971) seemed to indicate that lack of control was associated with elevation of systolic blood pressure (SBP) during an aversively motivated task, where controlling subjects were able freely to request rest periods, while rest periods were imposed by the experimenter for those without control. However, the majority of studies show opposite effects.

Light and Obrist (1980) examined cardiovascular responses in subjects performing auditory reaction times (RTs) to avoid aversive electric shock stimuli. They were specifically instructed 'to try to respond faster each trial, and that each time they did not react quickly enough, there was a chance that they would receive a shock' (p. 245). No-avoidance (or uncontrolling) subjects were yoked to avoidance subjects so that they received shock after the same trials as their yoking partner. They, too, were instructed to react faster and faster each time, but the instruction did not indicate any relationship between RT and shocks. Light and Obrist (1980), therefore, used an objective definition of controllability, and attempted to induce similar levels of RT performance in their two main groups. According to their results, this attempt was successful. Thus, the groups did not differ in RT, and according to self-reports subjects in both groups tried equally hard to improve their RT. However, practically all avoiding subjects attributed these efforts to their wish to avoid the shock, whereas only a quarter of the no-avoidance subjects attributed their efforts to the shock. The cardiovascular data demonstrated elevated heart rate (HR), SBP and pulse transit time (PTT) (time between R-wave of the electrocardiogram to peak pulse amplitude at the earlobe) in avoiding as compared to non-avoiding subjects. These data, therefore, support the notion that active control of an aversive stimulus is associated with increased cardiovascular activation, the pattern of which suggests β-adrenergic effects on the myocardium as the mediating factor (see also Obrist *et al.*, 1978).

Similar conclusions were reached by Contrada *et al.* (1982). They used a more complex visual choice RT task involving several stimulus–response relationships. Contingency subjects were led to believe (non-veridically) that they could detect a pattern in the complex sequence of stimulation that would allow improved performance. They could actually avoid some aversive stimuli (white noise or electric shock) by good performance and they were given feedback as to number of successful avoidance trials. Non-contingency subjects, on the other hand, were not instructed about any patterns in the sequence, and they were explicitly told that the relation between RT and noise/shock was random, which, for them, it actually was. Contingency subjects showed faster RTs, and improved their performance over time in comparison to the non-contingency subjects. They also showed reliably larger increases in SBP and diastolic blood pressure (DBP) from pre-experimental baselines. Both these measures were maximal at the beginning of the task and then declined. Such a decline was apparent also for HR, but for this measure there was no difference between contingency and non-contingency groups. Plasma adrenaline, but not noradrenaline, increased more from pre-experimental baseline levels in contingency than in non-contingency subjects. Thus, this study again demonstrated elevated cardiovascular levels in a situation involving controllable aversive stimuli. However, in contrast to the results reported by Obrist's group (Obrist, 1981; Obrist *et al.*, 1978), the physiological implications of these data are less clear as significant effects were observed for DBP but not for HR.

Smith *et al.* (1985) used a memory task and compared subjects instructed about controllable, uncontrollable or no-shock threat. Controllable shocks ostensibly related to performance failures whereas uncontrollable shocks were explained as random. In reality, no shocks were given. Subjects threatened with controllable shocks reported significantly greater sense of efficacy in avoiding shocks than did subjects in the uncontrollable condition. They also showed higher SBP than subjects in the uncontrollable situation, which, in turn, were above no-shock subjects. For HR, the controllability group was above the two others, whereas, for finger pulse volume responses, shock threat was uniquely associated with increased responsivity regardless of control.

In an ambitious study, Lovallo *et al.* (1985) examined a range of cardiovascular and neuroendocrine measures in subjects who either strived to control, or were passively exposed to, aversive stimuli (noises and shocks). Both conditions involved the same stimulus sequence, which was composed of light stimuli, half of which were followed by aversive stimuli. In the active condition the subjects were instructed to try to avoid aversive stimuli by pressing a telegraph key as fast as possible when the light appeared and were led to believe that fast RTs removed the punishing stimulus. They were told that slow responses might or might not get shocked. In the passive condition, the subjects were simply told that there was nothing they could do but to sit quietly and watch the lights. Thus, controllability was confounded with motor involvement. The order of the two task conditions was counterbalanced across subjects with a 20-minute rest period in between. As compared with passive exposure, the alleged avoidance task produced reports of greater control, sense of effort, tenseness, concentration and interest, and, in addition, this task was rated as more stimulating. Significant increases in cortisol, free fatty acids and noradrenaline were reported for both conditions, with no difference between conditions. Adrenaline did not change from baseline values. Corroborating the subjective reports of effort, the active task produced a regularly increasing gradient of muscle tension associated with task involvement (Malmo, 1965; Svebak, 1982), which clearly contrasted with the lack of a gradient in the passive condition. The active task produced higher HR, SBP and DBP as well as clear evidence of inotropic effects on the myocardium, for example shorter pre-ejection times and larger Heather contractility index (as derived from impedance cardiography). However, there were no task effects on stroke volume and total peripheral resistance. Some aspects of the results suggest that the cardiovascular findings were attributable to increased effort during the active task. For example, there was a significant inverse correlation between RTs, on the one hand, and subjective effort and muscle tension on the other. Muscle tension also was significantly associated with feelings of effort, concentration, tension and control. As already noted, both muscle tension and reported effort, concentration, control and tension were larger in the active group showing enhanced cardiovascular activation. However, differential motor involvement in the two conditions cannot be excluded as a contributing factor to the clear differences between the two groups.

In an attempt to resolve the discrepancy between DeGood's (1975) data and those of Obrist's (1976; 1981) group, Manuck *et al.* (1978) orthogonally manipulated perceived control of an aversive stimulus, and level of difficulty of a concept formation task in a factorial 2 × 2 design. Subjects' reports verified that all subjects judged the aversive 'tone shock' as equally probable (although none was received), that difficult problems were perceived as more difficult, and that subjects instructed about a contingency between good performance and avoidance perceived the task as more controllable. The results showed a clear interaction between the experimental variables in influencing SBP, so that enhanced levels were seen particularly in subjects instructed about control and given the difficult version of the task. For the easy task, there was actually a (nonsignificant) tendency for subjects instructed about control to be below no-control subjects in cardiovascular response. These data demonstrate that the nature of the coping response may be important for the controllability effect to appear. Thus, controllability may lead to enhanced cardiovascular activity only if the coping response is difficult.

The sample of studies reviewed so far seems reasonably consistent in demonstrating an association between increased cardiovascular (and β-adrenergically mediated) activity during attempts to control aversive stimulation. Thus, they support a direct relationship between controllability and evidence of stress on cardiovascular end-points (see Steptoe, 1983). However, with the possible exception of Light and Obrist (1980), the data are not particularly specific in attributing the effects to controllability. This is because effort is likely to be the crucial mediating factor, and effort is influenced by a host of other variables than control in several of the experiments. As documented particularly by Lovallo *et al.* (1985), there is a very clear relationship between various indices of effort and cardiovascular effects in an active avoidance task. If effort is the crucial variable, then similar results could be expected from different types of experimental settings where control is less clearly involved than in the present set of studies, which all involved active actual or perceived control of aversive stimulation. Below, therefore, we review a collection of studies examining effects of task difficulty on cardiovascular variables in different task settings.

Effects of task difficulty

As outlined above, there is a complex relation between task difficulty and controllability. Here, we will review a series of studies manipulating task difficulty to examine effects on cardiovascular responses. In each instance we shall note whether lack of control becomes an issue at extreme levels of task difficulty. However, the primary purpose is to examine whether increased task difficulty produces β-adrenergically mediated cardiovascular changes similar to those seen in situations of partial control over aversive stimuli, as would be expected from the effort interpretation given to such effects in the previous section.

In passing, it might be noted that task difficulty by itself is a complex variable, prone to introduce interpretational hazards. For example, manipulations of task difficulty often result in variations in motor output. Because of the cardiac–somatic coupling (Obrist, 1981), such variations may produce cardiac changes clouding the 'true' effects of task difficulty. Secondly, task difficulty is a multidimensional construct, the manipulation of which may be targeted at perceptual, cognitive or motor components of task performance. It cannot be taken for granted that the same psychophysiological effects will result from requiring faster and/or more accurate responses, as from making perceptual discriminations more difficult or from increasing the cognitive load of the task. Indeed, according to Lacey and Lacey (e.g. 1974), the latter two types of manipulations have dramatically different effects on the cardiovascular system.

Obrist *et al.* (1978) exposed subjects to an unsignalled auditory RT task where difficulty was manipulated by performance criteria to win a bonus and avoid aversive electric shocks. In the easy condition, subjects lost a quarter from a five-dollar bonus and received electric shock if their RT exceeded 400 ms. In the impossible condition, the performance criterion was 200 ms, but shocks were only presented on four trials chosen for slow RTs. The hard condition, finally, involved loss of a quarter each time the RT was slower than that on the previous trials, and instructions that they *might* receive a shock for slow RTs. The number of actual shocks was matched for the hard and impossible groups. This is clearly a complex procedure, and it could be questioned whether the hard condition is located on the same dimension as the two others, because it involved the unique manipulation of requiring faster RTs for each trial. Furthermore, lacking information about perceived controllability, its role in the experiment remains unclear. Nevertheless, similar to the study where controllability was directly manipulated (Light and Obrist, 1980), the results showed more sustained increases over time for HR, SBP, DBP and carotid dP/dt in the hard than in the easy and impossible conditions, which did not differ from each other. A subsequent experiment confirmed the β-adrenergic origin of these effects by documenting their abolition by β-blockade. However, given the impurity of the experimental manipulation, it remains in doubt whether these results demonstrate an inverted U-shaped relationship between task difficulty and cardiovascular activation, or merely that the specific manipulation of difficulty was effective in the hard condition.

Somewhat similar data were reported in a more recent experiment, using an appetitive RT task (Light and Obrist, 1983). Subjects in easy and impossible groups were given lax (370 ms) and extremely stringent (170 ms) RT criteria, respectively, for earning bonuses, whereas subjects in the hard condition were rewarded for improving performance from the previous trial. This manipulation of task difficulty obviously involves objective control, although, again, difficulty was manipulated by a different principle in the hard as compared to the easy and impossible conditions. The impossible condition resulted in less sustained changes in SBP and DBP, and longer pre-ejection periods and PTTs than the hard condition, which, however, did not differ from the easy condition. Thus, a clear difference from the aversively motivated task studied previously was the elevated levels seen in the easy condition.

However, the discrepancy between the data reported by Obrist *et al.* (1978) and Light and Obrist (1983) cannot be unequivocally attributed to the different types of motivation in the two studies, because data are inconsistent even for positively reinforced tasks. For example, van Schijndel *et al.* (1984) and Wright *et al.* (1986) obtained the same type of inverted U-shaped relation between SBP and level of difficulty for anagram solution and memory tasks, respectively, as previously claimed by Obrist *et al.* (1978). Carroll *et al.* (1986), on the other hand, found increases in HR from easy to difficult and practically impossible versions of mental arithmetic and Raven's matrices tasks, but no differences between the two more difficult conditions. Using relations between oxygen consumption and HR obtained from physical exercise, they were able to demonstrate that the HR increase was supplementary or additional to that required from metabolic considerations. Perkins (1984), finally, found weak effects of task difficulty on HR in a choice RT task manipulating response cost. Only with high response cost was there a tendency to lower HR with increased failure feedback. The effect of response cost was quite clear, however, with larger HR elevations when the loss involved money (high response cost) rather than points (low response cost).

Response cost may be related to a potentially critical variable in the context —that of goal valence (see Wright *et al.*, 1986). Light and Obrist (1983) discussed their failure to obtain differences between easy and hard versions of the appetitive RT task in terms of the larger attractiveness of earning money as compared to avoiding shock (see Obrist *et al.*, 1978), and the associated increases in effort occasioned by more attractive rewards. Wright *et al.* (1986) actually collected ratings of goal valence, and found the highest goal ratings in the hard condition which produced the largest SBP change. Thus, goal valence may be maximal in moderately difficult and hence challenging situations. This may promote maximal expenditure of effort to reach the goal, which, in turn, may activate cardiovascular responses. Thus, effort may be the psychological factor mediating both the effects of controllability and difficulty on the cardiovascular system.

Control under constant difficulty

The data reviewed so far quite unambiguously imply that subjects exerting effort to perform well either striving to control aversive stimuli or to master hard tasks show a patterned cardiovascular change related to β-adrenergic activation. However, there are very little data allowing conclusions as to how control affects cardiovascular responses at a given level of task difficulty. It could well be, for example, that subjects actively coping with a stressor would show less cardiovascular activation at a given level of task demand if their sense of control was high rather than low. To examine such possibilities it is necessary to design a task where subjects can be compared under conditions of high or low personal control, but where task demands would be constant across controllability conditions.

Such a task was devised by Bohlin *et al.* (1986a). They exposed subjects to a complex mental arithmetic task presented on slides. In the externally paced condition the duration of the slide, and thus the time available for solving the arithmetic problem, was controlled by the experimenter. In the self-paced condition, the subject advanced the slide tray himself by pressing a button. During external pacing, slide duration was changed over blocks from 15 to 10, 7, and 4 seconds. For one group of subjects these durations were constant within a block, whereas for another group it varied around these means within blocks. The subjects performed one series of externally paced and another of self-paced blocks in counterbalanced order. In this way, comparison between the two pacing conditions could be made for blocks having identical numbers of attempted problems, and thus being equivalent in terms of performance efforts. Subjects reported significantly more stress and irritation during external as opposed to self-pacing, and the quality of their performance became poorer as shown by more errors. However, the difference between conditions was less general in physiological measures. Only for DBP was there reliable evidence of a difference between the two pacing conditions, the externally paced task producing larger increases than the self-paced one. These data, then, demonstrate that lack of control of an important task parameter produces more subjective stress, poorer performance quality, and some evidence of enhanced cardiovascular activity. It would appear, therefore, that controllability under some circumstances can have stress-reducing effects on cardiovascular parameters that may counter the profound effort-mediated changes occasioned by active coping with stressors.

CONTROLLABILITY IN HYPERTENSION

Steptoe (1983) suggested that 'the deleterious consequences of lack of control (and helplessness) have been overstated; there may be psychophysiological reactions that are exacerbated rather than alleviated by behavioral control' (p. 362). He then went on to invoke the work of Obrist and Light reviewed above to argue that only during conditions of active coping would hypertensives be likely to differ from controls in cardiovascular reactivity. This theoretical argument was supported by data subsequently reported in detail by Steptoe *et al.* (1984). They selected mild hypertensives from screening of industrial employees and exposed them to three laboratory conditions: a Stroop colour–word interference task, a movie sequence illustrating anxiety, and a video game. The results indicated clear differences between mild hypertensive and controls in SBP and DBP reactivity both in terms of absolute and percentage change from baseline, but only during the two active tasks. While passively watching the movie, the subjects showed generally small responses that did not differ between groups. Although findings such as these are by no means universal (see, for example, Eliasson *et al.*, 1983), they are nevertheless supported by the statistical consensus of the literature. Thus, in a meta-analysis of the literature, Fredrikson and Matthews (in press) reported that, according to combined statistics, established hypertensives showed clearly enhanced SBP and DBP reactivity compared to controls for all types of laboratory tasks, whereas borderline hypertensives and normotensives with a family history of hypertension only showed elevated reactivity during active tasks. Similarly to the literature on normals, therefore, the data from studies of hypertensives appear to demonstrate that tasks forcing subjects to strive to perform well may be particularly effective in inducing strong cardiovascular responses, and particularly so for individuals with borderline, or at family risk for, hypertension.

However, these data do not demonstrate that it is control that exacerbates reactivity. Rather, imperfect or difficult control may be one of several manipulations that induces active, effortful coping attempts from the subjects, which then results in augmented cardiovascular responses. Thus, similar to the argument advanced above for normals, at a given level of task demand, control may still be beneficial in reducing cardiovascular response.

This possibility was directly examined by Bohlin *et al.* (1986b). They recruited borderline hypertensives and controls and exposed them to the task developed by

Bohlin *et al.* (1986a), where subjects solved arithmetic problems presented on slides. Half of the hypertensives and half of the controls had the task externally paced by the experimenter, with successively less and less time available to solve the problems across trial blocks. The remaining subjects paced the task themselves by advancing the slide tray when each problem was solved, but with instructions to work as fast as possible. Thus, again it was possible to find a work-pace where the externally paced and the self-paced groups worked at the same rate, thus keeping work-pace constant while allowing the effect of control to be determined. The results showed that control interacted with hypertensive versus normal status particularly for SBP (see Table 1). The table shows that the borderline hypertensives clearly surpassed the normotensives in the self-paced condition, but that the normotensives actually tended to show larger changes during externally paced work. Put in somewhat different terms, the borderline hypertensives did not differentiate the two conditions of control, whereas normotensives were able to attenuate their SBP responses when they had control over the work-pace. Thus, for normotensives, control had the attenuating effect on blood pressure that was reported in the previous study on normals (Bohlin *et al.* 1986a), although it was more clear for SBP this time and for DBP in the previous study.

The results reported for borderline hypertensives by Bohlin *et al.* (1986b) suggest that this group of subjects may benefit less from the stress-alleviating effects of control. Conceptually similar findings were reported for students with a family history of hypertension by Ditto (1986). His subjects went through two identical laboratory sessions spaced about one week apart, and including mental arithmetic, Stroop colour–word interference and isometric hand-grip as tasks. In the first session there were no differences between subjects with and without family history of hypertension. However, whereas the subjects without family history showed overall habituation of blood pressure reactivity from the first to the second session, subjects with a family history maintained the elevated SBP reactions to the psychologically active tasks during the second session. Consequently, for active tasks, their SBP reactivity was significantly above that of

TABLE 1. Systolic blood pressure (mmHg and % change from rest) in normotensives (NT) and borderline hypertensives (BHT) at rest and during self-paced and externally paced work (data from Bohlin *et al.*, 1986b)

Group	Self-paced			Externally paced		
	Rest	Task	% Change	Rest	Task	% Change
NT	108.2	115.1	6.3	108.8	127.3	17.0
BHT	130.0	146.3	12.5	130.6	144.5	10.6
$t(22)$			3.51**			−2.03*

* $p < 0.10$; ** $p < 0.01$.

subjects without family history during the second session. Thus, subjects at risk for hypertension were unable to utilize the stress-reducing effect of familiarity with the laboratory and the task (presumably associated with an increased sense of control) to attenuate their blood pressure responses to stress.

In a way, therefore, Steptoe (1983) may be right in his claim that control of aversive events rather than lack of control is critical in early stages of hypertension. However, control may not be critical because it generally augments cardiovascular reactivity, but because failure to use control to reduce stress may be a factor predisposing some individuals for hypertension. Thus, life events and circumstances requiring effort may induce slightly larger episodes of elevated pressure in individuals prone to develop hypertension, such as those with a family history (see Fredrikson and Matthews, in press). Because such individuals may be less able than normals to use whatever control that is available in the environment to dampen their reactions, their hypertensive episodes not only become more intense but also more frequent and prolonged. Over time this pattern may promote more stable elevated pressures. The ability to use control to alleviate stress responses must require psychological processes such as perception and judgement of controllability, as well as a connection between such processes and physiological reactivity. Whether persons at risk for hypertension differ from normals in such processes remains a moot point at present, but it is one that might well be worth pursuing empirically. Clearly, at the present time the notion advanced here is speculative and in need of further replication and empirical extensions.

CONCLUDING DISCUSSION

In this chapter we have argued that behavioural control is best defined objectively as a contingency between coping responses and reinforcing stimuli. Because such responses may be difficult to perform or may be completely absent from individuals' behavioural repertoires, controllability is closely intertwined with task difficulty. The fact that these two constructs are associated, however, does not imply that they are interchangeable. Although a difficult task in general may involve less potential for control, at a given level of difficulty, control may still make an important difference. From our review of the literature, we think that it is apparent that this distinction has often been neglected. It has generally been observed that difficult tasks engender effortful but imperfectly successful coping attempts, and induce strong cardiovascular responses. Such observations, however, do not legitimize the conclusion that control exacerbates cardiovascular reactivity. As pointed out by Steptoe (1983), 'control *per se* may not be crucial. Rather it is the coping behaviours demanded by different environmental contingencies that determine cardiovascular reactions' (p. 364). Thus, in some contexts, control or rather the potential for control, may be a factor promoting active coping attempts. However, control is neither necessary nor sufficient for effortful coping, which appears to be the most direct mediator of cardiovascular reactions.

Because of the conceptual complexities of the controllability area, laboratory studies allowing environmental control typically are preferable. The precision and control of the laboratory, however, are bought at a considerable cost in terms of threats to the external validity of the findings. Generalizing from laboratory to real life is always a risky business, and some problems are especially hard to cope with when the target of study is the effects of controllability. Ethical concerns dictate that the level of aversive stimulation must be modest, and, typically, that subjects are given the exclusive right to terminate their participation at any time. Thus, subjects always have the final control in the sense that they can simply leave the situation, however uncontrollable that it may appear within its own confines. Given these circumstances, one is sometimes surprised at the quite powerful laboratory findings reported in the literature (see, for example, Breier *et al.*, 1987).

A related shortcoming in the literature we have covered is the very limited time-span covered by most laboratory tasks. Establishing control takes time, particularly if the required response is difficult or the contingency hard to identify. Most studies examine only the initial reaction to the situation, where the novelty and unfamiliarity of the laboratory potentiate the general physiological response as participants strive to come to grips not only with the specific task they are exposed to but also with their general predicament as experimental subjects. If observations had been continued into phases where the necessary skills had been acquired to establish control, and subjects' general apprehension had been diminished, the conclusions might have been quite different. Such general habituation effects were brought home in the between-session effects reported by Ditto (1986), and in the effect of shock familiarity reported by Light and Obrist (1980). Indeed, it is quite obvious from the existing data that prolonging the session is likely to result in virtually a return to baseline of physiological responses. Even in highly stressful laboratory tasks such as Obrist's shock-avoidance procedures (Obrist *et al.*, 1978; Light and Obrist, 1980) or the choice RT used by Contrada *et al.* (1982) there is a very conspicuous decline in reactivity across time, and if these trends are extrapolated they suggest that eventually very little response would have been left.

This is exactly what is to be expected on theoretical grounds. According to Kahneman's (1973) influential theory of attention, effort mobilizes not only physiological responses but also cognitive resources to meet challenging situations. As cognitive schemata are developed to deal with challenges, and necessary action skills are acquired, effort subsides. And if the situation allows a consistent mapping of stimuli on responses (even though the mapping rule may be quite complex), actions may eventually become completely automatized, with no need for cognitive resources (Shiffrin and Schneider, 1977) and, most likely, a complete warning of physiological response. Thus, situations that are so controllable that they can be dealt with at the automatic level are likely to show a minimal cardiovascular or other sympathetically mediated response. However, if the situation precludes automatic routines, for example by inconsistent mapping of stimuli and responses, control necessarily becomes imperfect and effort-demanding. If important incentives are at stake, this situation becomes associated with a heavy investment of cognitive resources and elevation of sympathetic activation. Under such conditions, cardiovascular activity remains high for long periods of time, possibly resulting in lasting neuroendocrine changes and increased wear and tear on the organism. This is probably the situation encountered by the San Francisco bus drivers studied by Ragland *et al.* (1987). If attempts to control fail completely, individuals may give up coping attempts and become helpless, again with associated neuroendocrine changes, albeit different from those associated with striving (see, for example, Henry and Stephens, 1977). From these considerations, it is clear that control interacts with other processes and mechanisms to influence physiological states. Thus, although control by itself may alleviate, for instance, cardiovascular stress responses, the wider situation may be such that the net effect is still elevated cardiovascular reactivity.

Finally, as shown in our review of studies of control in hypertensives, individuals may differ in their capacity to benefit from control. While some individuals may be able to use control for constructive coping, with associated reductions in cardiovascular responses, others may lack the necessary coping ability and thus show an enhanced response even though the situation by itself may be controllable. Such coping failures may result in more frequent and enduring stress episodes, and thus may be a factor predisposing individuals to hypertension and associated syndromes such as coronary heart disease.

ACKNOWLEDGEMENT

Preparation of this chapter was facilitated by grants from the Bank of Sweden Tercentenary Foundation.

REFERENCES

Alfredsson, L., Karasek, R. A., and Theorell, T. (1982). Myocardial infarction risk and psychosocial work environment: An analysis of the male Swedish working force. *Social Science and Medicine*, **16**, 463–467.

Alloy, L. B., and Abramson, L. Y. (1979). Judgment of contingency in depressed and nondepressed students: Sadder but wiser? *Journal of Experimental Psychology: General*, **108**, 441–485.

Alloy, L. B., and Tabachnik, N. (1984). Assessment of covariation by humans and animals: The joint influence of prior expectations and current situation information. *Psychological Review*, **91**, 112–149.

Anisman, H., and Zacharko, R. M. (1982). Depression: The predisposing influence of stress. *Behavioral and Brain Sciences*, **5**, 89–137.

Averill, J. R. (1973). Personal control over aversive stimuli and its relationship to stress. *Psychological Bulletin*, **80**, 286–303.

Bandura, A. (1977). Self-efficacy: Toward a unifying theory of behavioral change. *Psychological Review*, **84**, 191–215.

Bohlin, G., Eliasson, K., Hjemdahl, P., Klein, K., and Frankenhaeuser, M. (1986a). Pace variation and control of work pace as related to cardiovascular, neuroendocrine, and subjective responses. *Biological Psychology*, **23**, 247–263.

Bohlin, G., Eliasson, K., Hjemdahl, P., Klein, K., Fredrikson, M., and Frankenhaeuser, M. (1986b). Personal control over work pace: Circulatory, neuroendocrine and subjective responses in borderline hypertension. *Journal of Hypertension*, **4**, 295–305.

Breier, A., Albus, M., Pickar, D., Zahn, T. P., Wolkowitz, O. M., and Paul, S. M. (1987). Controllable and uncontrollable stress in humans: Alterations in mood and neuro-endocrine and psychophysiological functions. *American Journal of Psychiatry*, **144**, 1419–1425.

Carroll, D., Turner, J. R., and Hellawell, J. C. (1986). Heart rate and oxygen consumption during active psychological challenge: The effects of level of difficulty. *Psychophysiology*, **23**, 174–181.

Contrada, R. J., Glass, D. C., Krakoff, L. R., Krantz, D. S., Kehoe, K., Isecke, W., Collins, C., and Elting, E. (1982). Effects of control over aversive stimulation and Type A behavior on cardiovascular and plasma catecholamine responses. *Psychophysiology*, **19**, 408–419.

DeGood, D. E. (1975). Cognitive control factors in vascular stress responses. *Psychophysiology*, **12**, 399–401.

Ditto, B. (1986). Parental history of essential hypertension, active coping, and cardiovascular reactivity. *Psychophysiology*, **23**, 62–70.

Eliasson, K., Hjemdahl, P., and Kahan, T. (1983). Circulatory and sympatho-adrenal responses to stress in borderline and established hypertension. *Journal of Hypertension*, **1**, 131–139.

Folkow, B. (1987). Psychosocial and central nervous influences in primary hypertension. *Circulation*, **76** (Suppl. I) 10–19.

Fredrikson, M., and Matthews, K. A. (in press). Cardiovascular responses to behavioral stress and hypertension: A meta-analytic review. *Annals of Behavioral Medicine*.

Garber, J., and Seligman, M. E. P. (eds) (1980). *Human Helplessness: Theory and Applications*. New York: Academic Press.

Henry. J. P., and Stephens, P. M. (1977). *Stress, Health, and the Social Environment*. New York: Springer-Verlag.

Hokanson, J. E., DeGood, D. E., Forrest, M. S., and Brittain, T. M. (1971). Availability of avoidance behaviors in modulating vascular stress responses. *Journal of Personality and Social Psychology*, **119**, 60–68.

Kahneman, D. (1973). *Attention and Effort*. Englewood Cliffs, NJ: Prentice-Hall.

Karasek, R. A., Russell, R. S., and Theorell, T. (1982). Physiology of stress and regeneration in job related cardiovascular illness. *Journal of Human Stress*, March, 29–42.

Krantz, D. S., and Munuck, S. B. (1984). Acute psychophysiologic reactivity and risk of cardiovascular disease. A review and methodologic critique. *Psychological Bulletin*, **96**, 435–464.

Lacey, B. C., and Lacey, J. I. (1974). Studies of heart rate and other bodily processes in sensorimotor behavior. In: P. A. Obrist, A. H. Black, J. Brener and L. V. DiCara (eds), *Cardiovascular Psychophysiology* (pp. 538–564). Chicago: Aldine.

Lefcourt, H. M. (1976). *Locus of Control*. Hillsdale, NJ: Lawrence Erlbaum.

Light, K. C. (1987). Psychosocial precursors in hypertension: Experimental evidence. *Circulation*, **76** (Suppl. I), 67–76.

Light, K. C., and Obrist, P. A. (1980). Cardiovascular response to stress: Effects of opportunity to avoid, shock experience, and performance feedback. *Psychophysiology*, **17**, 243–252.

Light, K. C., and Obrist, P. A. (1983). Task difficulty, heart rate reactivity, and cardiovascular responses to an appetitive reaction time task. *Psychophysiology*, **20**, 301–311.

Lovallo, W. R., Wilson, M. F., Pincomb, G. A., Edwards, G. L., Tompkins, P., and Brackett, D. J. (1985). Activation patterns to aversive stimulation in man: Passive exposure versus effort to control. *Psychophysiology*, **22**, 283–291.

Malmo, R. B. (1965). Physiological gradients and behavior. *Psychological Bulletin*, **66**, 367–386.

Manuck, S. B., Harvey, A. H., Lechleiter, S. L., and Neal, K. S. (1978). Effects of coping on blood pressure responses to threat of aversive stimulation. *Psychophysiology*, **15**, 544–549.

Mineka, S., and Tomarken, A. J. (1989). The role of cognitive biases in the origins and maintenance of fear and anxiety disorders. In: T. Archer and L.-G. Nilsson (eds), *Aversion, Avoidance and Anxiety: Perspectives on Aversively Motivated Behavior*. Hillsdale, NJ: Lawrence Erlbaum.

Obrist, P. A. (1976). The cardiovascular–behavioral interaction: As it appears today. *Psychophysiology*, **13**, 95–107.

Obrist, P. A. (1981). *Cardiovascular Psychophysiology: A Perspective*. New York: Plenum.

Obrist, P. A., Gaebelein, C. J., Teller, E. S., Langer, A. W., Grignolo, A., Light, K. C., and McCubbin, J. A. (1978). The relationship among heart rate, carotid dP/dt, and blood pressure in humans as a function of the type of stress. *Psychophysiology*, **15**, 102–115.

Perkins, K. A. (1984). Heart rate change in Type A and Type B males as a function of response cost and task difficulty. *Psychophysiology*, **21**, 14–21.

Ragland, D. R., Winkleby, M. A., Schwalse, J., Holman, B. L., Morse, L., Syme, S. L., and Fisher, J. M. (1987). Prevalence of hypertension in bus drivers. *Journal of Epidemiology*, **16**, 208–214.

Rodin, J. (1980). Managing the stress of aging: The role of control and coping. In: S. Levine and H. Ursin (eds), *Coping and Health*. New York: Plenum.

Rotter, J. B. (1966). Generalized expectancies for internal versus external control of reinforcement. *Psychological Monographs*, **80** (1, whole no. 609).

Seligman, M. E. P. (1975). *Helplessness: On Depression, Development and Death*. San Francisco: Freeman.

Seligman, M. E. P., Maier, S. F., and Solomon, R. L. (1971). Unpredictable and uncontrollable aversive events. In: F. R. Brush (ed.), *Aversive Conditioning and Learning*. New York: Academic Press.

Shiffrin, R. M., and Schneider, W. (1977). Controlled and automatic human information processing. II. Perceptual learning, automatic attention, and a general theory. *Psychological Review*, **84**, 127–190.

Sklar, L. S., and Anisman, H. (1981). Stress and cancer. *Psychological Bulletin*, **89**, 369–406.

Smith, T. W., Houston, B. K., and Stucky, R. J. (1985). Effects of threats of shock and control over shock on finger pulse volume, pulse rate and systolic blood pressure. *Biological Psychology*, **20**, 31–38.

Steptoe, A. (1983). Stress, helplessness and control: The implications of laboratory studies. *Journal of Psychosomatic Research*, **27**, 361–367.

Steptoe, A., Melville, D., and Ross, A. (1984). Behavioral response demands, cardiovascular reactivity, and essential hypertension. *Psychosomatic Medicine*, **46**, 33–48.

Svebak, S. (1982). *The significance of motivation for task-induced tonic physiological changes.* Doctoral dissertation, Department of Somatic Psychology, University of Bergen, Norway.

Theorell, T., Knox, S., Svensson, J., and Waller, D. (1985). Blood pressure variations during a working day at age 28: Effects of different types of work and blood pressure level at age 18. *Journal of Human Stress*, Spring, 36–41.

Thompson, S. C. (1981). Will it hurt less if I can control it? A complex answer to a simple question. *Psychological Bulletin*, **90**, 89–101.

van Schijndel, M., De Mey, H., and Näring, G. (1984). Effects of behavioral control and Type A behavior on cardiovascular responses. *Psychophysiology*, **21**, 501–509.

Weder, A. B., and Julius, S. (1985). Behavior, blood pressure variability, and hypertension. *Psychosomatic Medicine*, **47**, 406–414.

Weiss, J. M. (1977). Psychological and behavioral influences on gastrointestinal lesions in animal models. In: J. D. Maser and M. E. P. Seligman (eds) *Psychopathology: Experimental Models*. San Francisco: Freeman.

Wright, R. A., Contrada, R. J., and Patane, M. J. (1986). Task difficulty, cardiovascular response, and the magnitude of goal valence. *Journal of Personality and Social Psychology*, **51**, 837–843.

CHAPTER 13

Neuroendocrine correlates of control and coping

ROBERT DANTZER
INRA–INSERM U259, Bordeaux, France

CONCEPTUAL BACKGROUND: COPING, ACTIVATION AND BIOBEHAVIOURAL RESPONSES TO STRESSORS

Response to highly stressful conditions involves increased sympathetic activity, increased activation of the pituitary–adrenal axis, release of endogenous opiates, enhanced turnover of brain monoamines and suppression of the immune system. These physiological responses do not represent, however, an ineluctable and invariable outcome of the physical properties of the noxious stimulation, since their direction and intensity primarily depend on psychological factors such as the possibility that the organism can control and/or predict the occurrence of stressors. More specifically, individuals that are exposed to a stressful situation tend to display one pattern of physiological reactivity if they can engage in an appropriate coping response, whereas they show another pattern if coping responses are unavailable. This is an important concept, since it appears to provide a biological basis for the commonly held view that stress is not a consequence of the physical dimensions of stressors, but the result of the interaction between this factor and the organismic variables that the subject interposes between the stressor and responses to it. These organismic variables include perceptual and behavioural response styles, the characterization and study of which have long been confined to the realm of psychology.

For some authors, consideration of the biological dimension of the coping response is the only way to confer objectivity to this concept, and to decide whether the strategy adopted by an individual in a given condition is adaptive or

Stress, Personal Control and Health.   Edited by A. Steptoe and A. Appels.
Published by John Wiley & Sons Ltd.
© ECSC–EEC–EAEC, Brussels–Luxembourg, 1989

not. In other words, if a stressor elicits a physiological reaction A and if, in an individual engaged in a specific behavioural response, the observed physiological reaction is B, such as B < A, then by definition the response displayed by the subject is a coping response (Levine *et al.*, 1978). The underlying assumption is that coping responses are by definition adaptive, since they attenuate the (deleterious) physiological consequences of stressors. To account for the fact that various stressors actually elicit a number of different physiological responses, a useful concept is that of activation. Although activation has a long tradition both in psychology and in neurophysiology, this term is used in the coping literature to refer to a general, non-specific response to all situations in which there is a threat to the organism (Ursin, 1985). Within this theoretical framework, coping responses refer to the methods that are available to an individual for reducing activation. Several strategies are potentially relevant to this goal, but the important point is that a given strategy emerges and is retained if and only if it proves to be functional, in the sense of reducing affect and activation. At a descriptive level, the term coping may be used to refer either to the development of a pertinent strategy, in which case we usually speak of coping attempts, or to the organismic state achieved when the subject has found the correct way of dealing with the problems with which he or she is confronted. This distinction between a process or a state is not always evident in the way the term coping is used, in spite of the fact that the psychological and physiological responses accompanying coping are likely to be different in each case.

This review attempts to address the question of whether or not the data available on the physiological correlates of control in animals are consistent with the concept of decreased activation in coping individuals. Although most of the research in this area has concentrated on the hypothalamic–pituitary–adrenal system (HPA), the individual's response to stressful stimuli is known to involve different endocrine systems (Henry, 1986). We will therefore attempt to take into account the effect of coping on the multidimensional pattern of physiological activation whenever this information is available. Another dimension relevant to the influence of control on physiology and behaviour is that it can be assessed during or immediately after exposure to the stressful situation, or later, when subjects are back in their normal environments or when they are exposed to other aversive situations. This last case has been mainly studied within the framework of the 'learned helplessness' phenomenon, which refers to the fact that prior exposure to uncontrollable aversive stimulation impairs behavioural performance in a variety of situations (Anisman, 1978; Seligman, 1975; Weiss *et al.*, 1981). Since the effects of control sometimes differ according to whether they are assessed immediately after exposure to the stressful situation or later, in a context that is identical for coping and non-coping subjects, it is useful to distinguish between the immediate and proactive effects of control.

Coping responses are conveniently categorized into two different classes according to whether they aim at altering the stimulus situation (problem-focused coping) or whether they aim at controlling the emotion elicited by the stimulus situation (emotion-focused coping). Although this classification is mainly used in clinical psychology (Lazarus and Folkman, 1984), it has also a counterpart in animal experiments, in the form of the distinction between behavioural activities that enable the subject to change the situation (e.g. escape/ avoidance behaviour) and behavioural responses that are apparently irrelevant with respect to the eliciting conditions (e.g. displacement activities).

PHYSIOLOGICAL CORRELATES OF PROBLEM-FOCUSED COPING

There is ample evidence that the degree of behavioural control that an organism has over a stressor is a major determinant of the behavioural and physiological impact of this stressor. Nowhere is this more persuasively demonstrated than in the classic triadic design experiments in which Weiss compared the consequences of a session of escapable versus inescapable electric shocks in rats yoked together by electrodes attached to the same source. Rats in the escape/avoidance group were permitted to terminate electric shocks or to delay their occurrence by turning a wheel with their forepaws. Rats in the second group served as yoked controls, since their responses had no effect on the occurrence and duration of electric shocks; the shocks were in fact entirely dependent on the behaviour of their escape/avoidance partners. As a further control group, rats were placed in the same apparatus as rats of the first two groups, but were not exposed to electric shock. Avoidance animals had scores of gastrointestinal lesions that were identical to or slightly higher than those of non-shocked controls, whereas the yoked animals had more and larger lesions than both the avoidance and control groups. This appears to be the case, however, only when the situation can be easily mastered, since the ulceration scores of rats exposed to inescapable shocks were not different from those of yoked rats in the absence of a feedback safety signal (Weiss, 1971a,b).

Influence of control on pituitary–adrenal activity

In further studies using the triadic paradigm, HPA responses have been found to be lower in avoidance animals than in yoked controls. For example, rhesus monkeys trained to terminate an intense noise by depressing a retractable lever responded to a 1-hour session of noise presentation over which they had control by a smaller increase in plasma cortisol than monkeys having no control over noise (Hanson *et al.*, 1976). In addition, removal of the contingency between lever presses and noise termination resulted in an increase in plasma cortisol similar to that observed in animals having no control over noise. In a similar way, dogs exposed to a series of electric shocks which they could terminate or prevent showed less of an increase in plasma cortisol than yoked animals that had no control over shock (Dess *et al.*, 1983).

Several studies have, however, failed to find differential corticosteroid responses between escapable and inescapable shock exposure. For example, rats exposed to a free-operant avoidance–escape procedure in which they had to pull a disk in order to avoid or escape electric shocks delivered through tail electrodes had elevated levels of plasma corticosterone at the end of a shock session lasting for 3, 6 or 21 hours that did not differ from those of yoked rats (Tsuda and Tanaka, 1985). Some authors have suggested that the main difference between coping and non-coping animals is not in the peak level reached but the rate of decay, since plasma corticosterone levels remained elevated significantly longer in rats exposed to 60 minutes of inescapable foot-shock than in rats exposed to escapable shock (Swenson and Vogel, 1983). This finding could not be replicated, however, by Maier *et al.* (1986) in an experiment where rats were submitted to 80 trials of shock-escape training in wheel-turn boxes. Under these conditions, escapable and inescapable shocks led not only to equal rises of both plasma corticosterone and adrenocorticotrophic hormone (ACTH), but also to a similar decline in plasma levels of these two hormones after termination of the shock session.

The failure to find differences between escape/avoidance animals and yoked animals can be tentatively attributed to the use of a single test session rather than to shock parameters or procedural characteristics, by hypothesizing that on the first exposure to shock the possible beneficial effects of coping are obscured by the effort needed to gain control over the stressor. According to this interpretation, attenuation of the pituitary–adrenal response in avoidance animals should be easier to demonstrate under chronic than under acute conditions of exposure to shock. The plasma corticosterone levels of rats that had been exposed to a free operant schedule of avoidance responding on five occasions did not differ from those of non-shocked animals, whereas the corticosterone response was still maximal in yoked rats (Tsuda and Tanaka, 1985). In a similar way, rats with an extensive history of free-operant avoidance behaviour displayed lower corticosterone levels at the end of a 1-hour avoidance session than yoked animals (Herrman *et al.*, 1984). In this latter case, however, the plasma corticosterone of avoidance animals was significantly elevated above the levels of yoked and control subjects before the experimental session.

Attenuation of the pituitary–adrenal response to escape/avoidance sessions has been found to occur even in rats that do not improve their performance over the course of the experiment (Coover *et al.*, 1973). This phenomenon could obscure possible differences between avoidance and yoked subjects (Mormède *et al.*, 1988).

In summary, there is evidence to suggest that the ability to control aversive stressors can influence the intensity and duration of the pituitary–adrenal response, but the exact conditions leading to the manifestation of this effect have not yet been systematically investigated.

Influence of control on other hormonal systems

The influence of controllability on hormonal systems other than the HPA axis has received little attention. Chronically catheterized rats exposed to a single session of inescapable foot-shock were found to have significantly higher peak plasma noradrenaline and adrenaline concentrations than rats receiving escapable shock. Yoked rats also displayed significantly longer elevations of plasma catecholamines after foot-shock (Swenson and Vogel, 1983). Since these changes were observed in conditions where peak plasma corticosterone levels did not differentiate between the two groups, it is possible that circulating catecholamines are more sensitive to the influence of control than plasma corticosterone, but the generality of this finding remains to be tested.

The plasma prolactin levels of rats exposed to a free operant schedule of avoidance responding in a shuttle-box were not different from those of yoked controls after one to ten experimental sessions (Mormède *et al.*, 1988). There was, however, a significant habituation of the prolactin response over the course of the experiment in the groups exposed to electric shock. Rats submitted to five consecutive daily sessions of shock delivered through tail electrodes in wheel-turn boxes had similar levels of plasma luteinizing hormone (LH) and testosterone at the end of the last session, whether shock was escapable or not (Hellhammer *et al.*, 1984). The results of this last experiment are, however, difficult to interpret since the plasma corticosterone of non-shocked rats did not differ from the levels measured in shocked animals.

Influence of control on stress-induced analgesia

Exposure to a variety of stressors results in decreased responsiveness on a number of different measures of pain sensitivity or reactivity. This stress-induced analgesia (SIA) is not a unitary phenomenon, since different stressors activate different analgesic substrates, including opioid/non-opioid and hormonal/non-hormonal types (Lewis *et al.*, 1980; Watkins and Mayer, 1982). Opiate-mediated SIA is characterized by the fact that it is blocked by pretreatment with an opiate antagonist (naltrexone of naloxone) and that it is cross-tolerant with morphine analgesia. Cross-tolerance of SIA with morphine analgesia means that the decreased analgesic response that is observed following repeated treatment with morphine (tolerance to morphine) is also observed in animals exposed to the stressor. Inversely, animals that have repeatedly been exposed to a stressor producing an opiate-mediated SIA display a lower analgesic response to morphine than non-stressed animals or animals exposed to a non-opioid stressor. Hormone-dependent SIA is blocked by hypophysectomy, in contrast to hormone-independent SIA.

Exposure of rats to a series of inescapable electric shocks produced a naltrexone-insensitive analgesic reaction at the beginning of the session, which was replaced by a naltrexone-reversible analgesic reaction at the end of the shock session (Grau *et al.*, 1981). This might be interpreted as suggesting that learning that there is no escape from an aversive stimulus is an important factor in determining whether or not opiate systems are activated. In a direct test of this hypothesis, Drugan *et al.* (1985) observed that the early non-opioid analgesia was apparent in rats exposed to inescapable shock as well as in rats exposed to escapable shock, but that the late opiate-mediated analgesia was observed only in the former animals. In addition, the analgesia following inescapable electric shock persisted for a few hours after termination of the shock session, whereas the analgesia produced by escapable shock dissipated rapidly. Re-exposure to shock 24 hours after the initial stress session reinstated opioid analgesia only in rats' previously exposed to inescapable electric shock (Jackson *et al.*, 1979). This proactive effect of exposure to inescapable electric shock was found to be opioid in nature since it was completely blocked by opiate antagonists (Maier *et al.*, 1980) and was cross-tolerant with morphine (Drugan *et al.*, 1981). Analgesia upon re-exposure to shock can even be observed 48 hours after the initial stress session (Hemingway and Reigle, 1987). In this last study, however, the reinstated analgesia and the behavioural deficit exhibited by the animals of the inescapable group were not blocked by the administration of naloxone prior to the test session, suggesting that expression of these phenomena is not critically dependent on endogenous opiate systems. That the analgesia induced by inescapable electric shock and the learned helplessness phenomenon are simply coincidental but not causally related is further suggested by the observation that hypophysectomy or dexamethasone administration blocked the analgesic consequences of inescapable shock but did not reduce the magnitude of the escape deficit (MacLennan *et al.*, 1982).

The influence of controllability on stress-induced analgesia is not limited to electric shock, since rats that could obtain food by pressing a lever (controllable food) were found to display less analgesia at the end of the session than rats that received food independently of their behaviour (uncontrollable food) (Figure 1) (Tazi *et al.*, 1987). The possible involvement of endogenous opiates in this phenomenon was not tested.

In summary, exposure to uncontrollable appetitive as well as aversive events activates endogenous pain-inhibitory systems. In animals exposed to inescapable shock, this analgesic reaction can be reinstated by brief exposure to shock, even under shock conditions that do not induce SIA in previously non-shocked animals, but this phenomenon does not appear to play a significant role in the behavioral deficit that is observed in non-coping animals.

Influence of control on brain neurochemistry

Exposure to various stressors increases the turnover of most brain neurotransmitters. This increase is found in several projection areas in the brain, except for dopamine metabolism, which is enhanced only in the mesocortico-limbic area

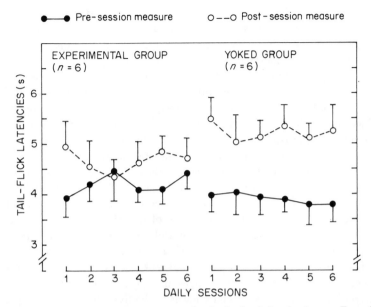

FIGURE 1. Uncontrollable food induces analgesia in food-deprived rats. Experimental animals were able to get food pellets by pressing a lever according to a continuous schedule of food reinforcement during six consecutive daily sessions, whereas yoked animals received the same amount and temporal distribution of food as their active partners. Each point represents tail-flick latencies (mean + SEM) measured before and after each session. (From Tazi *et al.*, 1987.)

(Blanc *et al.*, 1980; Thierry *et al.*, 1976). The influence of controllability has been mainly investigated on brain levels of noradrenaline, and lower concentrations of this neurotransmitter have been observed in whole brain, hypothalamus and brain stem for rats exposed to inescapable shock versus rats exposed to escapable shock (Glavin, 1985).

An important characteristic of the decreased noradrenaline levels observed in non-coping animals is that it is long-lasting and can be reinstated after re-exposure to only a small number of inescapable shocks, suggesting that the lack of control over an aversive stimulation can lead to sensitization of the neural structures involved. Since depletion of noradrenaline levels is closely associated with the behavioural depression induced by exposure to inescapable electric shock (the so-called 'learned helplessness' effect), and since the occurrence of this phenomenon is easier to demonstrate when cues present during exposure to inescapable shock are also present during the testing phase (cf. Minor and LoLordo, 1984), it is tempting to speculate that the neurochemical changes responsible for the behavioural deficit induced by prior stress exposure are conditioned to the environmental cues associated with inescapable shock. Although there are a few independent studies suggesting that such conditioned changes in neurotransmitter activity can take place (Cassens *et al.*, 1980; Herrmann *et al.*, 1984), the crucial experiments have not yet been carried out.

In a recent series of experiments, Weiss and Goodman Simson (1984) have proposed that the key factor in the series of events responsible for the development of behavioural depression following exposure to inescapable electric shocks is a functional blockade of α_2-receptors in the locus ceruleus. This hypothesis was based on the ability of local injections of clonidine, an α_2-agonist, to reverse both the behavioural deficit displayed by stressed animals and the depressing effects of α_2-antagonists, piperoxane and yohimbine in non-stressed animals.

The possibility that changes in neurotransmitter metabolism may help to differentiate coping efforts from mastering of the task is suggested by the results of two independent studies. Swenson and Vogel (1983) attributed the larger depletion of hypothalamic noradrenaline observed in non-coping rats compared with coping animals to the aversive nature of the stimulus, whereas the fall in hippocampal noradrenaline that was seen only in coping rats was attributed to the ability to cope with electric shocks. In rats exposed to a free operant schedule of avoidance responding, Tsuda and Tanaka (1985) found a higher turnover of noradrenaline, as measured by changes in noradrenaline and 3-methoxy-4-hydroxyphenylethylene glycol sulfate levels in the hypothalamus, amygdala and thalamus of avoidance rats compared to yoked controls after a 3-hour or 6-hour experimental session, but not after a 21-hour session. In this last case, only yoked rats displayed an increased noradrenaline turnover, whereas turnover rates were back to normal in avoidance rats. Significant avoidance performance was only achieved after at least 6 hours of exposure to the experimental conditions.

In summary, the data available on the effects of inescapable electric shocks on brain neurochemistry show that uncontrollability has profound and long-lasting influences on the metabolism of central neurotransmitters, especially noradrenaline, and that such changes mediate the proactive effects of uncontrollability on behaviour, possibly through aggravating phenomena such as sensitization and classical conditioning to environmental cues present during exposure to stress.

Influence of control on immune functions

In mice exposed to a single session of inescapable shock 24 hours following tumour cell transplantation, the rate of tumour growth was found to be accelerated, whereas mice exposed to escapable shock did not differ from non-shocked mice in tumour size and time of tumour appearance (Sklar and Anisman, 1979). This detrimental effect of uncontrollability on tumour development was no longer apparent, however, in animals exposed chronically to the stressor (Sklar *et al.*, 1981). In rats, a single session of inescapable, but not of escapable, shock significantly reduced the incidence of rejection of transplanted non-syngeneic tumour cells (Visintainer *et al.*, 1982). The possibility that such changes are mediated by suppression of the immune system is suggested by studies showing that inescapable but not escapable shock decreases cellular immune responses. Rats submitted to inescapable electric shocks on the first day and re-exposed to a few 'reminder' shocks on the second day displayed a lower proliferative response of blood lymphocytes to T-cell mitogens than rats submitted to escapable electric shocks or apparatus-control animals (Laudenslager *et al.*, 1983). This impairment of lymphoproliferative responses due to inescapable electric shock appears to carry over to chronic conditions, since it was also observed in yoked animals paired with rats exposed to ten sessions of free-operant avoidance learning in a shuttle-box (Mormède *et al.*, 1988). In this last experiment, however, uncontrollability did not have generalized immunosuppressive effects since, in contrast to the changes observed in lymphoproliferative responses, the primary antibody response against sheep erythrocytes was decreased in the avoidance rats, compared with yoked animals and apparatus-control animals. The factors responsible for these differential changes in humoral and cellular immune responses are not known.

PHYSIOLOGICAL CONSEQUENCES OF DISPLACEMENT ACTIVITIES

Characteristics of displacement activities

Early ethologists have long been puzzled by the behavioural patterns that appear in conflict situations. Displacement activities are of special interest since they occur at a high rate in spite of their apparent irrelevance to the eliciting situation. Tinbergen (1951) noted that displacement activities occur when 'there is a surplus of motivation, the discharge of which through the normal paths is somehow prevented'. By this formulation, he implied that displacement activities could release tension and act as outlets for nervous energy in situations where the ongoing behaviour was thwarted. Although this view seems to make intuitive sense, it was never proven and further studies actually showed that displacement activities could also be due to disinhibition, and have the function of diverting attention away from the stimuli normally controlling the ongoing behaviour (McFarland, 1985).

Experimental analogues of displacement activities have been found in the laboratory, in the form of adjunctive or schedule-induced behaviours that typically occur when hungry animals are exposed to an intermittent schedule of food reinforcement (Falk, 1971). Animals with water freely available at the same time develop excessive drinking within the intervals between successive food reinforcements. This behaviour is not regulatory with respect to thirst or dryness of the mouth induced by food ingestion, since it can be replaced by other activities such as wood-gnawing, air-licking or wheel-running, depending on the object available in the environment. In addition, it cannot qualify as superstitious

behaviour since it occurs with a maximum probability just after the ingestion of a
food pellet rather than immediately before it (Staddon, 1977).

Physiological correlates of schedule-induced behaviours

Like displacement activities, it has been proposed that schedule-induced behaviours serve a stabilizing or buffering function, by maintaining active engagement of the animal in situations where a strongly motivated behaviour is
interrupted or prevented (Falk, 1971, 1977). Support for this interpretation
comes from the observation of a significant drop in plasma corticosterone
concentration in rats that have developed schedule-induced polydipsia, in
contrast to the enhanced plasma corticosterone levels displayed by rats exposed
to intermittent distribution of food but without access to water (Figure 2) (Brett
and Levine, 1979). This decrease in pituitary–adrenal activity does not appear to
be due to the haemodilution which could result from reabsorption of the ingested

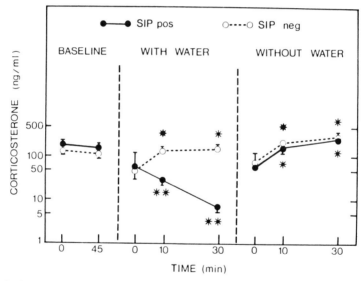

FIGURE 2. Schedule-induced polydipsia decreases pituitary–adrenal axis reactivity. Rats
were classified as positive (SIP-pos) or negative (SIP-neg) according to the amount of
water they ingested when submitted to an intermittent schedule of food delivery with
water freely available. The figure represents the time course of changes in plasma
corticosterone levels in SIP-pos rats and in SIP-neg rats during baseline conditions (left)
and intermittent distribution of food with access to water (middle) or no access to water
(right). Each point represents the mean ($+$SEM) of four animals. Note the decrease in
plasma corticosterone levels in SIP-pos animals having access to water and the contrasting
increase in plasma corticosterone levels in SIP-neg animals and in SIP-pos animals denied
access to water ($*p < 0.05$, $**p < 0.01$ compared to values measured on the start of the
session, at time $= 0$). (From Dantzer *et al.*, 1988a.)

water, since schedule-induced polydipsia is not accompanied by any significant haemodilution (Kenny *et al.*, 1976), and since decreased plasma corticosterone levels can be observed even when animals have ingested only a minimum amount of water (Brett and Levine, 1981). Similar findings have been obtained by other authors in polydipsic rats (Tazi *et al.*, 1986), but negative results have also been reported (Mittleman *et al.*, 1988; Wallace *et al.*, 1983). A possible explanation for these contradictory findings is that decreased pituitary–adrenal activity is a late phenomenon that appears only when schedule-induced polydipsia has fully developed.

The effects of schedule-induced polydipsia on other physiological indices are difficult to interpret. On the positive side, the analgesic response to intermittent distribution of food is blocked in polydipsic animals (Tazi *et al.*, 1987). In the same manner, the locomotor response to *d*-amphetamine, which can be taken as *in vivo* index of the activity of central dopaminergic neurones, is decreased after drinking in polydipsic animals (Tazi *et al.*, 1988). On the negative side, prolactin levels are elevated in animals having developed excessive drinking, in comparison to animals that do not drink (Dantzer *et al.*, 1988a). Plasma catecholamines levels are not affected by drinking (Dantzer *et al.*, 1988a), but polydipsia is accompanied by decreased heart rate and increased oxygen consumption (Mittleman *et al.*, 1987).

A few data are available on the possible generalization of the modulatory influences of schedule-induced polydipsia on pituitary–adrenal activity, to other schedule-induced behaviours and to species other than rats. Schedule-induced wheel-running in rats was found not to be accompanied by decreased plasma corticosterone but, instead, by increases which were proportional to the amount of running (Tazi *et al.*, 1986). Hungry pigs submitted to intermittent food delivery and given access to a nibbling chain gradually developed compulsive chain-nibbling during the intervals between successive food deliveries, and this behaviour was accompanied by a significant drop in plasma cortisol levels from pre-session levels (Dantzer and Mormède, 1981). However, this was secondary to an increase in pre-session cortisol levels and did not reflect a decrease in post-session cortisol levels. In addition, when pigs were given all their food at the beginning of the session rather than intermittently throughout the session, they still developed chain-nibbling and this behaviour was accompanied by an increase in cortisol levels instead of a decrease (Dantzer *et al.*, 1987).

It is difficult to conclude from this survey of the physiological correlates of schedule-induced behaviours whether these activities truly represent effective forms of coping with the situation. The main problem is that drinking behaviour already has potent inhibitory effects on pituitary–adrenal activity in rats maintained on deprivation schedules (Heybach and Vernikos-Danellis, 1979a). The elevated plasma levels of corticosterone that are displayed by such rats just before feeding or drinking are the result of an altered circadian rhythmicity in the circulating levels of corticosterone (Krieger, 1974). Upon presentation of food or water, plasma levels of corticosterone fall rapidly, within a few minutes. Whether this is due to a central nervous system mechanism that inhibits ACTH secretion independently of corticosteroid negative feedback, or to direct inhibitory neural influences on the adrenal cortex, is still controversial (Heybach and Vernikos-Danellis, 1979a; Wilkinson *et al.*, 1982). Whatever the case, this decrease in pituitary–adrenal activity during feeding or drinking results in an inhibition of the stress response that persists for 5–10 minutes after the initiation of the consummatory response (Heybach and Vernikos-Danellis, 1979b) and that could explain the apparent beneficial effects of consummatory activities during exposure to a stressful situation (e.g. Levine *et al.*, 1979).

Other forms of displacement activities have been observed to be accompanied by decreases in pituitary–adrenal activity. It is the case, for instance, of object-chewing in mice exposed to novelty (Hennessy and Foy, 1987), drinking in rats placed into a new environment (Weinberg *et al.*, 1980) and fighting in pairs of rats exposed to inescapable foot-shock (Conner *et al.*, 1971; Weinberg *et al.*, 1980). In the first case, shredding of cardboard or aluminium foil reliably occurred in mice placed into a novel cage, and this behaviour was accompanied by an attenuated corticosterone response to novelty. This was not the case, however, when mice had access to a highly palatable food. The reason for this difference is unknown and, in particular, the possible effects of feeding on pituitary–adrenal activity were not investigated.

The physiological consequences of the ability to engage in oral activities in face of aversive situations are certainly worth re-evaluating in view of the recent studies of Uvnas-Moberg (1987) on the effect of non-nutritive sucking on gastrointestinal hormones. Briefly, this author observed that somatostatin was decreased whereas insulin and gastrin were increased in infants allowed to suck a pacifier. She suggests that this pattern of change reflects a shift from sympathetic activation to parasympathetic activation. This would account for the enhanced gastrointestinal assimilation of nutrients, the improved growth and maturation of the gastrointestinal tract and the higher efficacy of the storing of ingested nutrients which are believed to lead to the increased growth rate reported to occur in response to non-nutritive suckling.

Displacement activities are not limited to oral activities. The administration of brief electric shocks to the feet of rats shocked by pairs induces an upright posture with both animals facing each other (boxing), striking with their forepaws, and very rarely biting. This targeting of defensive behaviour in response to shock on the other member of the pair is accompanied by a lower increase in post-session ACTH levels as compared with rats shocked alone (Conner *et al.*, 1971), a decrease in blood pressure from pre-shock levels instead of the increase seen in non-fighting rats (Williams and Eichelman, 1971) and a lower analgesic response (Tazi, 1987). These findings have been interpreted as showing that fighting in response to shock is a coping response. However, rats repeatedly exposed to electric shock in pairs displayed a stronger activation of the sympathetic–adrenal medullary system than rats shocked alone (Mormède *et al.*, 1984). These results suggest that the decreased pituitary–adrenal activity observed in rats exposed in pairs to electric shock reflects a shift in the pattern of physiological activation during fighting rather than physiological deactivation. Marked differences in the metabolism of noradrenaline in various regions of the brain were also observed, since fighting was accompanied by increased noradrenaline turnover after the shock session, whereas rats shocked alone displayed a rapid depletion of brain noradrenaline in response to shock (Stolk *et al.*, 1974). The social setting under which shock occurs had, however, no significant influence on brain dopamine turnover (Dantzer *et al.*, 1984).

Displacement activities and stereotypies: from coping to psychopathology

An important dimension of schedule-induced polydipsia is the existence of clear-cut individual differences in the propensity to develop this behaviour in the presence of appropriate stimulus conditions (Mittleman and Valenstein, 1984; Tazi *et al.*, 1987). In exploring what factors might be responsible for these differences, animals that display excessive drinking (SIP-pos) and those that do not (SIP-neg) have been compared both within SIP sessions as in other experimental paradigms. The main result of these studies has been the observation of a consistent relationship between the propensity to respond by eating or drinking to electrical stimulation of the lateral hypothalamus (ESLH) and the predisposition to develop SIP (Mittleman and Valenstein, 1984). As brain catecholamines, and specifically dopamine, have been implicated in the regulation of oral activities elicited by exposure to a wide variety of mild stressors, it has been suggested that the differences in the predisposition to display SIP and ESLH-induced drinking might be related to individual differences in the responsiveness of forebrain dopamine systems. In support of this hypothesis, SIP- or ESLH-positive animals have been found to develop sensitization to repeated injections of amphetamine and to display a more widespread activation of dopaminergic systems in response to foot-shock stress (Mittleman and Valenstein, 1985; Mittleman *et al.*, 1986). In addition, repeated injections of amphetamine can transform ESLH-negative animals into ESLH-positive animals (Mittleman and Valenstein, 1985). On the behavioural side SIP-pos animals learn more rapidly an active avoidance response and show less freezing when confronted with an aggressive resident male in a defeat test, than do SIP-neg subjects (Dantzer *et al.*, 1988b). These findings may be interpreted to suggest that the predisposition to develop SIP is another facet of a more general profile of behavioural and neurochemical reactivity to aversive situations. The basic factor underlying this characteristic could be a reduced ability to shift behavioural programmes, i.e. behavioural rigidity. SIP-pos animals may be individuals who easily develop routines and become more stereotyped in their way of responding to a given stimulus situation. This could be due to a greater sensitivity to sensitization processes of the neural structures underlying the behavioural response.

Similar mechanisms may account for the development of the compulsive oral or locomotor stereotypes displayed by farm and zoo animals under conditions of conflict and frustration. These abnormal behaviours are remnants of displacement activities or defensive reactions that are initially emitted in an attempt to control the eliciting situation. If such attempts have consummatory properties, in the sense that they put an end to a sequence of motivated behaviour, they can be functionally effective, by inhibiting the activity of the underlying neural command circuit. The problem with stereotypies is that because of a lack of a suitable goal-object in the situation, they stay within the appetitive repertoire and cannot become consummatory. Sensory feedback from appetitive oro-motor patterns normally enhances activity in the corresponding neural command system and this leads to increased activation in the absence of adequate consummatory behaviour. If the neuronal elements composing the repeatedly activated neural pathways are prone to sensitization, all the conditions are met for a positive feedback in which the sensory factors that normally guide behaviour trigger a behavioural sequence that becomes self-organized independently of further environmental guidance or any particular motivational state (cf. Dantzer, 1986).

CONCLUSION

Although classical concepts of coping emphasize the adaptive value of control gained by engaging in species-specific defence reactions (e.g. fight/escape) or related behaviours which aim at reducing the aversiveness of eliciting stimuli, it should be clear that this view is too simplistic. Coping attempts have a cost which can be bigger than the expected benefit, especially when the situation cannot be easily mastered. In addition, the dividing line between coping responses and abnormal behaviour is tenuous and depends both on individual factors and on environmental constraints. Studies of basic responses to life-threatening events have been decisive in deciphering the importance of controllability in response to aversive events. The time is now ripe to go beyond the coping concept and consider the richness of individual differences in adaptive strategies. This can be done not so much by describing the variety of options available to an individual in a given solution but by studying the mechanisms and functions underlying the emergence of a particular strategy.

REFERENCES

Anisman, H. (1978). Neurochemical changes elicited by stress: Behavioral correlates. In: H. Anisman and G. Bignami (eds), *Psychopharmacology of Aversively Motivated Behavior* (pp. 119–172). New York: Plenum Press.

Blanc, G., Hervé, D., Simon, H., Lisoprawski, A., Glowinsky, J., and Tassin, J. P. (1980). Response to stress of mesocortical-frontal dopaminergic neurons in rats after long-term isolation. *Nature*, **284**, 265–267.

Brett, L. P., and Levine, S. (1979). Schedule-induced polydipsia suppresses pituitary–adrenal activity in rats. *Journal of Comparative and Physiological Psychology*, **93**, 946–956.

Brett, L. P., and Levine, S. (1981). The pituitary–adrenal response to 'minimized' schedule-induced drinking. *Physiology and Behavior*, **26**, 153–158.

Cassens, G., Roffman, M., Kuruc, A., Orsulak, P. J., and Schildkraut, J. J. (1980). Alterations in brain norepinephrine metabolism induced by environmental stimuli previously paired with inescapable shock. *Science*, **209**, 1138–1140.

Conner, R. L., Vernikos-Danellis, J., and Levine, S. (1971). Stress, fighting and neuroendocrine function. *Nature*, **234**, 564–566.

Coover, G. D., Ursin, H., and Levine, S. (1973). Plasma corticosterone levels during active avoidance learning in rats. *Journal of Comparative and Physiological Psychology*, **82**, 170–174.

Dantzer, R. (1986). Behavioral, physiological and functional aspects of stereotyped behavior: A review and a reinterpretation. *Journal of Animal Science*, **62**, 1776–1786.

Dantzer, R., and Mormède, P. (1981). Pituitary–adrenal correlates of adjunctive activities in pigs. *Hormones and Behavior*, **16**, 78–92.

Dantzer, R., Guilloneau, D., Mormède, P., Herman, J. P., and Le Moal, M. (1984). Influence of shock-induced fighting and social factors on dopamine turnover in cortical and limbic areas in the rat. *Pharmacology, Biochemistry and Behavior*, **20**, 331–335.

Dantzer, R., Gonyou, H. W., Curtis, S. E., and Kelley, K. W. (1987). Changes in serum cortisol reveal functional differences in frustration-induced chain chewing in pigs. *Physiology and Behavior*, **39**, 775–777.

Dantzer, R., Terlouw, C., Mormède, P., and Le Moal, M. (1988a). Schedule-induced polydipsia experience decreases plasma corticosterone levels but increases plasma prolactin levels. *Physiology and Behavior*, **43**, 275–279.

Dantzer, R., Terlouw, C., Tazi, A., Koolhas, J. M., Bohus, B., Koob, G. F., and Le Moal, M. (1988b). The propensity for schedule-induced polydipsia is related to differences in conditioned avoidance behaviour and in defense reactions in a defeat test. *Physiology and Behavior*, **43**, 269–273.

Dess, N. K., Linwick, D., Patterson, J., Overmier, J. B., and Levine, S. (1983). Immediate and proactive effects of controllability and predictability on plasma cortisol responses to shock in dogs. *Behavioral Neuroscience*, **97**, 1005–1016.

Drugan, R. C., Grau, J. W., Maier, S. F., Madden, J., and Barchas, J. D. (1981). Cross-tolerance between morphine and the long-term analgesic reaction to inescapable shock. *Pharmacology, Biochemistry and Behavior*, **14**, 677–682.

Drugan, R. C., Ader, D. N., and Maier, S. F. (1985). Shock controllability and the nature of stress-induced analgesia. *Behavioral Neuroscience*, **99**, 791–801.

Falk, J. L. (1971). The nature and determinants of adjunctive behavior. *Physiology and Behavior*, **6**, 577–588.

Falk, J. L. (1977). The origin and functions of adjunctive behavior. *Animal Learning and Behavior*, **5**, 325–335.

Glavin, G. B. (1985). Stress and brain noradrenaline: A review. *Neuroscience and Biobehavioral Reviews*, **9**, 233–243.

Grau, J. S., Hyson, R. L., Maier, S. F., Madden, J., and Barchas, J. D. (1981). Long-term stress-induced analgesia and activation of the opiate system. *Science*, **203**, 1409–1412.

Hanson, J. D., Larson, M. E., and Snowdon, C. T. (1976). The effect of control over high intensity noise on plasma cortisol levels in rhesus monkeys. *Behavioral Biology*, **16**, 333–340.

Hellhammer, D. H., Rea, M. A., Bell, M., Belkien, L., and Ludwig, M. (1984). Learned helplessness: Effects on brain monoamines and the pituitary–gonadal axis. *Pharmacology, Biochemistry and Behavior*, **21**, 481–485.

Hemingway, R. B., and Reigle, T. G. (1987). The involvement of endogenous opiate systems in learned helplessness and stress-induced analgesia. *Psychopharmacology*, **95**, 353–357.

Hennessy, M., and Foy, T. (1987). Nonedible material elicits chewing and reduces the plasma corticosterone response during novelty exposure in mice. *Behavioral Neuroscience*, **101**, 237–245.

Henry, J. P. (1986). Neuroendocrine patterns of emotional response. In: R. Plutchik and H. Kellerman (eds), *Emotion: Theory, Research and Experience. Vol. 3: Biological Foundations of Emotion* (pp. 37–60). Orlando: Academic Press.

Herrmann, T. F., Hurwitz, H. M. B., and Levine, S. (1984). Behavioral control, aversive stimulus frequency and pituitary–adrenal response. *Behavioral Neuroscience*, **98**, 1094–1099.

Heybach, J. P., and Vernikos-Danellis, J. (1979a). Inhibition of adrenocorticotrophin secretion during deprivation-induced eating and drinking in rats. *Neuroendocrinology*, **28**, 329–338.

Heybach, J. P., and Vernikos-Danellis, J. (1979b). Inhibition of the pituitary–adrenal response to stress during deprivation-induced feeding. *Endocrinology*, **104**, 967–973.

Jackson, R. L., Maier, S. F., and Coon, D. J. (1979). Long-term analgesic effects of inescapable shock and learned helplessness. *Science*, **209**, 91–94.

Kenny, T. J., Wright, J. W., and Reynolds, T. J. (1976). Schedule-induced polydipsia: The role of oral and plasma factors. *Physiology and Behavior*, **17**, 939–945.

Krieger, D. T. (1974). Food and water restriction shifts corticosterone, temperature, activity and brain amine periodicity. *Endocrinology*, **95**, 1195–1201.

Laudenslager, M. L., Ryan, S. M., Drugan, R. C., Hyson, R. L., and Maier, S. F. (1983). Coping and immunosuppression: Inescapable but not escapable shock suppresses lymphocyte proliferation. *Science*, **221**, 568–570.

Lazarus, R. S., and Folkman, S. (1984). Coping and adaption. In W. D. Gentry (ed.), *Handbook of Behavioral Medicine* (pp. 282–325). New York: Guilford Press.

Levine, S., Weinberg, J., and Ursin, H. (1978). Definition of the coping process and statement of the problem. In: H. Ursin, E. Baade and S. Levine (eds), *Psychobiology of Stress: A Study of Coping Men* (pp. 3–21). New York: Academic Press.

Levine, S., Weinberg, J., and Brett, L. P. (1979). Inhibition of pituitary–adrenal activity as a consequence of consummatory behavior. *Psychoneuroendocrinology*, **4**, 275–286.

Lewis, J. W., Cannon, J. T., and Liebeskind, J. C. (1980). Opioid and nonopioid mechanism of stress analgesia. *Science*, **208**, 623–625.

MacLennan, A. J., Drugan, R. C., Hyson, R. L., Maier, S. F., Madden, J., IV, and Barchas, J. D. (1982). Dissociation of long-term induced analgesia and the shuttle-box escape deficit caused by inescapable shock. *Journal of Comparative and Physiological Psychology*, **96**, 904–912.

Maier, S. F., Davies, S., Grau, J. W., Jackson, R. L., Morrison, D. H., Moye, T., Madden, J., IV, and Barchas, J. D. (1980). Opiate antagonists and long-term analgesic reaction induced by inescapable shock in rats. *Journal of Comparative and Physiological Psychology*, **94**, 1172–1183.

Maier, S. F., Ryan, S. M., Barksdale, C. M., and Kalin, N. H. (1986). Stressor controllability and the pituitary–adrenal system. *Behavioral Neuroscience*, **100**, 669–674.

McFarland, D. J. (1966). The role of attention in the disinhibition of displacement activity. *Quarterly Journal of Experimental Psychology*, **18**, 19–30.

McFarland, D. J. (1985). *Animal Behaviour*. London: Pitman.

Minor, T., and LoLordo, V. (1984). Escape deficits following inescapable shock: The role of contextual odor. *Journal of Experimental Psychology: Animal Behavior Processes*, **10**, 168–181.

Mittleman, G., and Valenstein, E. S. (1984). Ingestive behavior evoked by hypothalamic stimulation and schedule-induced polydipsia are related. *Science*, **224**, 415–417.

Mittleman, G., and Valenstein, E. S. (1985). Individual differences in non-regulatory ingestive behavior and catecholamine systems. *Brain Research*, **348**, 112–117.

Mittleman, G., Castaneda, E., Robinson, T. E., and Valenstein, E. S. (1986). The propensity for nonregulatory ingestive behavior is related to differences in dopamine systems: Behavioral and biochemical evidence. *Behavioral Neuroscience*, **100**, 213–220.

Mittleman, G., Brener, J., and Robbins, T. W. (1987). Metabolic correlates of schedule-induced polydipsia. *Neuroscience Abstracts*, **7**, 253.

Mittleman, G., Jones, G. H., and Robbins, T. W. (1988). The relationship between schedule-induced polydipsia and pituitary–adrenal activity: Pharmacological manipulations and individual differences. *Behavioral Brain Research*, **28**, 315–324.

Mormède, P., Dantzer, R., Montpied, P., Bluthé, R. M., Laplante, E., and Le Moal, M. (1984). Influence of shock-induced fighting and social factors on pituitary–adrenal activity, prolactin and catecholamine synthesizing enzymes in rats. *Physiology and Behavior*, **32**, 723–729.

Mormède, P., Dantzer, R., Michaud, B., Kelley, K. W., and Le Moal, M. (1988). Influence of stressor predictability and behavioral control on lymphocyte reactivity, antibody responses and neuroendocrine activation in rats. *Physiology and Behavior*, **43**, 577–583.

Seligman, M. E. P. (1975). *Helplessness: On Depression, Development and Death*. San Francisco: Freeman.

Sklar, L. S., and Anisman, H. (1979). Stress and coping factor influence tumor growth. *Science*, **205**, 513–515.

Sklar, L. S., Bruto, V., and Anisman, H. (1981). Adaptation to the tumor-enhancing effects of stress. *Psychosomatic Medicine*, **43**, 331–342.

Staddon, J. E. R. (1977). Schedule-induced behavior. In: W. K. Honig and J. E. R. Staddon (eds), *Handbook of Operant Behavior*, (pp. 125–152). New York: Prentice Hall.

Stolk, J. M., Conner, R. L., Levine, S., and Barchas, J. D. (1974). Brain norepinephrine metabolism and shock-induced fighting behavior in rats: Differential effects of shock and fighting on the neurochemical response to a common footshock stimulus. *Journal of Pharmacology and Experimental Therapeutics*, **190**, 193–209.

Swenson, R. M., and Vogel, W. H. (1983). Plasma catecholamine and corticosterone as well as brain catecholamine changes during coping in rats exposed to stressful footshock. *Pharmacology, Biochemistry and Behavior*, **18**, 689–693.

Tazi, A. (1987). *Psychobiologie des activités de déplacement chez le rat*. Thèse de Doctorat d'Etat ès-Sciences, Université de Bordeaux II, no. 59.

Tazi, A., Dantzer, R., Mormède, P. and Le Moal, M. (1986). Pituitary–adrenal correlates of schedule-induced polydipsia and wheel-running in rats. *Behavioral Brain Research*, **19**, 249–256.

Tazi, A., Dantzer, R., and Le Moal, M. (1987). Prediction and control of food rewards modulate endogenous pain inhibitory systems. *Behavioral Brain Research*, **23**, 197–204.

Tazi, A., Dantzer, R., and Le Moal, M. (1988). Schedule-induced polydipsia experience decreases locomotor response to amphetamine. *Brain Research*, **445**, 211–215.

Thierry, A. M., Tassin, J. P., Blan, G., and Glowinsky, J. (1976). Selective activation of the mesocortical DA system by stress. *Nature*, **263**, 242–244.

Tinbergen, N. (1950). Derived activities: Their causation, biological significance, origin and emancipation during evolution. *Quarterly Review of Biology*, **27**, 1–32.

Tinbergen, N. (1951). *The Study of Instinct*. Oxford: Oxford University Press.

Tsuda, A., and Tanaka, M. (1985). Differential changes in noradrenaline turnover in specific regions of rat brain produced by controllable and uncontrollable shocks. *Behavioral Neuroscience*, **99**, 802–817.

Ursin, H. (1985). The instrumental effects of emotional behavior. In: P. P. G. Bateson and P. H. Klopfer (eds), *Perspectives in Ethology* (Vol. 6, pp. 45–62). New York: Plenum.

Uvnas-Moberg, K. (1987). Gastrointestinal hormones and pathophysiology of functional gastrointestinal disorders. *Scandinavian Journal of Gastroenterology*, **22** (Suppl. 128), 138–148.

Visintainer, M. A., Volpicelli, J. R., and Seligman, M. E. P. (1982). Tumor rejection after inescapable or escapable shock. *Science*, **216**, 437–439.

Wallace, M., Singer, G., Finlay, J., and Gibson, S. (1983). The effect of 6-OHDA lesions of the nucleus accumbens system on schedule-induced drinking, wheel running and corticosterone levels in the rat. *Pharmacology, Biochemistry and Behavior*, **18**, 129–136.

Watkins. L. R., and Mayer, D. J. (1982). Organization of endogenous opiate and non-opiate pain control systems. *Science*, **216**, 1185–1192.

Weinberg, J., Erskine, M., and Levine, S. (1980). Shock-induced fighting attenuates the effect of prior shock experience in rats. *Physiology and Behavior*, **25**, 9–16.

Weiss, J. M. (1971a). Effects of coping behavior in different warning signal conditions on stress pathology in rats. *Journal of Comparative and Physiological Psychology*, **77**, 1–13.

Weiss, J. M. (1971b). Effects of coping behavior with and without a feedback signal on stress pathology in rats. *Journal of Comparative and Physiological Psychology*, **77**, 22–30.

Weiss, J. M., and Goodman Simson, P. (1984). Neurochemical mechanisms underlying stress-induced depression. In: T. M. Field, P. M. McCabe and N. Schneiderman (eds), *Stress and Coping* (pp. 93–116). Hillsdale, NJ: Lawrence Erlbaum.

Weiss, J. M., Goodman, P., Losito, B., Corrigan, S., Charry, J., and Bailey, W. (1981). Behavioral depression produced by an uncontrollable stressor. Relationship to norepinephrine, dopamine and serotonin levels in various regions of rat brain. *Brain Research Review*, **3**, 167–205.

Wilkinson, C. W., Shimsako, J., and Dallman, M. F. (1982). Rapid decreases in adrenal and plasma corticosterone concentrations are not mediated by changes in plasma adrenocorticotropin concentrations. *Endocrinology*, **110**, 1599–1606.

Williams, R. B., and Eichelman, B. (1971). Social setting: Influence on the physiologic response electric shock in the rat. *Science*, **174**, 613–614.

CHAPTER 14

Social control in relation to neuroendocrine and immunological responses

JAAP KOOLHAAS AND BÉLA BOHUS
Department of Animal Physiology, University of Groningen, The Netherlands

INTRODUCTION

A general biological requirement for the survival of living organisms is the ability to adapt to changes in the environment. The behavioural, physiological and neuroendocrine mechanisms underlying this ability has been the focus of research in many scientific disciplines for decades. The early studies by Cannon (1915) and Selye (1935) laid the foundations of modern stress research by emphasizing the role of the adrenal medulla and the adrenal cortex as major organizers of body reactions to environmental demands. The results of these studies were summarized by Selye (1950) in his formulation of the 'general adaptation syndrome'. This theory, that emphasized the non-specificity of the physiological and neuroendocrine responses to stressors, was mainly based upon studies using physical stressors such as tissue damage and extreme temperatures.

More recently, the importance of psychological factors as stimuli activating physiological, neuroendocrine and behavioural adaptation mechanisms has been recognized (Lazarus, 1966). Animal experiments led to the reinforcement of this view. Using a shock-avoidance situation, Weiss (1968) showed that rats that could perform a response to avoid the aversive electric shock developed less severe stomach ulcers than yoked controls that received the same amount of shocks, but could not perform such a coping response. In a series of subsequent studies by a variety of authors it became clear that the controllability and predictability of environmental stressors is of fundamental value to the organism (Weiss, 1971; Seligman *et al.*, 1980; Overmier *et al.*, 1980). In particular, the absence of control

Stress, Personal Control and Health.   Edited by A. Steptoe and A. Appels.
Published by John Wiley & Sons Ltd.
© ECSC–EEC–EAEC, Brussels–Luxembourg, 1989

over a stressor has been shown to induce a variety of stress pathologies. Inescapable electric shock results in more stomach ulcers, higher levels of plasma corticosterone and a stronger reduction of food intake than escapable shock (Weiss, 1968). Similarly, uncontrollable stressors induce immunosuppression as measured by the reduced lymphocyte proliferation response, whereas exposure to similarly intense but controllable stressors failed to affect this response (Laudenslager *et al.*, 1983). Sklar and Anisman (1979) demonstrated the importance of controllability on enhanced tumour development after uncontrollable shock relative to the controllable one. In these experiments, control over the environment is achieved instrumentally by enabling the animal to switch off a painful electric shock by pressing a lever. Here, pressing the lever is the behavioural coping response to achieve control. However, in the everyday life of people and animals living in complex social environments, it is far more difficult to characterize what is to be controlled and what behavioural possibilities there are to achieve control. The present chapter will focus on the question of the extent to which the concept of control is helpful in understanding the (patho)physiological changes induced by the social environment of rats. Our observations on male rats and mice living in a social structure serve as the experimental basis for investigating this question.

SOCIAL POSITION AND STRESS PATHOLOGY

Under natural conditions, many animal species live in rather complex social structures in which individuals differ in their social relations to other group members. A number of studies have demonstrated a relationship between position in the social hierarchy and the incidence of certain stress pathologies. For instance, the appearance of hypertension and cardiovascular (e.g. arteriosclerosis) abnormalities have been demonstrated in dominant male mice (Ely, 1981) and in subdominant male cynomolgous monkeys (Manuck *et al.*, 1983). Severely subordinate social outcasts in rat colonies suffer from stomach ulcers (Calhoun, 1962; Barnett, 1975), whereas subordinate male tupaias have been reported to die from renal failure (von Holst, 1986). In the past few years, a number of studies have been performed at our department to study the relationship between position in the social structure of male rats and cardiovascular, immunological and neuroendocrine parameters. These studies have been performed on colonies of male rats housed with five sterilized females in an enriched environment of 6 m². In these colonies a stable social structure usually develops, in which one male has the dominant position, i.e. it is continuously socially active and never loses an interaction with other colony members. A second group of males that can be distinguished is the group of subdominants. These animals were also socially very active, but they occasionally lose fights, in particular with the dominant and sometimes with other subdominants. Next there is a group of subordinate males

TABLE 1. Summary of physiological changes observed in the different social positions of male rats living in a complex colony structure

Social position	Mean blood pressure	Stomach ulcers	Thymus	Spleen prolifer.	$T_{Helper}/T_{cyt.}$
Dominant	Normal	No			
Subdominant	High	No	Involuted	Normal	High
Subordinate	Normal	No	Normal	Reduced	Low
Outcast		Present			

that display very little social behaviour. They are rather passive, and other colony members do not pay much attention to them. Finally, in some colonies, a social outcast may be present. This animal is frequently attacked and chased away by both the dominant and the subdominants. Often this social outcast is a dominant that has lost its leading position.

Table 1 summarizes the results we have obtained so far on the relation between position in the hierarchy, blood pressure and immune system. There are a number of empty cells in this table because it is hard to collect data from a sufficient number of dominants and outcasts. Each colony has only one dominant, whereas outcasts may occur only in every two or three colonies.

As can be seen in Table 1, the subdominants have the highest baseline blood pressures, whereas dominants and subordinates are normotensive (Fokkema, 1986). The social structure is also reflected in the various compartments of the immune system. Subdominants have low levels of lymphocytes in peripheral blood and an involuted thymus, but a normal *in vitro* proliferation response of the spleen to mitogenic stimulation with ConA and PHA. The subordinates, on the other hand, have a normal thymus, normal blood lymphocyte levels, but a reduced *in vitro* proliferation response of the spleen. There seems to be a shift within the subpopulation of T-lymphocytes towards a higher T-helper/T-cytotoxic ratio in the subdominants (Koolhaas *et al.*, in preparation).

Finally, the few social outcasts that occurred in our rat colonies all suffered from stomach ulcers.

These results show that each type of position in the social structure, and possibly each individual animal, has its characteristic cardiovascular and immunological profile after three months of colony housing. Although these profiles cannot always be considered as pathological, it is conceivable that they reflect a differential susceptibility for somatic, cardiovascular and immunological diseases.

COPING STRATEGIES

The main question is to what extent the incidence of stomach ulcers, the relationship between social position and cardiovascular and immunological profile, and the consequent susceptibility for pathology is due to a different degree of social control. If control is defined as successful coping, we have to consider the possibility that the different positions in the social structure are in fact based upon different coping strategies. This possibility was studied extensively in individually housed male rats and mice. In these studies the tendency to perform aggressive behaviour in the presence of a standard unfamiliar male intruder into the home cages was related to physiological parameters as well as behaviour in a wide variety of other social and non-social situations. It appeared that the individual variation in social (aggressive) behaviour is related to behaviour in the presence of a dominant male, maze performance and active shock avoidance (Bohus *et al.*, 1987). The individual variation in behaviour and the related physiological differences are summarized in Figure 1. Basically, the extremes of the variation represent two different behavioural strategies, i.e. an active and a passive one. The active strategy is characterized by a strong

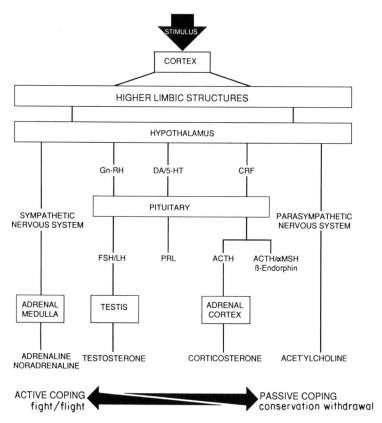

FIGURE 1. Summary of the physiologial differences between the two behavioural strategies.

tendency to defend the home territory against unfamiliar intruders, whereas these animals readily escape in the presence of a dominant. Physiologically, the active strategy has high baseline levels of testosterone and plasma noradrenaline and also a high reactivity of the sympathetic nervous system as indicated by the responsiveness of plasma catecholamines and blood pressure (Bohus *et al.*, 1987; Fokkema *et al.*, 1988). The passive strategy reflects very little social activity, and the animal mostly reacts with immobility upon approach by a dominant male. Physiologically, these males react predominantly with a parasympathetic response in stressful situations, have a more reactive pituitary adrenocortical system and have lower levels of plasma testosterone. The relationships between behaviour and physiology are based upon correlations between both dependent and independent measurements. Accordingly, the individual differentiation in active and passive behavioural strategies represents the individual appraisal of the animals' environment in general. The behavioural strategy as defined in an individually housed animal appears to have predictive value for the social position when group-housed in a colony later on. Animals with an active strategy take the dominant and subdominant positions, whereas passive animals remain passive in the colony and take the subordinate positions.

The next question to address is whether these behavioural characteristics can be considered as coping strategies that may lead to control of the social environment. This question can only be answered with an operational definition of control in terms of successful coping. In a social situation, control may be defined as the successful avoidance of attacks by a dominant male. Figure 2 shows a behavioural analysis of the success of the two strategies during a confrontation with a dominant male. By definition, the two strategies differ in escape and immobility. However, despite this difference the degree in which these animals are attacked by the dominant is the same. Accordingly, escape from the dominant works just as well in avoiding attacks as hiding immobile in a corner of the test cage.

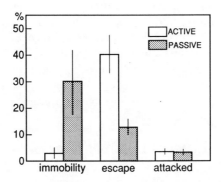

FIGURE 2. Percentage of total time spent on various behaviours by male rats characterized by either an active strategy (open bars) or a passive strategy (shaded bars) during a social interaction with a dominant male.

In a number of behavioural experiments in non-social situations, we have found evidence that the two strategies are in fact successful under different environmental conditions. This is best illustrated with the performance of active (aggressive) and passive (non-aggressive) male rats and mice in various mazes. The animals had to run in a Hebb–Williams type of maze in order to obtain a small pellet of food. In this case control is defined as the ability to solve the maze and obtain the food. This can be measured as number of food pellets obtained, latency of the run or the number of errors made during the run in the maze. The first task was a problem-solving task developed by Rabinovitch and Rosvold (1951). Basically, this task consisted of three consecutive trials in a certain maze configuration. Subsequently, the configuration was changed for the next three trials, etc. In fact the animals are confronted with a frequently changing environment. There was a highly significant negative correlation between aggressive (active) behaviour and maze performance (Benus *et al.*, 1987). This means that animals with an active strategy have serious problems in obtaining food in a continuously changing environment. In a second maze experiment, animals were first trained until a stable good performance was reached in one and the same maze configuration. After reaching an arbitrary criterion, a small change in either intra-maze or extra-maze cues was applied. Males with an active strategy hardly noticed the change, whereas the passive males reacted with a strong increase in latency and errors (Benus *et al.*, 1987). Apparently, under stable environmental conditions active males have a superior performance because they do not pay attention to minor environmental changes. Passive males seem to depend strongly on environmental cues. Hence, if we measure the success of a strategy on the bases of errors in the maze or speed of obtaining the food reward, it is obvious that the active strategy is better under stable conditions whereas the passive strategy is more successful under changing environmental conditions. This conclusion is supported by a study on the population dynamics of wild house mice by van Oortmerssen and Busser (1988), showing that active and passive behavioural strategies are differentially successful in different population densities. This means that the two behavioural strategies can be considered as coping strategies suited to different environmental conditions. If we accept the view that control is successful coping, then both strategies lead to a different type of control. When coping is successful, animals using the active strategy obtain objective control by taking some action whereas the animals with a passive strategy seem to adjust themselves to the environment; the latter may be considered as perceived control.

CONTROL AND PATHOLOGY

In most animal experimental studies, the occurrence of stress pathologies such as stomach lesions and immune deficiencies are related to conditions that are considered to involve lack or loss of control, e.g. inescapable shock or restraint. In social situations, loss of control might mean being confronted, attacked and defeated by another (dominant) male despite of using a strategy which is considered subjectively as successful (e.g. flight or immobility). In a number of experiments we studied the behavioural and physiological consequences of such a loss of control situation. In these experiments the behaviour was measured in social and non-social situations both before and after an inescapable confrontation with a trained, dominant fighter rat. This confrontation resulted almost by definition in defeat of the experimental animal. The social defeat results in a strong behavioural change that can be observed in a variety of social and non-social situations. Figure 3 shows that the exploratory behaviour in an unfamiliar complex maze was strongly reduced after defeat. This behavioural change outlasted the defeat for at least three weeks. There are long-lasting physiological changes as well. The total number of lymphocytes is significantly reduced for at least three weeks after termination of the uncontrollable social stress (Koolhaas *et al.*, in preparation). Preliminary measurements on the primary and secondary antibody response to sheep red blood cells suggest that losing fights also reduces the secondary antibody response.

These data show that a loss of control experience in a social situation can induce long-lasting behavioural and physiological changes that are comparable to the results obtained with uncontrollable non-social stress situations reported in the literature. Along this line, the high incidence of stomach ulcers observed in the social outcasts of rat colonies might also be explained by loss of control. These outcasts are regularly attacked and defeated by other colony members.

However, not all stress pathologies can be explained by loss of control. Buchholz *et al.* (1981) reported that a cardiovascular disease such as hypertension cannot be induced by using the inescapable shock paradigm as described by Weiss (1968). On the contrary, recent experiments suggest that loss of control in a social situation may result in a decrease rather than an increase in blood pressure.

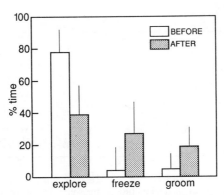

FIGURE 3. Percentage of total time spent on various behaviours in a complex, unfamiliar maze both before and after social defeat.

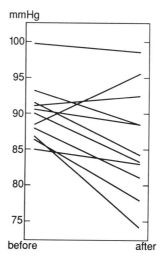

FIGURE 4. Change in mean arterial blood pressure in individual normotensive male rats measured 24 hours after social defeat.

Figure 4 shows the decline in mean blood pressure under resting conditions in individual male rats that lost a single fight 24 hours earlier. This decline is even more pronounced in hypertensive rats. Figure 5 shows the results of repeated daily social defeat in Doca salt-hypertensive rats and their normotensive controls. In these hypertensive animals loss of control results in a highly significant decrease in mean blood pressure. Similar findings have been reported by Adams and Blizard (1987) using the Dahl salt-sensitive strain of rats. Although the mechanisms underlying this drop in blood pressure are far from clear, it is clear that loss of control does not invariably induce hypertension.

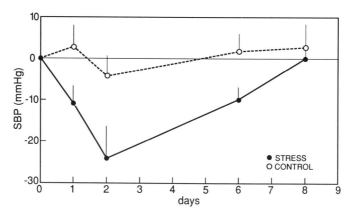

FIGURE 5. Change in mean arterial blood pressure in normotensive $(N = 6)$ and Doca salt-hypertensive male rats $(N = 6)$ measured 24 hours after social defeat on day 1 and day 2.

A number of experiments indicate that it is threat to control rather than loss of control that causes elevated blood pressures. Herd *et al.* (1969) reported an experiment using a conditioned avoidance paradigm in squirrel monkeys. In the initial learning trials during which the animals did not yet control the task, i.e. received most noxious stimuli, there was no change in arterial blood pressure. As training progressed, the number of aversive electric shocks received by the animals declined, but blood pressure increased even under the resting conditions present between the test sessions. Since finally the animals perfectly controlled the situation, this experiment suggests that the crucial factor in hypertension is the continuous threat to control, rather than loss of control. This hypothesis is consistent with our own observations on the relationship between blood pressure and position in the social structure of rat colonies. In these colonies, we observed a significant correlation between the amount of threatening behaviour and flight performed by individuals during colony aggregation and the mean arterial blood pressure under resting conditions (Fokkema, 1986). The individual score on this threatening and flight behaviour is in fact an indication of subdominance and reflects the active behavioural strategy. The explanation of this correlation may be that these subdominant males, despite the fact that they actively control the situation by flight behaviour, live under a continuous threat to control due to the presence of the dominant. Dominant males, on the other hand, are usually normotensive. However, a consequence of this way of reasoning is that one may expect higher blood pressures in dominants as well, under conditions in which they have difficulty in maintaining their position. Indeed, we have observed hypertension in the dominant in one socially very unstable rat colony. Similarly, Ely (1981) found hypertension was common in the dominant in mice colonies. The reason for this apparent discrepancy with the rat data is that mice have a slightly different social organization from rats. Mice live in deme structures in which the dominant only tolerates females and some juvenile males. Moreover, the construction of the colony cages used by Ely was such that it was difficult for the dominant to control all the small alleys of the cage. Hence, here too it seems likely that threat to control is the important factor in the development of hypertension.

CONCLUDING REMARKS

The notion that control of the situation is of fundamental value to animals and humans has been a major step forward in understanding stress pathology. However, control cannot be separated from the situation under investigation, and hence depends on the aims and goals of the organism. In this chapter we have presented some evidence that rats and mice show individual differences in behavioural strategy in reaction to environmental changes. We argued that these strategies can be considered as coping 'styles' that may lead to either objective control in the case of the active strategy or adjustment or perceived control in the passive strategy. This way of reasoning brings us to the conclusion that animals also may have different goals. The different coping strategies are associated with different physiological and neuroendocrine mechansims. These may be the basis for a differential susceptibility to certain stress pathologies. In understanding the detailed relationship between environment, behaviour, the neuroendocrine and immune systems and pathology, we have to think in degrees and/or kinds of control rather than only the two extremes, namely control and loss of control.

REFERENCES

Adams, N. and Blizard, D. A. (1987). Defeat and cardiovascular response. *Psychological Record*, **37**, 349–368.

Barnett, S. A. (1987). *The Rat: A Study in Behavior*. Chicago: University of Chicago Press.

Benus, R. F., Koolhaas, J. M., and van Oortmerssen, G. A. (1987). Individual differences in behavioural reaction to a changing environment in mice and rats. *Behaviour*, **100**, 105–122.

Bohus, B., Benus, R. F., Fokkema, D. S., Koolhaas, J. M., Nyakas, C., van Oortmerssen, G. A., Prins, A. J. A., de Ruiter, A. J. H., Scheurink, A. J. W., and Steffens, A. B. (1987). Neuroendocrine states and behavioral and physiological stress responses. *Progress in Brain Research* **72**, 57–70.

Buchholz, R. A., Lawler, J. E., and Parker, G. F. (1981). The effect of avoidance and conflict schedules on blood pressure and heart rate of rats. *Physiology and Behavior* **26**, 853–863.

Calhoun, J. B. (1962). *The Ecology and Sociology of the Norway Rat*. Washington, DC: Government Printing Office.

Cannon, W. B. (1915). *Bodily Changes in Pain, Hunger, Fear and Rage*. New York: Appleton.

Ely, D. L. (1981). Hypertension, social rank and aortic arteriosclerosis in CBA/J mice. *Physiology and Behavior* **26**, 655–662.

Fokkema, D. S. (1986). *Social behavior and blood pressure: A study of rats*. Thesis, State University, Groningen.

Fokkema, D. S., Smit, K., van der Gugten, J., and Koolhaas, J. M. (1988). A coherent pattern among social behavior, blood pressure, corticosterone and catacholamine measures in individual male rats. *Physiology and Behavior*, **42**, 485–489.

Herd, J. A., Morse, W. H., Kelleher, R. T., and Jones, L. G. (1969). Arterial hypertension in the squirrel monkey during behavioral experiments. *American Journal of Physiology*, **217**, 24–29.

Koolhaas, J. M., Kamstra, A., Bohus, B., Ballieux, R., and Heijnen, C. J. Position in the social structure determines the state of the immune system in male rats (in preparation).

Laudenslager, M. L., Ryan, S. M., Drugan, R. C., Hyson, R. L., and Maier, S. F. (1983). Coping and immunosuppression: Inescapable but not escapable shock suppresses lymphocyte proliferation. *Science*, **211**, 568–570.

Lazarus, R. (1966). *Psychological Stress and the Coping Process*. New York: McGraw-Hill.

Manuck, S. B., Kaplan, J. R., and Clarkson, T. B. (1983). Behaviorally induced heart rate reactivity and atherosclerosis in cynomolgous monkeys. *Psychosomatic Medicine*, **45**, 95–108.

Oortmerssen, G. A. van, and Busser, J. (1988). Studies in wild house mice. 3: Disruptive selection and aggression as a possible force in evolution. In: P. F. Brain (ed.), *House Mouse Aggression: A Model for Understanding the Evolution of Social Behaviour*. London: Harwood.

Overmier, B., Patterson, J., and Wielkiewicz, R. M. (1980). Environmental contingencies as sources of stress in animals. In: S. Levine and H. Ursin (eds), *Coping and Health*. New York: Plenum Press.

Rabinowitch, M. S., and Rosvold, H. E. (1951). A closed-field intelligence test for rats. *Canadian Journal of Psychology*, **5**, 122–128.

Seligman, M. E. P., Weiss, J. M., Weinraub, M., and Schulman, A. (1980). Coping behavior, learned helplessness, physiological change and learned inactivity. *Behaviour Research and Therapy*, **18**, 459–512.

Selye, H. (1935). A syndrome produced by diverse nocuous agents. *Nature*, **138**, 32–33.

Selye, H. (1950). *Stress: The Physiology and Pathology of Exposure to Stress*. Montreal: Acta Medica.

Sklar, L. S., and Anisman, H. (1979). Stress and coping factors influence tumor growth. *Science*, **250**, 513–515.

von Holst, D. (1986). Psychosocial stress and its pathophysiological effects in tree shrews. In: T. H. Schmidt, T. M. Dembroski and G. Blümchem (eds), *Biological and Psychological Factors in Cardiovascular Disease*. Berlin: Springer.

Weiss, J. M. (1968). Effects of coping responses on stress. *Journal of Comparative and Physiological Psychology*, **65**, 251–260.

Weiss, J. M. (1971). Effects of coping behavior with and without a feedback signal on stress pathology in rats. *Journal of Comparative and Physiological Psychology*, **77**, 22–30.

Postscript

CHAPTER 15

The significance of personal control in health and disease

ANDREW STEPTOE
Department of Psychology, St George's Hospital Medical School, University of London, UK

INTRODUCTION

Earlier chapters in this book have discussed the relevance of the concepts of personal control and lack of control for the understanding of health-related phenomena. The very fact that scientists from so many disciplines find some merit in describing their data in terms of personal control testifies to the value of the construct. However, such widespread use of the concept of control may give an impression of consensus that is spurious, because the observations made in different domains may in fact have little in common. The purpose of this chapter is not to provide a summary of material detailed elsewhere, nor to attempt an integration of data from the diverse scientific fields related to control. Rather, the aim is to highlight certain themes that have emerged through the contributions to this book.

CONTROL IN RELATION TO STRESS AND DISEASE

Several definitions of personal control have been offered in previous chapters, and a further taxonomy would be superfluous. Nevertheless, it is interesting to note that in all the main areas of study—occupational, clinical and laboratory —three broad aspects of control are defined: behavioural or objective control over environmental contingencies or events, subjective or perceived control, and

Stress, Personal Control and Health.   Edited by A. Steptoe and A. Appels.
Published by John Wiley & Sons Ltd.
© ECSC–EEC–EAEC, Brussels–Luxembourg, 1989

an element of individual differences variously described as need for control or belief in control.

Most of the research related to health has focused specifically on control over aversive stimulation, and on conditions in which the goal of control is the elimination or diminution of noxious events. The concept of control might equally apply to actions that increase the aversiveness of situations, although the psychobiological consequences of such behaviours is unknown. It is important to bear in mind that control over positive experiences may also be significant. The studies of young primates described by Mineka and Kelly (Chapter 8) demonstrate that high levels of appetitive control have generalized beneficial effects on later social integration, fear and exploratory behaviour patterns. Rodin (1986) has argued that control should be viewed as one facet of a broader concept such as self-determination, to denote that it may apply to positive and negative situations, and that people may choose not to exercise control in certain situations, but nevertheless feel a sense of autonomy in their decision.

Control is, of course, only one factor in the interplay between psychosocial demands and personal resources that defines whether or not an interaction is stressful, as can be seen in the general model outlined in Figure 1. When resources are inadequate for enabling the individual to adapt competently to the level or quality of psychosocial stimulation, a variety of psychobiological responses may emerge. Stress responses may also be elicited when demands are low or insufficient to match the person's capacity. Several of the dimensions of psychosocial stimulation that are known to influence stress responses are listed in Figure 1, as are the characteristics of the individual's capability and social context that are relevant to the interaction (see Steptoe, 1989, for fuller details).

Behavioural control occupies an important position relative to these other factors, in that it is genuinely interactive. It is neither an element of the environment, nor is it a property of the individual. Behavioural control will only emerge through an interaction between certain dispositions of the environment, perceived in such a light by the organism that appropriate behavioural responses are mobilized.

It is apparent from earlier chapters that behavioural control is itself a complex notion, since it is often difficult to characterize the responses involved in achieving control. Even when the parameters can be systematically manipulated, as in experimental studies of pain, different effects are observed depending on whether control is exerted over the initiation, termination or rate of change of stimulation (Arntz and Schmidt, Chapter 7). In laboratory studies of physiological responses in humans, control is varied in several ways, including comparisons of self and external task pacing, rapid psychomotor performance, or the avoidance of aversive stimulation by accurate cognitive processing (Phillips, Chapter 11; Öhman and Bohlin, Chapter 12). In occupational settings, skill discretion and authority over decisions have been distinguished, and again these may have

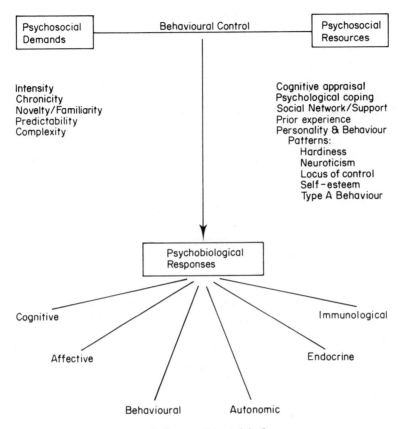

FIGURE 1. Interactive model of stress.

different effects on biological parameters (Theorell, Chapter 3). Furthermore, behavioural control does not simply alter the transient aversiveness of a situation, but may increase perceived capability and coping efficacy in general. One message to emerge from the analyses presented in this book is that the notion of behavioural control may be too general adequately to define the interactions between person and environment that influence health-related responses. In order to understand any particular observation, it is necessary to know precisely in what ways events are amenable to control.

The concept of perceived control is also hard to pin down, since it is used in two rather different senses by authors in this volume: first as perceived control over events, and second as perceived control over emotional reactions which may leave the stimulus array unchanged. The first use is related to behavioural control, in order to account for the fact that belief in control over events often has similar effects to actual control, even when that perception is non-veridical. The distinction between this form of perceived control and actual behavioural control can be specious at an analytical level, in that if the belief in control is never tested there is no phenomenological difference between the two as far as the subject is concerned. There are many cases in which perceived control over the source of aversive stimulation evidently reduces distress, even though the controlling response is not mobilized, as in investigations of dental pain and distress (e.g. Wardle, 1983). Nevertheless, the importance of this form of perceived behavioural control is highlighted by studies showing that the benefits of control depend on the individual's certainty that the behavioural response will have a favourable impact (Arntz and Schmidt, Chapter 7). There are also circumstances in which events are perceived as controllable, yet no action is taken since people lack (or believe they lack) appropriate behavioural competencies. Bandura (1977) has postulated a distinction between outcome expectancies and efficacy expectancies to account for this effect. High levels of perceived behavioural control are engendered when positive outcome expectancies are accompanied by expectations that the person will be able to carry out the response effectively.

The second use of perceived control describes belief in strategies designed to regulate the impact of aversive situations by attenuating emotional and behavioural responses. In the past, the term 'cognitive control' has been used to denote the way in which information about impending events or access to knowledge about coping strategies might modify reactions (see Cohen *et al.*, 1986). The distinction between this type of perceived control and that described in the previous paragraph is important, since there are many settings (such as surgery) in which little can be done to alter aversive events themselves, whereas perceived control over distress and discomfort may contribute to the person's well-being (Miller, Combs and Stoddard, Chapter 6). However, there is a danger that when perceived control is used to describe techniques for regulating reactions, it becomes synonymous with psychological coping, and therefore redundant as an explanatory variable. Consequently, it may be valuable to draw a distinction between the coping strategies that modify aversive reactions and discretion over the deployment of these strategies. Control would then refer to the belief that these strategies are available, and that the person has choice over when they are utilized. Conversely, lack of perceived control over ways of regulating emotional responses and their manifestations is implicated in the maintenance of a variety of anxiety-related disorders (Mineka and Kelly, Chapter 8).

Perceived control over reactions can best be viewed as a superordinate construct. Its importance is highlighted in cases where people have a coping response available for blunting their psychobiological reactions, but choose not to mobilize it. For example, the technique of 'applied tension' has been successfully developed for the management of fainting in patients with phobias of blood and injury (Öst and Sterner, 1987). The method is based on the physiological rationale that tension in major muscle groups will increase venous return to the heart, countering the hypotension and bradycardia that characterize the fainting response. Patients are therefore trained to tense their muscles for short periods when they begin to feel faint. The interesting aspect in the present context is that, following training, patients are frequently able to view phobic stimuli and even observe major surgery with little anxiety or faintness, but also without actually employing the tension technique. They perceive that they have a coping response available for controlling their reactions, and this is sufficient. The same effect is present among anxious patients who carry a benzodiazepine or other tranquilizer about with them, without ever using it.

It can be argued almost by definition that adaptive emotion-focused coping responses promote a sense of control over reactions to aversive situations. It is also possible that perceived control may be the final common pathway for a range of different coping responses (relaxation, self-statements, cognitive restructuring, distraction, etc.), and that these strategies are only effective in as much as they engender a belief in control. There are, however, alternative candidates for this central role, such as distraction from the aversive properties of the situation or enhanced self-efficacy, and it is possible that different coping strategies operate through separate mechanisms.

MECHANISMS UNDERLYING THE EFFECTS OF CONTROL

Several processes through which control and lack of control may affect health have been described in this volume. At the biological level, changes in autonomic function, endocrine responses and immunological activity have been documented. Subjective responses, including modifications in cognition and affect, are present in many situations, while health-related behaviours may also be influenced. One of the major issues that remains unresolved is the interaction between these levels, and the extent to which concordant or independent responses are observed. The mechanisms responsible for health outcomes are also far from being well defined.

The biological responses associated with control and lack of control present a complex pattern in themselves. It has repeatedly been observed that behavioural control that can be exerted competently with low response costs tends to reduce stress-related reactions in many systems (Dantzer, Chapter 13). Situations in which control is difficult to exert, and where the organism has low efficacy expectancies, may on the other hand have activating properties (Öhman and Bohlin, Chapter 12). However, even when control is reliable, there may be differences between the immediate and longer-term physiological responses. Furthermore, it cannot necessarily be inferred that the stress-related reactions associated with uncontrollable aversive stimulation are maladaptive. A good example of this is the stress-induced analgesia characteristic of uncontrollable conditions (Kelly, 1986). Many challenges require perseverance in the face of adversity, and premature termination of efforts because of pain or discomfort may be disadvantageous. It can be argued therefore that an endogenous mechanism that permits organisms to endure stressful stimulation at a reduced level of physical discomfort may be adaptive (Bandura *et al.*, 1988). More generally, Phillips (Chapter 11) has argued that at the level of energy expenditure and biological efficiency, the behavioural inertia produced in conditions of uncontrollable stress may be adaptive in eliminating wasteful ineffective responding.

It is also true to say that behavioural coping responses which attenuate reactions in some systems may have the reverse effect on other processes. Thus administration of brief electric shocks to rats in pairs induces a form of fighting that is associated with diminution in corticosteroid reactions and stress-induced analgesia (Dantzer, Chapter 13). However, this 'coping response' also leads to increased catecholamine production in the adrenal medulla, suggesting a shift in pattern rather than generalized physiological deactivation.

Control and lack of control also have a profound effect at the subjective level, altering perceptions concerning the outcome of different behaviours as well as affective variables such as anxiety and depression. These subjective experiences are frequently paralleled by biological changes, and a recent study on experimental pain suggests that cognitive responses mediate at least some of the physiological effects of control manipulation (Bandura *et al.*, 1988). Volunteers participated in an experimental study in which half could regulate the presentation of a sequence of mental arithmetic problems, while the remainder were presented with problems at a pace that exceeded their capacity. This manipulation affected subjects' expectancies (or self-efficacy perceptions) that they could solve such tasks. Subsequently, a series of cold pressor tests were performed, following administration of the opioid antagonist naloxone or a placebo. Subjects with low mathematical self-efficacy perceptions (low control) showed high pain tolerance (a form of stress-induced analgesia). This response was blocked by naloxone, suggesting mediation through opioid mechanisms. However, the effects of cognitive responses to the arithmetic task generalized beyond the immediate situation, so within the high perceived self-efficacy (behavioural control) group increases in self-efficacy were correlated with greater pain tolerance, evidently through non-opioid pathways.

Affective responses are, of course, important end-points in themselves, since control and lack of control have been implicated in depression, anxiety and related states (see Chapters 6–10). But it seems that while cognitive processes may be related to biological responses the same cannot be said of affective changes. Parkes (Chapter 2) has concluded from studies in occupational settings that lack of control is associated with behavioural changes and biological responses indicative of increased health risk, but that specific affective responses such as depression do not generally develop. Similarly, in situations in which people attempt to cope actively with high work demands despite having very restricted autonomy, adverse effects may be recorded at the biological level without emotional distress being reported (see Siegrist and Matschinger, Chapter 4). Consequently, it cannot be assumed that affective reports are adequate markers of the biological responses that may determine health; people may show pronounced physiological reactions without feeling distressed.

The third level at which control may affect health is through changes in behaviour. Lack of control may be associated with coping responses that themselves carry health risk, such as heavy drinking and smoking. To the individual, these actions may be seen as beneficial and valuable components of their behavioural repertoire, enabling them to manage situations that might otherwise be overwhelming or lead to unacceptable distress. Appels (Chapter 10) has argued that lack of control may promote vital exhaustion and its attendant cardiac risks, not simply through some psychobiological mechanism, but by altering the environmental conditions impinging on the person (for example through increasing workload). On the positive side, there is considerable evidence that people with a strong sense of personal control maintain higher levels of active involvement in their own health care, adhering to medical advice concerning lifestyle change more rigorously than those with low perceived control (Strickland, 1978; Wallston *et al.*, 1987).

The fact that several different mechanisms may mediate associations between control and health has important methodological as well as theoretical implications. One issue to emerge concerns the appropriate ways of assessing interventions that are expected to increase personal control. As Wallston (Chapter 5) illustrates, well-constructed and (on the face of them) valuable manipulations designed to modify patients' sense of control in health-care settings are not always effective. There may be several reasons for this, such as the meaningfulness of the response provided; if control is available over only minimal components of the interaction, it may not be beneficial, and may indeed have adverse effects by highlighting the generally helpless situation of the patient (Miller and colleagues, Chapter 6). The point here is that measures of control (either behavioural or subjective), and not only health measures, should be among the dependent variables in any intervention study. If experimental manipulations of control are assessed only in terms of affective or physiological responses, then in the situation in which differences between conditions are absent it is impossible to know whether the manipulation was ineffective in altering control, or control had no relevance to the setting. It is all too tempting in field and laboratory studies only to measure the variables that are directly relevant to health, rather than those which will confirm the success (or otherwise) of the intervention.

INDIVIDUAL DIFFERENCES AND CONTROL

An important theme to emerge through this volume is that individual differences in behaviour, beliefs and preferences for control are now recognized in many disciplines. In the past this was not the case; in animal studies of control, for example, failure to perform the behavioural response would have been regarded as a failure to learn, rather than as an expression of individual preferences (Phillips, Chapter 11). The individual differences relevant to control are of at least three distinct types.

The first dimension of individual differences concerns behavioural strategy and competence. This is demonstrated most vividly in animal studies in which variations in the behavioural strategies adopted in response to challenge are associated with different psychobiological reactions (Koolhaas and Bohus, Chapter 14). In occupational settings, Parkes (Chapter 2) concludes that having control over various aspects of working conditions may not be adaptive if the necessary skills are not available. In the health context, people may know what they ought to do to improve their condition, but nevertheless fail to take appropriate action; one reason for this may be that they do not believe that they have the requisite behaviours in their repertoires (Wallston, Chapter 5).

The second aspect of individual differences concerns variations in a person's need, preference or desire to control. Siegrist and Matschinger (Chapter 4) document the way in which need for control influences the emotional distress elicited by unsatisfactory work demands. In this case, need for control seems to have components related to control over work output, preference for involvement in all aspects of the working situation, and desire for recognition by others. Clinically, it might be argued that the most extreme manifestation of need for control is seen in obsessive-compulsive patients who display elaborate checking and cleaning rituals. At a more general level, it has been argued that preferences for control is likely to be associated with information-seeking behaviour (Miller and colleagues, Chapter 6; Phillips, Chapter 11). Indeed, individual variations in preference for information may be more fundamental than control needs, since they operate at a wider level. However, it should be borne in mind that a low need or desire for control may imply an active preference for not having control, or else a complete indifference to whether control is available or not.

Thirdly, belief in control (or locus of control) is an important individual difference construct. Generalized expectancies for control may arise through childhood experiences (Mineka and Kelly, Chapter 8). They subsequently influence the individual's appraisal of events, although their precise role may vary. Ormel and Sanderman (Chapter 9) argue that locus of control is a vulnerability factor mediating the specific association between loss events and depression, and making its most important contribution in situations that are ambiguous (Benassi et al., 1988). The notion that people will be better off when beliefs in control are congruent with environmental conditions and demands is attractive, but has yet to be documented extensively in the literature (Folkman, 1984; Warr, 1987). Furthermore, the possibility of non-linear associations between beliefs in controls and outcome is suggested in both occupational and medical settings (Parkes, Chapter, 2; Wallston, Chapter 5).

These dimensions of individual differences may exert independent effects on responses to stressful events, although there are important similarities between locus of control and behavioural self-efficacy expectancies (Strecher *et al.*, 1986). Literature from a variety of sources suggests that the most adaptive responses may emerge from those at intermediate levels on these dimensions. Both very high and very low beliefs in personal control may represent cognitive distortions of the real world, leading to the persistence of maladaptive behaviours in inappropriate settings. Similarly, animals who adopt an actively aggressive (as opposed to passive, non-aggressive) response to events may be successful in stable environments, but poor at adapting to changes in conditions (Koolhaas and Bohus, Chapter 14).

CONCLUSIONS: IMPLICATIONS FOR HEALTH PROMOTION AND HEALTH CARE

The value of designing management and treatment strategies that increase personal control has been identified in several fields, notably in relation to job satisfaction (Parkes, Chapter 2), ageing (Baltes and Baltes, 1986) and behaviour therapy (Mineka and Kelly, Chapter 8). In other settings, control has been postulated as a central mechanism without having been studied systematically. Thus there is a dearth of investigations that have specifically manipulated control in medical settings (Miller and colleagues, Chapter 6). The management of problems such as chronic pain or the psychological state following myocardial infarction may also involve procedures intended to enhance personal control, but these are generally deployed as part of a broader programme, so the specific contribution of control is difficult to evaluate (Ormel and Sanderman, Chapter 9; Appels, Chapter 10). There is a pressing need to develop rigorous tests of control from a multidisciplinary perspective, so that the value and limitations of the concept can be defined more precisely.

REFERENCES

Baltes, M. M., and Baltes, P. B. (1986). *The Psychology of Control and Aging*. Hillsdale, NJ:Erlbaum.

Bandura, A. (1977). Self-efficacy: Toward a unifying theory of behavior change. *Psychological Review*, **84**, 191–215.

Bandura, A., Cioffi, D., Taylor, C. B., and Brouillard, M. E. (1988). Perceived self-efficacy in coping with cognitive stressors and opioid activation. *Journal of Personality and Social Psychology*, **55**, 479–488.

Benassi, V. A., Sweeney, P. D., and Dufour, C. L. (1988). Is there a relation between locus of control orientation and depression? *Journal of Abnormal Psychology*, **97**, 357–367.

Cohen, S., Evans, G. W., Stokols, D., and Krantz, D. S. (1986). *Behavior, Health and Environmental Stress*. New York: Plenum.

Folkman, S. (1984). Personal control and stress and coping processes: A theoretical analysis. *Journal of Personality and Social Psychology*, **46**, 839–852.

Kelly, D. D. (1986). *Stress-Induced Analgesia*. Annals of the New York Academy of Sciences, Vol. 467.

Öst, L.-G., and Sterner, U. (1987). Applied tension: A specific behavioral method for treatment of blood phobia. *Behaviour Research and Therapy*, **25**, 25–29.

Rodin, J. (1986). Aging and health: Effects of the sense of control. *Science*, **233**, 1271–1276.

Steptoe, A. (1989). Psychobiological stress responses. In: M. Johnston and L. Wallace (eds), *Stress and Medical Procedures*. Oxford: Oxford University Press.

Strecher, V. J., DeVellis, B. M., Becker, M. H., and Rosenstock, I. M. (1986). The role of self-efficacy in achieving health behavior change. *Health Education Quarterly*, **13**, 73–91.

Strickland, B. R. (1978). Internal–external expectancies and health-related behaviors. *Journal of Consulting and Clinical Psychology*, **46**, 1192–1211.

Wallston, K. A., Wallston, B. S., Smith, M. S., and Dobbins, C. J. (1987). Perceived control and health. *Current Psychology Research and Reviews*, **6**, 5–25.

Wardle, J. (1983). Psychological management of anxiety and pain during dental treatment. *Journal of Psychosomatic Research*, **27**, 399–402.

Warr, P. (1987). *Work, Unemployment and Mental Health*. Oxford: Oxford University Press.

Index